Clinical Hemodialysis

Clinical Hemodialysis

Editor: Sean Eastwood

hayle medical

New York

Hayle Medical,
750 Third Avenue, 9th Floor,
New York, NY 10017, USA

Visit us on the World Wide Web at:
www.haylemedical.com

ISBN 978-1-64647-575-9 (Hardback)

Cataloging-in-publication Data

Clinical hemodialysis / edited by Sean Eastwood.
p. cm.
Includes bibliographical references and index.
ISBN 978-1-64647-575-9
1. Hemodialysis. 2. Blood--Filtration. 3. Dialysis. 4. Therapeutics.
5. Kidneys--Diseases--Treatment. 6. Clinical medicine. 7. Nephrology.
I. Eastwood, Sean.
RC901.7.H45 C55 2023
617.461 059--dc23

Contents

Preface

This book has been an outcome of determined endeavour from a group of educationists in the field. The primary objective was to involve a broad spectrum of professionals from diverse cultural background involved in the field for developing new researches. The book not only targets students but also scholars pursuing higher research for further enhancement of the theoretical and practical applications of the subject.

Hemodialysis is a machine-aided process that purifies blood for people suffering from acute kidney disease. It is one of the three types of renal replacement therapies. A person requires dialysis if their kidneys are not able to remove the wastes and fluids from their bloodstream. Dialysis utilizes a dialysis machine and a specific filter known as an artificial kidney to filter creatinine, urea, potassium and free water from the blood in the same way as the kidneys work in healthy conditions. There are three major types of hemodialysis: conventional hemodialysis, daily hemodialysis and nocturnal hemodialysis. This process aids in controlling the blood pressure and maintaining essential minerals and fluids in the blood. Some of the prominent complications associated with hemodialysis include fluid shifts, bacterial infections, venous needle dislodgement, anti-coagulation-related issues, cardiovascular issues, electrolyte imbalances and vitamin deficiency. This book outlines the processes and uses of hemodialysis in detail. It consists of contributions made by international experts. This book will provide comprehensive knowledge to the readers.

It was an honour to edit such a profound book and also a challenging task to compile and examine all the relevant data for accuracy and originality. I wish to acknowledge the efforts of the contributors for submitting such brilliant and diverse chapters in the field and for endlessly working for the completion of the book. Last, but not the least; I thank my family for being a constant source of support in all my research endeavours.

Editor

1

Biomarkers in Chronic Kidney Disease - The Linkage Between Inflammation, Ventricular Dysfunction and Overhydration

Olimpia Ortega
Hospital Severo Ochoa, Leganés, Madrid
Spain

1. Introduction

Since 1970s several studies have shown a significant prevalence of cardiovascular disease (CVD) among patients with end-stage renal disease (Linder et al., 1974). Among patients treated by hemodialysis and peritoneal dialysis, the prevalence of CVD is approximately 40%. Even after stratification by age, sex, race, and diabetes, CVD mortality in chronic kidney disease (CKD) patients is 10 to 20 times higher than in the general population (Foley et al., 1998). End-stage-renal-disease patients often have a high prevalence of cardiovascular risk factors as hypertension, diabetes and dyslipemia. Nevertheless, previous studies have shown that the high prevalence of CVD in hemodialysis patients is only partly explained by traditional risk factors (Cheung et al., 2000). Non-traditional risk factors have been emerged in the last decade. One of this non-traditional risk factor is C-reactive protein (CRP).

In this chapter, it is tried to explain the results of several studies supporting an association between inflammation (measured by high levels of CRP), left-ventricular dysfunction and volume overload among patients with CKD and how volume overload, which is present at the very early stages of CKD, could be the main underlying factor contributing to the worse CV prognosis among these patients.

2. Inflammation (C-reactive protein) in patients with chronic kidney disease: prevalence and prognostic factor

CRP is considered the prototypical acute-phase reactant in man. Plasma CRP is produced by hepatocytes although other sites of local CRP synthesis have been suggested.

The plasma half-life of CRP is about 19 hours and is constant under all conditions of health and disease, so that the sole determinant of circulating CRP concentration is the synthesis rate, which thus directly reflects the intensity of the pathological process stimulating CRP production. In most disease, the circulating value of CRP reflects ongoing inflammation and/or tissue damage much more accurately than other laboratory parameters of the acute-phase response. The CRP concentration is thus a very useful nonspecific biochemical marker of inflammation, measurement of which contributes importantly to screening for organic disease, monitoring of the response to treatment of inflammation and infection and detection of intercurrent infection (Pepys et al., 2003).

Elevated CRP levels have been described in a significant proportion of end-stage-renal-disease patients on hemodialysis or peritoneal dialysis (Arici et al., 2001). About one-third of patients with chronic renal failure have serum CRP concentration > 10 mg/l (Owen et al., 1998). In healthy men, high CRP level has been identified as a risk factor for cardiovascular disease (Ridker et al., 2001). As occurs in the general population, prospective studies point to a correlation between CRP plasma levels and overall and cardio-vascular mortality also in end-stage-renal disease patients (Arici et al., 2001; Ikizler et al., 1999; Noh et al., 1998; Owen et al., 1998; Panichi et al., 2008; Wang et al., 2009; Yeun et al. 2000; Zimmermann et al., 1999).

3. Inflammation and anemia

In dialysis patients, inflammation expressed by high levels of CRP is also associated with low blood hemoglobin and/or resistance to eritropoyesis-stimulating agents (Barany et al., 1997; Bradbury et al., 2009; Gunnel et al., 1999; Owen et al., 1998). This has been attributed to the inhibition of erythropoietin secretion by pro-inflammatory cytokines. Inflammation also contributes to anemia by inducing functional iron deficiency probably blocking the delivery of iron from the reticuloendothelial cells to the hemathopoietic cells. Cytokines may also induce ferritin synthesis directly or by increasing iron uptake into hepatocytes. The increase in ferritin synthesis by hepatocytes and reticuloendothelial cells underlies in the iron storage pool during inflammation. Thus, inflammation among patients with CKD can contribute to anemia and impaired response to erythropoietin. Erythropoietin resistance by itself has been associated with higher short-term mortality in CKD patients (López-Gómez et al., 2008).

4. Inflammation and malnutrition

High concentration of acute phase protein is correlated with low serum albumin in malnourished hemodialysis patients (Kaysen et al., 1997; Qureshi et al., 1998). Low serum albumin concentrations are highly associated with increased mortality risk in patients with renal replacement therapy (Lowrie et al., 1990). Hypoalbuminemia has been traditionally been assumed to result from inadequate protein and calorie intake. However, albumin is a negative acute-phase protein. The synthesis of this protein decreases during inflammation independently of nutritional state. Albumin concentration in dialysis patients is negatively correlated with levels of positive acute-phase protein. Moreover, inflammation and malnutrition data has been associated with the presence of atherosclerotic carotid plaques (Stenvinkel et al., 1999) describing the so called MIA (malnutrition-inflammation-atherosclerosis) syndrome in patients with advanced renal failure.

In summary, inflammation is high prevalent among patients with chronic kidney disease and predicts anemia, malnutrition and CV death. An intriguing question is whether CRP is just a sensitive marker of systemic inflammation or actively contributes to the development and progression of atherosclerotic lesions and, therefore, to the CV damage. Some authors have demonstrated CRP content inside the atherosclerotic lesions, suggesting the active participation in the inflammatory process (Zhang et al., 1999) what hints that inflammation could be the cause rather than the consequence of CV damage. Based on the bad prognosis of patients with markers of inflammation, it is important to try to known the possible causes of inflammation in this population in order to prevent morbidity and mortality.

5. Possible causes of inflammation

The causes of inflammation in patients with CKD patients remained unclear over time. Several studies have attempted to address the question as to whether some factors related to the dialysis technique by itself could induce the inflammatory response. Activation of monocytes with the subsequent enhanced release of inflammatory cytokines can be caused by membrane-induced complement activation, by direct cell-membrane interaction and by dialysis fluids containing endotoxins (Carracedo et al., 2006; Honkanen et al., 1991; Kerr et al., 2007; Schouten et al. 2000).

However, a similar prevalence of inflammation has been described in patients with advanced renal failure not yet on dialysis (Ortega et al., 2002; Panichi et al., 2002; Stenvinkel et al., 1999). An inverse correlation between CRP levels and clearance of creatinine has been observed (Panichi et al., 2002); thus, CRP levels increase as renal function declines. This finding suggests the possibility of a decreased renal clearance of CRP as a cause of an activated acute-phase response in patients with chronic kidney disease. Another possibility could be that uremia by itself could be the cause of inflammation among these patients. However, in another study performed in pre-dialysis patients with a more homogeneous clearance of creatinine (Ortega et al., 2002), a non-normal distribution of CRP levels were detected. That means that only a group of patients with advanced renal failure shows high levels of CRP, whereas other patients with the same degree of renal insufficiency have even normal CRP values. Hence, it seems that uremia by itself is not the unique cause of inflammation. Probably, inflammation could be related to some factors, frequently associated with renal failure, which can worsen with the worsening of renal function. In this study (Ortega et al., 2002), CRP levels were higher in those patients with a previous history of CVD. Comparing with patients with normal CRP levels at baseline, patients with higher levels maintained significant higher levels on follow-up. This group of inflamed patients showed during the study period persistently lower serum albumin, lower blood hemoglobin, needed higher doses of erythropoietin stimulating agents and showed higher hospitalization rate (table 1).

	Group I (CRP>6 mg/dL) n = 23	Group II (CRP<6 mg/dL) n = 43	*P* value
CRP (mg/L)*	21.6 (12.9 - 32.6)	2 (2 - 4.6)	0.00001
Albumin (g/dL)	3.5 ± 0.4	3.8 ± 0.4	0.017
Hemoglobin (g/dL)	11.6 ± 1.1	12.2 ± 0.8	0.045
Epo (IU/kg/week)	67 ± 32	43 ± 20	0.025
Hemoglobin/Epo	0.19 ± 0.08	0.32 ± 0.13	0.004
Hospitalization (n)	0.52 ± 0.8	0.03 ± 0.19	0.004

Table 1. Comparison of the evolution of analytical and clinical data between patients with high (Group I) or low (Group II) CRP levels at baseline. Mean ± standard deviation.
*Median (interquartile range).

In summary, at this point we know that inflammation is high prevalent among patients with CKD, that the prevalence is higher among patients with associated CVD, that inflammation tends to increase with the decline of renal function but that only about one third of patients with advance renal function shows persistently high levels of inflammatory markers. Thus, we could argue that uremia by itself is not the cause of inflammation. It seems that another factor, usually associated with uremia and which usually worsens with the decline of renal function could be the responsible of inflammation in patients with CKD. In the past decade, it has been observed that circulating inflammatory cytokines are elevated in patients with chronic heart failure (Levin et al., 1990) and it has been suggested that cytokines can be in part responsible for cardiac disease progression in these patients (Seta et al., 1996). Some authors have detected elevated plasma levels of endotoxins and cytokines during the acute phase of heart failure and that normalization of endotoxins and cytokines concentration can be achieved using intensive diuretic treatment (Niebauer et al. 1999, Peschel et al. 2003). The authors hypothesized that during acute cardiac decompensation, acute mesenteric venous congestion with subsequently altered gut permeability for endotoxins would lead to translocation of these materials into the circulation inducing the inflammatory response. Thus, the authors highlight that inflammation could be the consequence, rather than the cause of heart failure.

6. Association between inflammation, overhydratacion and cardiac disease: B-type natriuretic peptide

Cardiac disease is high prevalent among patients with CKD (Foley et al. ,1995; Hayashi et al., 2006; Levin et al., 1996; Zocali et al., 2004). The typical feature of uremic cardiomyopathy is left ventricular diastolic dysfunction related to left ventricular hypertrophy and left ventricular fibrosis (Ahmed et al., 2007; Losi et al., 2010; Mark et al., 2006). Left ventricular hypertrophy is particularly highly prevalent in end-stage renal disease patients because of hypertension, hyperparathyroidism and increased volume. However, myocardial fibrosis is a specific finding among patients with CKD comparing with patients with isolated hypertension as revealed autopsy studies (Sharer et al., 1999). Probably, volume overload could be a main cause of myocardial fibrosis among these patients as volume overload can produce mechanical stress on the ventricular wall and it has been demonstrated that mechanical factors can induce the activation of the fibroblasts of the myocardium synthesizing the extracellular matrix (MacKenna et al., 2000). Volume overload is present very early in the course of CKD and is the consequence of the inability of the insufficient kidney to eliminate the excess of water and salt. Usually, the increase in extracellular water in the very early course of CKD is modest and may easily be underestimated by clinical examination and can only be proved by accurate measurement of body water volume, as with bioimpedance. Extracellular water excess increases when glomerular filtration rate declines and has emerged as an independent factor in the structural cardiac damage, as a direct relation between extracellular water excess and left ventricular mass has been demonstrated as well as with left ventricular data of diastolic dysfunction (Essig et al., 2008). The authors also highlighted that cardiac remodeling was present at the very early stages of CKD. Over time, structural myocardial alterations progress, leading to diastolic dysfunction. The central disturbance in diastolic dysfunction involves abnormalities in myocardial relaxation and ventricular compliance (Martos et al., 2007). Thus, in order to complete ventricular filling and achieve a sufficient end-diastolic volume, which will provide adequate stroke volume, the left ventricle needs filling pressure higher than normal. Diastolic dysfunction, in fact, means that the left ventricle fills at higher pressure. Echocardiographic data of diastolic dysfunction are the most frequent findings among patients with CKD (Hayashy et al., 2006).

Based on the association between inflammation and heart failure in the general population and as myocardial dysfunction is high prevalent among patients with CKD, several authors tried to find an association between inflammation and cardiac disease also in this population. Furthermore, this hypothesis could explain why only some patients (those with more ventricular damage) show high levels of CRP, whereas other patients with similar clearance of creatinine (those with less cardiac disease) could present even normal values of CRP.

Some authors (Ates et al., 2005; Kim et al., 2005) have observed an association between CRP and left ventricular hypertrophy or dysfunction among patients with CKD. However, most authors have employed in their studies the measurement of a biochemical marker of ventricular dysfunction such as B-type natriuretic peptide.

B-type natriuretic peptide (BNP) is a cardiac neurohormone specifically secreted from cardiac ventricles in response to an increased left-ventricular wall tension (Maeda et al., 1998). When end-diastolic filling pressure is increased (related to ventricular dysfunction, hypervolemia or both conditions), the release of BNP is induced. BNP is a potent natriuretic peptide by enhancing renal sodium excretion, reducing so the intravascular volume and, therefore, the end-diastolic volume and pressure. BNP is a strong predictor of systolic and diastolic abnormalities and is a powerful marker for prognosis and risk stratification in the setting of heart failure (Tabbibizar et al., 2002). In the general population, a cut point of about 100 pg/ml can discriminate patients with heart failure from patients without it.

BNP is increased among patients with CKD and an inverse correlation between BNP levels and glomerular filtration rate has been observed (McCullough et al., 2003). This increased BNP level among these patients is in part related to the decreased renal clearance as well as the accompanying increased intravascular volume which is usually present in these patients. However, values above a cut-point reflect ventricular dysfunction and predict heart failure also among patients with CKD. In general, as CKD stage advances, a higher cut point of BNP is implied. BNP levels higher than 500 pg/ml usually predict heart failure even in patients with renal failure. Diastolic dysfunction is the most frequent cardiac disease among patients with CKD. In this setting, a small increment in end-diastolic volume lead to an exaggerated increase in diastolic pressure (Mandinov et al., 2000), inducing the release of natriuretic peptide. Probably, this pathophysiological mechanism partly explains the high levels of BNP detected among patients with CKD. In fact, several studies have observed an association between natriuretic peptide levels and echocardiographic data of left ventricular hypertrophy and dysfunction among patients with CKD (Guo et al., 2009; Paniagua et al., 2010; Zocali et al., 2001). Natriuretic peptide levels among patients with CKD predict death, as it occurs in patients with heart failure and normal renal function. Otherwise, some authors (Jacobs et al., 2010) have demonstrated a direct correlation between extracellular water, measured by bioelectrical impedance, and natriuretic peptide in CKD patients, explaining how volume overload can increase end-diastolic volume and, therefore, end-diastolic pressure favoring the release of BNP. Probably both mechanisms, volume overload and myocardial damage, both high prevalent among patients with CKD, could explained the high levels of natriuretic peptides detected in this population.

NT-proBNP is the amino-terminal peptide fragment of the precursor of BNP and shows a close correlation to BNP (Masson et al., 2002). A non-normal distribution of NT-proBNP levels was observed among patients with advanced renal failure, as previously observed with CRP (Ortega et al., 2004). Newly, it means that only a group of patients with advanced renal failure shows high levels of natriuretic peptides, whereas other patients with similar creatinine clearance show even normal values. This finding probably reflects the presence of a mixed population among patients with advanced CKD with a group of patients with more severe cardiac disease whereas other patients can achieve the end-stage disease phase with less myocardial damage. But most importantly, a strong correlation between NT-proBNP and CRP levels is found (figure 1), suggesting an association between left-ventricular filling pressure and inflammation among patients with CKD.

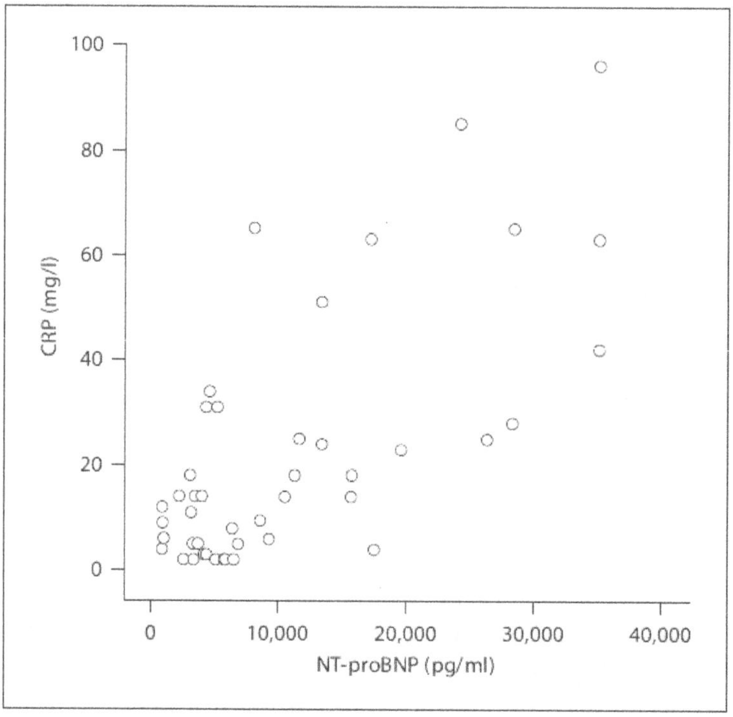

Fig. 1. Regression graph demonstrating the correlation between NT-proBNP and C-reactive protein values at baseline (r: 0.7; $p < 0.001$)

This association between left-ventricular filling pressure and inflammation among CKD patients has been confirmed in subsequent years (Guo et al., 2009; Jacobs et al., 2010; Paniagua et al., 2010). Otherwise, the same studies and other authors (Booth et al., 2010) observed a relationship between cardiac and inflammatory biomarkers and volume overload. An association between volume overload and inflammation had been previously observed among patients on peritoneal dialysis (Woodrow, 2006). Overhydration by itself has emerged as an independent predictor on mortality in chronic hemodialysis patients (Wizemann et al., 2009).

Thus, all these findings show the complex relation between overhydration, malnutrition, inflammation and cardiac biomarkers in CKD patients. Although CRP can actively participate in the atherosclerotic process inducing CV damage, it has also been suggested that inflammation among patients with CKD could be the consequence, rather than the cause, of an increased left-ventricular filling pressure, related to ventricular dysfunction, hypervolemia or both conditions (Ortega, 2005).

The complex relation between ventricular dysfunction, overhydration and inflammation highlights the importance of strict volume control in patients with CKD. Usually, ventricular dysfunction progress over time. In an interesting longitudinal study performed in hemodialysis patients, a progressive deterioration of left ventricular filling pressure (an index of diastolic dysfunction) was observed in parallel with the progression of left ventricular hypertrophy and a progressive increment in levels of NT-proBNP (Kim et al., 2011). Thus, these results suggest that diastolic dysfunction progress over time among patients with chronic kidney disease. In another longitudinal study performed in hemodialysis patients (Ortega et al., 2009), the effect of strict volume control on the evolution of cardiac biomarker levels over time was analyzed. In this study, the strategy of strict volume control permitted the stabilization of cardiac biomarker levels over time, suggesting that this strategy may prevent further progression of left ventricular hypertrophy, cardiac fibrosis and diastolic dysfunction. Patients with higher biomarker levels at baseline, probably those with more severe myocardial damage, were the most beneficed as NT-proBNP levels could even be reduced over time (figure 2). In these high risk patients, continuous prevention of fluid overload diminished the inflammatory parameters on follow-up, confirming the importance of volume control for preventing inflammation in dialysis patients (figure 3).

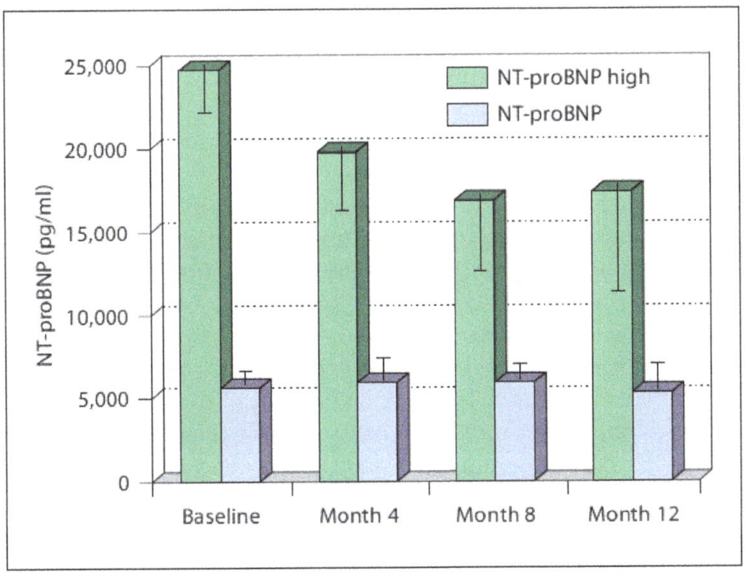

Fig. 2. Evolution over time of NT-proBNP values among patients distributed in high quartile at baseline (NT-proBNP high) and those distributed in other basal quartiles (NT-proBNP). Data expressed as mean ± standard error.

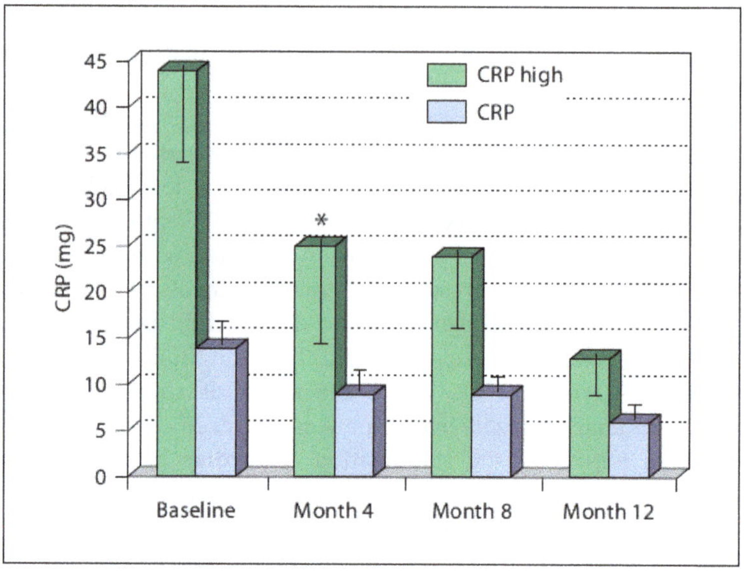

Fig. 3. Evolution over time of CRP values among patients distributed in high quartile at baseline (CRP high) and those distributed in other basal quartiles (CRP). * $p<0.05$ vs baseline levels. Data expressed as mean ± standard error.

7. Other cardiac biomarkers: Troponin T

Cardiac troponins are regulatory proteins within the myocardium that are released into the circulation when damage to the cardiomyocite has occurred. Therefore, serum troponin is an exquisitely sensitive marker of myocardial injury during the acute coronary syndrome and is necessary for establishing the diagnosis of myocardial infarction (Daubert et al., 2010).

Cardiac troponins control the calcium-mediated interaction of actin and myosin, which results in contraction and relaxation of striated muscle. The troponin complex is made up to three subunits: troponin C, troponin I and troponin T. Troponin C is expressed by cells in both cardiac and skeletal muscle. In contrast, troponin I and T are unique to cardiac muscle.

Among patients with acute coronary syndrome, cardiac troponin has not only diagnostic value, but yield prognostic information as well. It has been proven to be a potent independent indicator of recurrent ischemic events and an estimate for the risk of death among patients presenting with acute coronary syndrome (Heidenreich et al., 2001).

Persistently elevated cardiac troponin is frequently observed among asymptomatic patients with end-stage-renal-disease and is associated with increased mortality (Apple et al., 2002; de Fillipi et al., 2003; Ogi et al., 2001). There has been proposed several mechanisms for explaining the high levels of troponin among patients with CKD. Although troponin is a relative large molecule which is believed to be cleared by the reticuloendothelial system, more recent evidence suggest that troponin T is fragmented into molecules small enough to be renally excreted, which may partly explain the high prevalence of troponin T elevation in patients with renal failure (Diris et al., 2004).

Cardiac microinfarctions and arrhythmia have also been suggested as possible causes of elevations of troponin among patients with CKD.
More recently, it has been observed that CKD patients with high troponin T concentrations had clear evidence of myocardial dysfunction and raised left ventricular filling pressure (Sharma et al., 2006), supporting that volume and pressure overload can cause excessive ventricular wall tension with resultant myofibrillary damage or cardiomyocites death (Horwich TB et al., 2003). In this way, a strong association between troponin T and NT-proBNP has been observed in hemodialysis patients (figure 4) (Ortega et al., 2009) and both troponin T and NT-proBNP levels has been observed to be higher in volume-overloaded CKD patients (Sommerer et al., 2007).

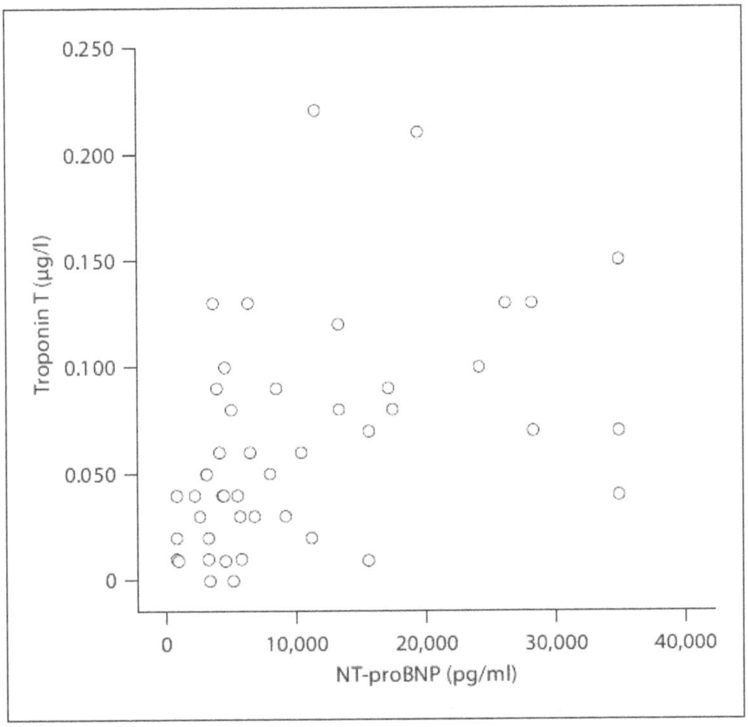

Fig. 4. Regression graph demonstrating the correlation between NT-proBNP and troponin T values at baseline (r: 0.4; p= 0.002)

Thus, it seems that the increased troponin T in a high proportion of patients with CKD could be related to myocardial injury induced by an increased left ventricular volume especially in those patients with diastolic dysfunction, in whom a small increase in end-diastolic volume produces an exaggerated increment in end-diastolic pressure with the subsequent myocardial damage. Furthermore, in hemodialysis patients, a strategy of strict volume control over time could significantly reduce the troponin T levels especially in those patients with higher biomarker levels at baseline, probably those with more severe myocardial dysfunction (figure 5) (Ortega et al., 2009).

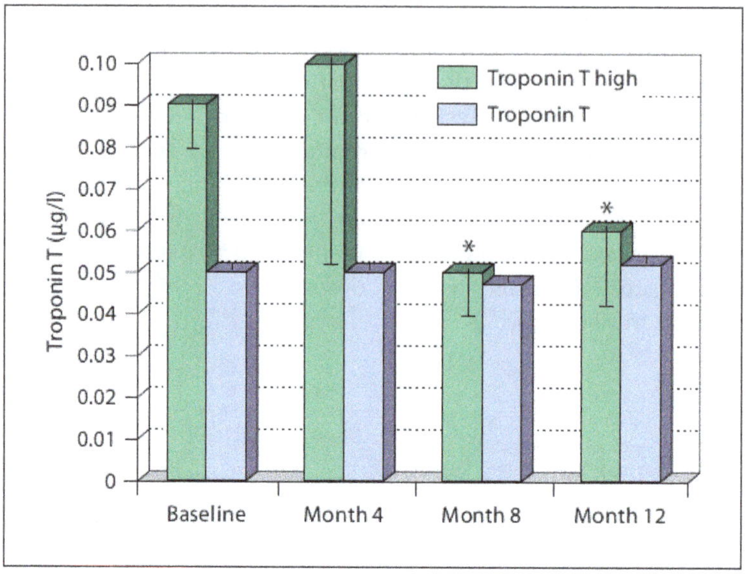

Fig. 5. Evolution over time of troponin T values among patients distributed in the high quartile at baseline (Troponin T high) vs those distributed in the other basal quartiles (Troponin T). * $p<0.05$ vs baseline levels. Data expressed as mean ± standard error.

8. Summary and future perspectives

There is a complex association between ventricular dysfunction, cardiac biomarkers, malnutrition, inflammation and overhydration among patients with CKD, which could partly explain the high CV morbidity and mortality among these patients, comparing with the general population.

Probably, these alterations begin in the very early stages of CKD and volume overload could be an important underlying factor. The inability of the insufficient kidney for excreting water and salt induces an increase in extracellular volume, which may be underestimated in the early phases of CKD. Persistently volume overload can induce an increment in blood pressure, myocardial hypertrophy and myocardial fibrosis. Over time, diastolic dysfunction develops. In this setting, further small increments in end-diastolic volume produce an exaggerated increment in end-diastolic pressure favoring the release of BNP and also, myocardial damage and cardiac remodeling. During cardiac remodeling, death of cardiomyocites is produced inducing a serum increment in troponins, and normal myocardium is progressively substituted by a fibrotic matrix, worsening so diastolic dysfunction. In this situation, systemic inflammation is produced by a yet non clear mechanism.

Thus, in this chapter, it is tried to highlight the importance of early intervention for controlling volume excess in the very early stages of CKD in order to prevent future cardiac dysfunction and inflammation, reducing so the bad CV prognosis of these patients.

It is noteworthy that at this early stage of CKD some patients can show normal plasma creatinine, especially older patients or patients with low muscle mass, but they may be subclinically overhydrated. A prescription of low sodium diet and the carefully use of diuretics at this phase of CKD could be the main tool for preventing volume overload and future CV damage.

9. References

Ahmed A, Rich MW, Sanders PW, Perry GJ, Bakris GL, Zile MR, Love TE, Aban IB, Shlipak MG (2007). Chronic kidney disease associated mortality in diastolic versus systolic heart failure; a propensity matched study. *Am J Cardiol* 99, 3 (Feb 2007): 393-398

Apple FS, Murakami MM, Pearce LA, Herzog CA (2002). Predictive value of cardiac troponin I and T for subsequent death in end-stage renal disease. *Circulation* 106, 23 (Dec 2002): 2941-2945

Arici M, Walls J (2001). End-stage renal disease, atherosclerosis and cardiovascular mortality: is C-reactive protein the missing link? *Kidney Int* 59, 2 (Feb 2001): 407-414.

Ates K, Yilmaz O, Kutlay S, Ates A, Nergizoglu G, Erturk Sl (2005). Serum C-reactive protein level is associated with renal function and it affects echocardiographic cardiovascular disease in pre-dialysis patients. *Nephron Clin Pract* 101, 14 (Aug 2005): c190-c197

Barany P, Divino Filho JC, Bergstrom J (1997). High C-reactive protein is a strong predictor of resistance to erythropoietin in hemodialysis patients. *Am J Kidney Dis* 29, 4 (Apr 1997): 565-568

Booth J, Pinney J, Davenport A. N-terminal proBNP. Marker of cardiac dysfunction, fluid overload, or malnutrition in hemodialysis patients? (2010) *Clin J Am Soc Nephrol* 5, 6 (Jun 2010): 1036-1040

Bradbury BD, Critchlow CW, Weir MR, Stewart R, Krishnan M, Hakim RH (2009). Impact of elevated C-reactive protein levels on erythropoiesis-stimulating agents (ESA) dose and responsiveness in hemodialysis patients. *Nephrol Dial Transplant;* 24, 3 (Mar 2009): 919-925

Carracedo J, Merino A, Nogueras S, Carretero D, Berdud I, Ramirez R, Tetta C, Rodriguez M, Martin-Malo A, Aljama P (2006). On-line hemodiafiltration reduces the proinflammatory CD14+CD16+monocyte-derived dendritic cells: a prospective, crossover study. *J Am Soc Nephrol* 17, 8 (Aug 2006): 2315-2321

Cheung AK, Sarnek MJ, Yan G, Dwyer JT, Heyka RJ, Rocco MV, Teehan BP, Levey AS (2000). Atherosclerotic cardiovascular disease risks in chronic hemodialysis patients. *Kidney Int* 58, 1 (Jul 2000): 407-414

Daubert MA, Jeremias A (2010). The utility of trponin measurement to detect myocardial infarction: review of the current findings. *Vasc Health Risk Manag* 6 (Sep 2010): 691-699

deFillipi C, Wasserman S, Rosanio S, Tiblier E, Sperger H, Tocchi M, Christenson R, Uretsky B, Smiley M, Gold J, Muniz H, Badalamenti J, Herzog C, Henrich W (2003). Cardiac troponin T and C-reactive protein predicting prognosis, coronary atherosclerosis, and cardyomyopathy in patients undergoing long-term hemodialysis. *JAMA* 290, 3 (Jul 2003): 353-359

Diris JH, Hackeng CM, Kooman JP, Pinto YM, Hermens WT, van Dieijen-Visser MP (2004). Impaired renal clearance explain elevated troponin T fragments in hemodialysis patients. *Circulation* 109, 1 (Jan 2004): 23-25

Essig M, Escoubet B, de Zuttere D, Blanchet F, Arnoult F, Dupuis E, Michel C, Mignon F, Mentre F, Clerici C, Vrtovsnik F (2008). Cardiovascullar remodelling and extracellular fluid excess in early stages of chronic kidney disease. *Nephrol Dial Transplant* 23, 1 (Jan 2008): 239-248

Foley RN, Parfrey PS, Harnett JD, Kent GM, Murray DC, Barré PE (1995). The prognosis of left-ventricular geometry in uremic cardiomyopathy. *J Am Soc Nephrol* 5, 12 (Jun 1995): 2024-2031

Foley RN, Parfrey PS, Sarnek MJ. Epidemiology of cardiovascular disease in chronic renal disease (1998). *J Am Soc Nephrol* 9, suppl 12 (Dec 1998): S16-S23

Gunnell J, Yeun JY, Depner TA, Kaysen GA (1999). Acute-phase response predicts erythropoietin resistance in hemodialysis and peritoneal dialysis patients. *Am J Kidney Dis* 33, 1 (Jan 1999): 63-72

Guo Q, Barany P, Qureshi AR, Snaedal S, Heimburger O, Stenvinkel P, Lindholm B, Axelsson J (2009). N-terminal pro-brain natriuretic peptide independently predicts protein energy wasting and is associated with all-cause mortality in prevalent HD patients. *Am J Nephrol* 29, 6 (2009): 516-523

Hayashi SY, Rohani M, Lindholm B, Brodin LA, Lind B, Barany P, Alvestrand A, Seeberger A (2006). Left ventricular function in patients with chronic kidney disease evaluated by colour tissue Doppler velocity imaging. *Nephrol Dial Transplant* 21, 1 (Jan 2006): 125-132

Heidenreich PA, Alloggiamento T, Melsop K, McDonald KM, Go AS, Hlatky MA (2001). The prognostic value of troponin in patients with non-ST elevation acute coronary syndromes: a meta-analysis. *J Am Coll Cardiol* 38, 2 (Aug 2001): 478-485.

Horwich TB, Patel J, MacLellan WR, Fonarow GC (2003). Cardiac troponin I is associated with impaired hemodinamics, progressive left ventricular dysfunction and increased mortality rates in advanced heart failure. *Circulation* 108, 7 (Aug 2003): 833-838

Honkanen E, Gronhagen-Riska C, Teppo AM, Maury CP, Meri S (1991). Acute-phase proteins during hemodialysis: correlations with serum interleukin-1 levels and differents dialysis membranes. *Nephron* 57, 3 (1991): 283-287

Ikizler TA, Wingard RL, Harvell J, Shyr Y, Hakim RM (1999). Association of morbidity with markers of nutrition and inflammation in chronic hemodialysis patients: a prospective study. *Kidney Int* 55, 5 (May 1999): 1945-1951.

Jacobs LH, Van de Kerkhof JJ, Mingels AM, Passos VL, Kleijnen VW, Mazairac AH, van der Sande FM, Wodzig WK, Konings CJ, Leunissen KM, van Dieijen-Visser MP, Kooman JP (2010). Inflammation, overhydration and cardiac biomarkers in hemodialysis patients: a longitudinal study. *Nephrol Dial Transplant* 25, 1 (Jan 2010): 243-248

Kaysen GA, Stevenson FT, Depner TA (1997). Determinants of albumin concentration in hemodialysis patients. *Am J Kidney Dis* 29, 5 (May 1997): 658-668

Kerr PG, Sutherland WH, de Jong S, Vaithalingham I, Williams SM, Walker RJ (2007). The impact of standard high-flux polysulfone versus novel high-flux polysulfone dialysis membranes on inflammatory biomarkers: a randomized, single-blinded, controlled clinical trial. *Am J Kidney Dis* 49, 4 (Apr 2007): 533-539

Kim BS, Jeon DS, Shin MJ, Kim YO, Song HC, Lee SH, Kim SY, Choi EJ, Chang YS, Bang BK (2005). Persistent elevation of C-reactive protein may predict cardiac hypertrophy and dysfunction in patients maintained on hemodialysis. *Am J Nephrol* 25, 3 (May-Jun 2005): 189-195

Kim YK, Shin SJ, Ihm SH, Park CS, Kim HY, Hong TY, Song HC, Yang CW, Kim YS, Choi EJ (2010). Longitudinal changes of left ventricular filling pressure and N-terminal pro-brain natriuretic peptide on chronic hemodialysis. *Clin Nephrol* 74, 3 (Sept 2010): 190-197

Levin A, Singer J, Thompson CR, Ross H, Lewis M (1996). Prevalent left-ventricular hypertrophy in the predialysis population: identifying opportunities for intervention. *Am J Kidney Dis* 27, 3 (Mar 1996): 347-354

Levine B, Kalman J, Mayer L, Fillit HM, Packer M. (1990) Elevated circulating levels of tumor necrosis factor in severe chronic heart failure. *N Eng J Med* 323, 4 (Jul 1990): 236-241

Lindner A, Charra B, Sherrard DJ, Scribner BH (1974). Accelerated atherosclerosis in prolonged maintenance hemodialysis. *N Engl J Med* 290, 13 (Mar 1974): 697-701

López-Gómez JM, Portolés JM, Aljama P (2008). Factors that condition the response to erythropoietin in patients on hemodialysis and their relation to mortality. *Kidney Int* 74, S111 (Dec 2008): S75-S81

Losi MA, Memoli B, Contaldi C, Barbati G, Del Prete M, Betocchi S, Cavallaro M, Carpinella G, Fundaliotis A, Parrella LS, Parisi V, Guida B, Chiariello M (2010). Myocardial fibrosis and diastolic dysfunction in patients on chronic hemodialysis. *Nephrol Dial Transplant* 25, 6 (Jun 2010): 1950-1954

Lowrie EG, Lew NL (1990). Death risk in hemodialysis patients: The predictive value of commonly measured variables and an evaluation of death rate differences between facilities. *Am J Kidney Dis* 15, 5 (May 1990): 458-482

Maeda K, Tsutamoto T, Wada A, Hisanaga T, Kinoshita M. Plasma brain natriuretic peptide as a biochemical marker of high left ventricular end-diastolic pressure in patients with symptomatic left ventricular dysfunction. *Am Heart J* 135, 5 (May 1998): 825-832

MacKenna D, Summerour SR, Villarreal FJ (2000). Role of mechanical factors in modulating cardiac fibroblast function and extracellular matrix synthesis. *Cardiovasc Research* 46, 2 (May 2000): 257-263

Mandinov L, Eberli FR, Seiler C, Hess OM (2000). Diastolic heart failure. *Cardiovasc Res* 45, 4 (Mar 2000): 813-825

Mark PB, Johnston N, Groenning BA, Foster JE, Blyth KG, Martin TN, Steedman T, Dargie HJ, Jardine AG (2006). Redefinition of uremic cardiomyopathy by contrast-enhanced cardiac magnetic resonance imaging. *Kidney Int* 69, 10 (May 2006): 1839-1845

Martos R, Baugh J, Ledwidge M, O'Loughlin C, Conlon C, Patle A, Donnelly SC, McDonald K (2007). Diastolic heart failure: evidence of increased myocardial collagen turnover linked to diastolic dysfunction. *Circulation* 115, 7 (Feb 2007): 888-895

Masson S, Vago T, Baldi G, Salio M, De Angelis N, Nicolis E, Maggioni AP, Latini R, Norbiato G, Bevilacqua M (2002). Comparative measurement of N-terminal pro-brain natriuretic peptide and brain natriuretic peptide in ambulatory patients with heart failure. *Clin Chem Lab Med* 40, 8 (Aug 2002): 761-763

McCullough PA, Duc P, Omland T, McCord J, Nowak RM, Hollander JE, Herrmann HC, Steg PF, Westheim A, Knudsen CW, Storrow AB, Abraham WT, Lamba S, Wu AH, Perez A, Clopton P, Krishnaswamy P, Kazanegra R, Maisel AS; Breathing Not Properly Multinantional Study Investigators (2003). B-type natriuretic peptide and renal function in the diagnosis of heart failure: an analysis from the Breathing Not Properly Multinational Study. *Am J Kidney Dis* 41, 3 (Mar 2003): 571-579

Niebauer J, Volk HD, Kemp M, Dominguez M, Schumann RR, Rauchhaus M, Poole-Wilson PA, Coats AJ, Anker SD (1999). Endotoxin and immune activation in chronic heart failure: a prospective cohort study. *Lancet* 353, 9167 (May 1999): 1838-1842

Noh H, Lee SW, Kang SW, Shin SK, Choi KH, Lee HY, Hans DS (1998). Serum C-reactive protein: a predictor of mortality in continuous ambulatory peritoneal dialysis patients. *Perit Dial Int* 18, 4 (Jul-Aug 1998): 387-394

Ooi DS, Zimmerman D, Graham J, Wells GA (2001). Cardiac troponin T predicts long-term outcomes in hemodialysis patients. *Clin Chem* 47, 3 (Mar 2001): 412-417

Ortega O, Rodriguez I, Gallar P, Carreño A, Ortiz M, Espejo B, Jimenez J, Gutierrez M, Oliet A, Vigil A (2002). Significance of high C-reactive protein levels in pre-dialysis patients. *Nephrol Dial Transplant* 17, 6 (Jun 2002): 1105-1109

Ortega O, Gallar P, Munoz M, Rodríguez I, Carreño A, Ortiz M, Molina A, Oliet A, Lozano L, Vigil A (2004). Association between C-reactive protein levels and N-terminal pro-B-type natriuretic peptide in pre-dialysis patients. *Nephron Clin Pract* 97, 4 (Aug 2004): c125-c130

Ortega O (2005). Could we reduce the prevalence of inflammation among patients with chronic kidney disease? *Nephron Clin Pract* 101, 4 (Aug 2005): c198-c199

Ortega O, Rodriguez I, Gracia C, Sanchez M, Lentisco C, Mon C, Gallar P, Ortiz M, Herrero JC, Oliet A, Vigil A (2009). Strict volume control and longitudinal changes in cardiac biomarker levels in hemodialysis patients. *Nephrol Clin Pract* 113, 2 (Jul 2009): c96-c103

Owen WF, Lowrie EG (1998). C-reactive protein as an outcome predictor for maintenance hemodialysis patients. *Kidney Int* 54, 2 (Aug 1998): 627-636

Paniagua R, Ventura MD, Avila-Diaz M, Hinojosa-Heredia H, Mendez-Duran A, Cueto-Manzano A, Cisneros A, Ramos A, Madonia-Juseino C, Belio-Caro F, Garcia-Contreras F, Trinidad-Ramos P, Vazquez R, Ilabaca B, Alcantara G, Amato D (2010). NT-proBNP, fluid overload and dialysis modality are independent predictors of mortality in ESRD patients. *Nephrol Dial Transplant* 25, 2 (Feb 2010): 551-557

Panichi V, Migliori M, de Pietro S, Taccola D, Bianchi AM, Giovannini L, Norpoth M, Metelli MR, Cristofani R, Bertelli AA, Sbragia G, Tetta C, Palla R (2002). C-reactive protein and interleukin-6 levels are related to renal function in predialytic chronic renal failure. *Nephron* 91, 4 (Aug 2002): 594-600

Panichi V, Rieza GM, Paoletti S, Bigazzi R, Aloisi M, Barsotti G, Rindi P, Donati G, Antonelli A, Panicucci E, Tripepi G, Tetta C, Palla R; RISCAVID Study Group (2008). Chronic inflammation and mortality in hemodialysis: effect of different renal replacement therapy. Results from the RISCAVID study. *Nephrol Dial Transplant* 23, 7 (Jul 2008): 2337-2343

Pepys MB, Hirschfield GM (2003). C-reactive protein: a critical update. *J Clin Invest* 111, 12 (Jun 2003): 1805-1812

Peschel T, Schonauer M, Thiele H, Anker S, Schuler G, Niebauer J (2003). Invasive assessment of bacterial endotoxin and inflammatory cytokines in patients with acute heart failure. *Europ J of Heart Fail* 5, 5 (Oct 2003): 609-614

Qureshi AR, Alvestrand A, Danielsson A, Divino-Filho JC, Gutierrez A, Lindholm B, Bergstrom J (1998). Factors influencing malnutrition in hemodialysis patients: A cross-sectional study. *Kidney Int* 53, 3 (Mar 1998): 773-782

Ridker PM (2001). High-sensitivity C-reactive protein: potential adjunt for global risk assessment in the primary prevention of cardiovascular disease. *Circulation* 103, 13 (Apr 2001): 1813-1818.

Schouten WE, Grooteman MP, van Houte AJ, Schoorl M, van Limbeck J, Nube MJ (2000). Effects of dialysers and dialysate on the acute phase reaction in clinical bicarbonate dialysis. *Nephrol Dial Trnsplant* 15, 3 (Mar 2000): 379-384

Seta Y, Shan K, Bozkurt B, Oral H, Mann DL (1996). Basic mechanism in heart failure: the cytokine hypothesis. *J Card Fail* 2,3 (Sep 1996): 243-249

Sharer K, Schmidt KG, Soergel M (1999). Cardiac function and structure in patients with chronic renal failure. *Pediatr Nephrol* 13, 9 (Nov 1999): 951-965

Sharma R, Gaze DC, Pellerin D, Mehta RL, Gregson H, Streather CP, Collinson PO, Brecker SJ (2006). Cardiac structural and functional abnormalities in end stage renal disease patients with elevated cardiac troponin T. *Heart* 92, 6 (Jun 2006): 804-809

Sommerer C, Beimler J, Schwenger V, Heckele N, Katus HA, Giannitsis E, Zeier M (2007). Cardiac biomarkers and survival in hemodialyisis patients. *Eur J Clin Invest* 37, 5 (May 2007): 350-356

Stenvinkel P, Heimburger O, Paultre F, Diczfalusy U, Wang T, Berglund L, Jogestrand T (1999). Strong association between malnutrition, inflammation and atherosclerosis in chronic renal failure. *Kidney Int* 55, 5 (May 1999): 1899-1911

Tabbibizar R, Maisel A (2002). The impact of B-type natriuretic peptide levels on the diagnoses and management of congestive heart failure. *Curr Opin Cardiol* 17, 4 (Jul 2002): 340-345.

Wang AY, Lam CW, Chan IH, Wang M, Lui SF, Sanderson JE (2009). Long-term mortality and cardiovascular risk stratification of peritoneal dialysis patients using a combination of inflammation and calcification markers. *Nephrol Dial Transplant* 24 12 (Dec 2009): 3826-3803

Wizemann V, Wabel P, Chamney P, Zaluska W, Moissl U, Rode C, Malecka-Masalska T, Marcelli D (2009). The mortality risk of overhydration in hemodialysis patients. *Nephrol Dial Transplant* 24, 5 (May 2009): 1574-1579

Woodrow G (2006). Extracellular water expansion; part of the malnutrition-inflammation-atherosclerosis syndrome? *Peri Dial Int* 26, 5 (Sep-Oct 2006):566-570

Yeun JY, Levine RA, Mantadilok V, Kaysen GA (2000). C-reacive protein predicts all-cause and cardiovascular mortality in hemodialysis patients. *Am J Kidney Dis* 35, (Mar 2000): 469-476

Zhang YX, Cliff WJ, Schoefl GI, Higgins G (1999). Coronary C-reactive protein distribution: its relation to development of atherosclerosis. *Atherosclerosis* 145, 2 (Aug 1999): 375-379

Zimmermann J, Herrlinger S, Pruy A , Metzger T, Wanner C (1999). Inflammation enhances cardiovascular risk and mortality in hemodialysis patients. *Kidney Int* 55, 2 (Feb 1999): 648-658

Zoccali C, Mallamaci F, Benedetto FA, Tripepi G, Parlongo S, Cataliotti A, Cutrupi S, Giacone G, Bellanuova I, Cottini E, Malatino LS (2001). Cardiac natriuretic peptides are related to left ventricular mass and function and predict mortality in dialysis patients. *J Am Soc Nephrol* 12, 7 (Jul 2001): 1508-1515.

Zoccali C, Benedetto FA, Mallamaci F, Tripepi G, Giacone G, Stancanelli B, Cataliotti A, Malatino LS (2004). Left ventricular mass monitoring in the follow-up of dialysis patients: prognostic value of left ventricular hypertrophy progression. *Kidney Int* 65, 4 (Apr 2004): 1492-1498.

2

Hemodialysis Principles and Controversies

Parin Makadia, Payam Benson, Filberto Kelly and Joshua Kaplan
New Jersey Medical School,
United States of America

1. Introduction

The incidence rates of End-stage renal disease (ESRD) have increased steadily internationally since 1989. The United States has the highest incident rate of ESRD, followed by Japan; Japan has the highest prevalence per million population, with the United States second (1). Of the 490,000 patients with ESRD in the United States, more than 380,000 are currently on hemodialysis (HD) (2).

ESRD on HD disproportionately affects minority populations. Whites represent the majority of the HD population (59.8%), while African Americans (33.2%), Asians (3.6%), and Native Americans (1.6%) comprise the rest of the ESRD population. However, the incidence rate of ESRD among African Americans is 4-fold higher and Native Americans 2-fold higher than that for whites. ESRD is slightly more prevalent in men than in women (male-to-female ratio, 1.2:1) and more prevalent in older adults (3).

2. Morbidity/mortality

Chronic renal failure is associated with a very high morbidity and hospitalization rate, likely due to existing comorbid conditions, such as hypertension, coronary artery disease, and peripheral vascular disease. The first-year age-adjusted mortality rate of patients on dialysis is 9.4%, the two-year mortality rate is 32.3%, and the 5-year mortality rate is 60.8% (3). ESRD patients with diabetes have a first-year mortality rate of 23% (3). In patients with ESRD, cardiovascular disease is the primary cause of death, followed by sepsis and cerebrovascular disease. The dialysis population in the United States has a 10- to 20-fold higher risk of death due to cardiovascular complications than the general population after adjusting for age, race, and sex. The relative risk with respect to the general population is much higher in younger patients, with cardiovascular event rates in ESRD patients in their 20s equivalent to the event rates in the general population in their 80s (3). Increased understanding of the disease process, new insights into pathogenic mechanisms, and new therapeutic options are emerging that may improve survival rates and quality of life for patients with ESRD.

3. The need for dialysis

Given the poor outcomes for patients on HD, every effort should be undertaken to preserve residual renal function, which is associated with improved survival (4). Early nephrology referrals, patient education, and consideration of transplant options may be helpful in decreasing the progression to ESRD. Preparation for dialysis therapy is critical for the smooth transition from CKD care to ESRD. Poor planning for initiation of dialysis is a major cause of increased morbidity and mortality. The use of temporary or tunneled dialysis catheters contributes to dialysis mortality by increasing the incidence of sepsis, acting as a stimulus for chronic inflammation, and damaging the central veins, thereby preventing or shortening the survival of more permanent vascular access once created. The chapter will discuss in detail regarding type of dialysis access.

3.1 Indications for initiation of dialysis

The appropriate time to initiate dialysis for a patient is not clearly defined. The decision to initiate dialysis in a patient with CKD involves the consideration of subjective and objective parameters by the physician and the patient. Over the past decade a trend of increasing estimated glomerular filtration rate (eGFR) at the initiation of dialysis for treatment of ESRD has been noted in the United States. In 1996, only 19% of patients began dialysis therapy with an eGFR of greater than 10 ml/min/1.73 m^2 (denoted as 'early start'), but by 2005 the fraction of early start dialysis patients had risen to 45% (5). It is not known whether early start of dialysis is beneficial, harmful or neutral with respect to the outcome of dialysis treatment for ESRD (5). The timing of initiation of dialysis for ESRD is a matter of clinical judgment guided by values of residual renal function and symptoms and signs present in the patients, including those related to comorbidity. By the time the eGFR falls below 10 ml/min/1.73 m^2, most patients require dialysis. However, many patients appear to function quite well until the eGFR approaches 5 ml/min/1.73 m^2. As a general rule, patients with diabetes require earlier intervention (eGFR<15 ml/min/1.73 m^2) than do those with other etiologies for renal failure (6). Clearly, dialysis must be initiated before the uremic symptoms of peripheral neuropathy, encephalopathy, malnutrition, or serositis (including pericarditis) become evident (See Table 1).

• Pericarditis or pleuritis (urgent indication)
• Progressive uremic encephalopathy or neuropathy, with signs such as confusion, asterixis, myoclonus, wrist or foot drop, or, in severe cases, seizures (urgent indication)
• A clinically significant bleeding diathesis attributable to uremia (urgent indication)
• Fluid overload refractory to diuretics
• Hypertension poorly responsive to antihypertensive medications
• Persistent metabolic disturbances that are refractory to medical therapy; these include hyperkalemia, metabolic acidosis, hypercalcemia, hypocalcemia, and hyperphosphatemia
• Persistent nausea and vomiting
• Evidence of malnutrition

Table 1. Clinical indications to initiate dialysis in patients with CKD. (7)

3.2 'Early' versus 'Late' dialysis

There is conflicting evidence concerning the effect of the early initiation of dialysis on survival. Some retrospective and uncontrolled prospective studies have reported no survival benefits with early dialysis while others have found that early start of dialysis may be harmful (8). After a comprehensive review of the published literature by the National

Kidney Foundation (NKF) workgroup in 1997, they recommended that initiation of dialysis be considered when the arithmetic mean of the urea and creatinine clearances fell below approximately 10.5 ml/min/1.73 m^2 except in well-nourished, asymptomatic patients (9). In 1999 Obrador *et al.*, observed that 23% of the US ESRD population, between 1995 and 1997, started dialysis at an eGFR less than 5 ml/min/1.73 m^2. They opined that this 'late start' of dialysis needed further examination, including studies of the impact on outcomes and cost of ESRD treatment (10).

In 2006, the NKF work group updated the guidelines for initiation of hemodialysis and stated that 'at CKD Stage 5, when the eGFR is < 15 ml/min/1.73 m^2, that nephrologists should evaluate the benefits, risks and disadvantages of beginning renal replacement therapy'. They also suggested that initiation of dialysis therapy before CKD Stage 5 (an eGFR of > 15 ml/min/1.73 m^2) may be appropriate in patients who have symptoms believed to be related to both their comorbidities and their level of residual kidney function (11). Only one study has reported the outcomes of patients with CKD who initiated dialysis only after the onset of symptoms due to uremia. In this prospective cohort study of 233 consecutive patients with advanced uremia, 151 were elective starters on dialysis, while 82 initially declined dialysis. Among the initial refusers, 55 percent developed a uremic emergency, while 48 percent were eventually established on maintenance dialysis. In this study, one year mortality was significantly higher among the initial refusers than the elective starters (18 versus 7 percent). However, these results are confounded by lack of randomization and by three deaths among the initial refusers resulting from treatment withdrawal (12).

Additional published studies have not been able to demonstrate any clear-cut survival benefits for early start of dialysis. The only randomized controlled trial that examined mortality and time of dialysis initiation, the IDEAL study (13), found no difference in survival between early or late initiation of dialysis. In this study, 828 patients with progressive CKD and an estimated GFR between 10.0 and 15.0 mL/min/1.73 m2 (as determined by the Cockcroft-Gault equation) were randomly assigned to dialysis initiation when the estimated GFR was either 10 to 14 mL/min/1.73 m2 or 5 to 7 mL/min/1.73 m^2. The median time to the initiation of dialysis was 1.8 and 7.4 months in the early and late start groups, respectively. At a median follow-up period of 3.6 years, the authors noted no significant difference in survival (38 and 37 percent mortality, hazard ratio of 1.05 with early initiation, 95% CI of 0.83 to 1.30) as well as no difference in cardiovascular events, infections, or dialysis complications between the late start group and early start group.

However, these results do not imply that the initiation of dialysis can be delayed until the GFR is between 5 to 7 mL/min/1.73 m^2 in all patients. The design of the IDEAL study permitted clinicians to initiate dialysis based upon the presence of symptoms due to uremia as well as on the estimated GFR. As a result, 76 percent of patients assigned to the late start arm initiated dialysis when the GFR was much greater than 5 to 7 mL/min/1.73 m^2. This resulted in a mean GFR of 9.8 mL/min/1.73 m^2 at the start of dialysis for the late start group, which was only 2.2 mL/min/1.73 m^2 less than the mean start GFR for the early group (12.0 mL/min/1.73 m^2). Thus, approximately 88 percent of all enrolled patients had initiated dialysis with an estimated GFR of approximately 10 mL/min/1.73 m^2 or more, either because of symptoms or enrollment in the early dialysis arm (13).

A recent study published in *Canadian Medical Association Journal* examined trends in initiation of hemodialysis within Canada and compared the risk of death between patients with early and late initiation of dialysis (14). Using the Canadian Organ Replacement

Registry from 2001 to 2007, the investigators identified a cohort of 25,910 patients 18 years or older who began hemodialysis. Dialysis was defined as beginning early if the eGFR exceeded 10.5 mL/minute/1.73 m^2. Mean eGFR at initiation of dialysis increased from 9.3 mL/minute/1.73 m^2 in 2001 to 10.2 mL/minute/1.73 m^2 in 2007 ($P < .001$). During the same period, the proportion of early dialysis initiations increased from 28% (95% confidence interval [CI], 27% - 30%) to 36% (95% CI, 34% - 37%). Among those starting dialysis early, mean GFR at initiation was 15.5 mL/minute/1.73 m^2 vs 7.1 mL/minute/1.73 m^2 among those who started dialysis late. For early vs late initiation of dialysis, the unadjusted hazard ratio (HR) for death was 1.48 (95% CI, 1.43 - 1.54). This suggests that early initation is associated with higher mortality. After adjustment for demographic factors, serum albumin, primary cause of end-stage renal disease, type of vascular access, comorbid conditions, late referral, and transplant status, the hazard ratio for death decreased to 1.18 (95% CI, 1.13 - 1.23). Difference in mortality per 1000 patient-years between starting dialysis early vs late decreased after 1 year of follow-up but persisted and began increasing again after 24 months of follow-up, with significant differences at 6, 12, 30, and 36 months. (14)

There may be two additional advantages to early dialysis: control of hypertension and increased dietary intake. Reversal of volume overload with dialysis often leads to a reduction in blood pressure, which is typically volume-dependent in CKD. Perhaps more important, patients on dialysis patients require at least 1 g/kg of protein per day to replace dialysis losses and maintain nitrogen balance. Thus, early institution of dialysis can allow a more liberal diet in terms of both food and fluid.

The overall conclusion of these trials largely supports current practice that dialysis initiation should be based upon clinical factors rather than the estimated GFR alone. Patients with progressive CKD require close follow up, early nephrology referral, and adequate advance dialysis planning (including the presence of a functioning peritoneal or vascular access and referral for transplantation). Among patients with progressive CKD, clinicians must be vigilant for the presence of symptoms and/or signs of uremia and dialysis should be initiated in the patient with these symptoms.

4. Dialysis modality selection

Although the life expectancy of patients with end-stage renal disease has improved since the introduction of dialysis in the 1960s, it is still far below that of the general population. As an example, the mean life span at age 49 in the United States is 33 years in the general population but only approximately seven years in patients receiving maintenance dialysis (15), in whom the overall five-year survival rate is about 30 to 50 percent in nondiabetics (depending upon the co-morbid diagnoses) and 25 percent in diabetics (15). Despite improvements in technology and patient care, the mortality rate of patients on maintenance dialysis remains alarmingly high, at approximately 15 to 20 percent per year (16).

There are two principal choices for maintenance dialysis: hemodialysis (HD) and peritoneal dialysis (PD). Selecting one of these modalities is influenced by a number of considerations such as availability and convenience, comorbid conditions, socioeconomic and dialysis center factors, the patient's home situation, method of physician reimbursement, and the ability to tolerate volume shifts (17-23). Most studies suggest a better survival rate in PD than in HD patients during the first few years after starting therapy (24). However, after 2 or 3 years, outcome on PD becomes equal to HD, or worse (25-28). This section mainly focuses on different means of receiving hemodialysis.

The European Best Practice Guidelines for Hemodialysis recommends the standard hemodialysis dose should be delivered as three times per week for 4 hours each session (29). In an attempt to improve outcomes, it was postulated that a higher dialysis dose than commonly provided during conventional dialysis may increase survival among patients undergoing renal replacement therapies (30).
However, this hypothesis was refuted in two large well-designed studies in both hemodialysis and peritoneal dialysis patients:

- The HEMO study found that increasing the dialysis dose within the general restrictions of a thrice weekly regimen failed to decrease patient mortality (31).
- In the ADEMEX study, no decrease in mortality was seen with peritoneal dialysis doses greater than a weekly Kt/V of 1.7 (32)

In light of these negative studies, significant attention has turned to alternative dialysis schedules, such as, short-daily HD (SHD), nocturnal HD (NHD), and long, intermittent hemodialysis (LHD). It is suggested that more frequent dialysis may be associated an improvement in health-related quality of life (HRQoL) and with improved survival (33-34).
The first successful use of short daily, or "quotidian" hemodialysis was first reported by DePalma in 1969 (35). This approach was based upon the premise that improved patient outcomes, compared with conventional three times per week hemodialysis, would occur with a dialysis schedule that consisted of the same number of hours of dialysis per week but delivered over twice as many sessions. More specifically, it involves five to seven treatments per week, each lasting 1.5 to 2.5 hours. The rationale for short daily hemodialysis is based upon a strategy that is proposed to enhance both dialysis efficiency and hemodynamic stability. With short daily dialysis, shortening the dialysis time while increasing the frequency of dialysis allows more time to be spent dialyzing against higher uremic solute concentration gradients. This enhances the efficiency of solute removal (36). More frequent dialysis allows for less interdialytic fluid accumulation. This is likely to improve hemodynamic stability during dialysis with increased potential for normalizing the extracellular fluid volume. This form of therapy has been associated with significant improvement in serum albumin, calcium phosphate, and volume control in small scale studies. However, no mortality data is available.
A recent study, Frequent Hemodialysis Network (FHN) Daily Trial, was a multicenter, randomized trial that included 245 patients assigned to either frequent hemodialysis (six times weekly) or conventional hemodialysis. Two primary composite outcomes were determined at one year, including death or one-year change from baseline in left ventricular (LV) mass as assessed by cardiac resonance imaging, and death or one-year change in physical health as assessed by a RAND health survey. Both composite outcomes showed significant benefit to the frequent-dialysis group compared with the conventional-dialysis group (with hazard ratios of 0.61, 95% CI, 0.46-0.82 for death or change in LV mass; and 0.70, 95% CI, 0.53-0.92, for death or change in physical health) (37). This study also demonstrated benefits in pre-determined secondary outcomes to the frequent dialysis group such as a decrease in LV mass, improved blood pressure control and phosphate balance but not on cognitive performance, depression, serum albumin concentration, or use of erythropoiesis-stimulating agents.
Nocturnal hemodialysis (e.g, long nightly home hemodialysis) was introduced as a potentially more desirable alternative to conventional dialysis, since it provides superior dialysis based upon dose, duration, and frequency (38). This can be accomplished because it is performed during nightly sleep, an otherwise unproductive time (39). The late Robert

Uldall started the first quotidian (daily) nocturnal hemodialysis program in 1994 at the Wellesley Hospital in Toronto (40). Since then, its use has been extended to more centers in Canada, the United States, Australia, and several European countries (41-44). This hemodialysis modality is performed five to seven times per week, with each treatment lasting 6 to 8 hours. Although the number of patients studied has been rather limited, but these evidence suggest signficant improvements in caloric intake and serum albumin results.
Long intermittent hemodialysis is given three times a week and a dialysis time of 6 to 8 hours. This procedure is practiced in Tassin, France, and has been associated with improvements in blood pressure control and better overall nutritional status.
Although, no data on randomized controlled trials are available on home hemodialysis, some recent well-conceived cohort studies have indicated that outcome of home (daily) HD is superior to conventional in-centre dialysis, and even equal to cadaveric transplantation, when differences in case mix are taken into account (45).

4.1 Hemofiltration and hemodiafiltration

Hemodiafiltration is a form of chronic renal replacement therapy used most in Europe, particularly Germany and Belgium, and very rarely used currently in the United States (46). Based upon relatively better clearance of larger "middle" molecules through solvent drag, some claim that replacement therapy with hemodiafiltration may be superior to that with hemodialysis, including improved hemodynamics.
For chronic renal replacement therapy, the two principal regimens used to provide substantial removal of larger MW uremic toxins via convection are intermittent hemofiltration (HF) and intermittent hemodiafiltration (HDF). Daily convective therapy has also been used.

- Hemofiltration — With HF, fluid is removed by the dialysis machine through increased transmembrane pressure and the replacement solution is infused intravenously at equal volume minus the desired fluid volume removal. The clearance of the method for a particular solute is dictated by the ultrafiltration volume and the sieving coefficient. As the sieving coefficient for low MW unbound solutes equals 1, the clearance for small molecules equals the ultrafiltrate volume. Although hemofiltration is effective in the removal of the larger MW solutes, it is less effective in the removal of small molecules as it is restricted by the ultrafiltration volume.
- Hemodiafiltration — HDF is a combination of hemodialysis and hemofiltration devised to overcome the low clearance of small solutes by hemofiltration by adding a diffusive component.

For chronic renal replacement therapy, the standard regimen for both HF and HDF includes three sessions per week for three to five hours, as with conventional intermittent hemodialysis. A typical conservative (or high dose) regimen for HDF includes a post dilution configuration with a blood flow of 300 mL/min (500 mL/min for high dose), a dialysate flow of 500 mL/min, a flow of a substitution volume of 60 mL/min (120 mL/min for high dose) and a high flux dialyzer of 1.4 m^2 (2.2 m^2 for high dose) (47).
Several small studies using daily HF/HDF have been published.

- One study that addressed the short term effects of daily HF reported that predialysis beta-2-microglobulin levels decreased by 40 percent (48).
- In one study in which 12 patients switched from HD to HF at home on a daily basis for one month, HF was associated with a lower blood pressure, higher caloric intake, and

improved quality of life, findings consistent with previous reports on short daily HD (49-50). A trend toward a decrease in serum beta-2-microglobulin could be ascribed to the HF alone. The infusion volume used was 40 percent of total body water, which offered a standard Kt/V of approximately 2.0.

- In another study of eight patients undergoing in center daily hemodiafiltration for six months, there were lower serum levels of predialysis BUN and creatinine (which were expected by the change to a daily schedule), as well as lower levels of other solutes including beta-2-microglobulin and homocysteine (51). Additional benefits included improved phosphate control, discontinuation of all antihypertensive agents, and a 30 percent regression in left ventricular mass. Although some of these results can be attributed to the daily treatment schedule, the decrease in the pretreatment levels of beta-2-microglobulin and the improvement in phosphate control are clearly attributable to both convection and the increased treatment frequency.

4.2 Adequacy of hemodialysis

For greater than 50 years hemodialysis (HD) has been performed in some form or another. Outcomes for dialysis patients expressed in terms of quality of life (QOL), mortality, and hospitalization, is reportedly similar to those seen in patients with solid organ cancer. Despite improvements in long-term outcomes demonstrated with all dialysis modalities, the adjusted annual mortality of dialysis patient remains high at 19% (52-53). There are many factors (dialysis and non-dialysis) that determines outcome. One such influential factor is "adequacy" of dialysis. Adequate dialysis was originally used to describe dialysis dosing measured by small solute removal, but is now deemed as the amount of dialysis required to keep a patient symptoms free, functional, with a life expectancy similar to that of healthy individuals. Since its inception, there have been numerous approaches to quantify the delivered dialysis dose in a reproducible manner, and to link the dialysis dose with clinical outcomes.

4.3 Importance of urea and its use as a surrogate marker of uremic toxicity

Solute removal during hemodialysis focuses on urea. Urea is produced from the anabolism, catabolism of proteins and is the principal way by which nitrogenous substances are excreted from the body. Urea is a small water soluble molecule (molecular weight 60 daltons) that is slightly toxic. Recent studies have demonstrated that urea removal does not closely parallel that of other small water-soluble compounds, protein-bound solutes, or middle molecules. (54) Despite this information, adequacy of HD dosing is predominantly evaluated by removal of urea. During the development of the uremic syndrome, losses of kidney function are accompanied by deteriorating organ function attributable to the accumulation of uremic retention solutes or uremic toxins. (54) Uremic toxins are diverse and complex, they include inorganic compounds (phosphate water, potassium, water and trace elements), as well as organic compounds that comprises small water-soluble solutes (<500 d), middle molecules (>500 d), and protein-bound solutes. These peptides can be altered by glycosylation, oxidization or carbamylation, and they can provoke inflammation, hypertrophy, oxidative stress, coagulation, constriction, thus uremia is more than the retention and accumulation of urea or water-soluble compounds alone. (54) Mortality has repeatedly been shown to be associated with the clearance of urea. Of commonly measured protein-derived substances, only the serum concentration of $ß_2$-microglobulin correlates with mortality. Recently, a higher free concentration of the protein-bound solute *p*-cresol has also been reported to be associated with mortality. (55) Current dialysis and dialysis-related treatments do not remove any significant quantity of substances larger than 10 to 15 kd. Future means of removing higher molecular weight toxins or protein-bound substances may include the use of sorbents in addition to traditional diffusive and convective dialysis strategies.

4.4 Urea kinetic modeling, URR and KT/V

The mathematical model known as urea kinetics can be used to calculate the rate of production and removal of urea. Measurement of the dialysis dose has, for the most part, relied on estimation of clearance of the small, water-soluble, and nitrogenous waste product urea, and hence the mathematical model is referred to as urea kinetic modeling (UKM). Formal (UKM) is the most accurate method for assessment of delivered dialysis dose. It assumes that urea is distributed in a single, well-mixed pool. UKM presumes that full equilibration occurs immediately between blood and tissue compartments. However, in vivo there is a delay in redistribution and it takes 30 to 60 minutes for equilibration between blood and tissue compartments post dialysis. UKM also assumes that urea is generated at a constant rate by protein metabolism and is removed at a constant rate by residual renal function, and intermittently by dialysis. Hence, in a person with negligible renal function, the extent of urea removal provides a measure of dialysis adequacy, and the rate of production correlates with dietary protein intake. (56) Thus, it's inappropriate to follows predialysis blood urea nitrogen (BUN) or serum urea only; because low serum urea could be attributed to malnutrition (insufficient protein diet) rather than adequate dialysis urea removal. UKM has formed the basis for retrospective interpretation of the National Cooperative Dialysis Study and for prescription and control of the HEMO and the Frequent Hemodialysis Network studies. (60) Due its mathematical intricacy, UKM requires advanced computer support. UKM is the most rigorous available method for prescribing and evaluating dialysis dose and is widely used in the United States. Current methods for assessment of dialysis dose are based on the predialysis and postdialysis difference in BUN and include the urea reduction ratio (URR), the single-pool *Kt/V* (*spKt/V*), the equilibrated *Kt/V* (*eKt/V*), and the weekly standard *Kt/V* (*std-Kt/V*).

Kt/V is a dimensionless ratio representing fractional urea clearance, where *K* is the dialyzer urea clearance (liters per hour), *t* is the length of HD session (hours), and *V* is the volume of distribution of urea (liters). It is the most widely used parameter to assess dialysis dose. Kt/V is derived from single-pool urea kinetics and is referred to as spKt/V. A value of spKt/V of 1 indicates that the total volume of blood completely cleared of urea during a dialysis session is equivalent to the volume of distribution of urea. Solute disequilibrium occurs when dialysis time is decreased in addition to increasing dialysis and blood flow rates. Solute disequilibrium can be corrected by adjusting the Kt/V for the rebound in urea, which happens mainly in the 30–60 minutes immediately post dialysis. The resultant Kt/V is termed equilibrated Kt/V or eKt/V. Numerous equations have been developed by Daugirdas and others to help derive the eKt/V from spKt/V.(57-59) With a conventional 4-hour HD treatment, eKt/V is usually about 0.2 units lower than spKt/V. The difference is even larger with short, high-efficiency HD or hemodiafiltration, in which urea rebound is higher. Single-pool *Kt/V* or, even better, *eKt/V* should be assessed monthly, and dialysis prescription should be adapted accordingly. In large cross-sectional studies, mortality increases when *spKt/V* falls below 1.2, and international guidelines (e.g., KDOQI) recommend a target *spKt/V* of 1.3 for a conventional dialysis schedule of three times per week.

Online clearance is the term used when the dialysis dose is calculated by measuring conductivity or ionic clearance across the dialysis membrane. Multiple ions can be tracked at the same time to minimize error, and the delivered Kt/V can be predicted in real time before the treatment is over. Although sound in theory, the practical application is limited. UKM is also used to calculate the protein catabolic rate (PCR) and the protein catabolic rate normalized to body weight (nPCR), both of which are useful measures of nutrition.

Urea reduction ratio (URR) is another way of quantifying the delivered dialysis dose. However, it's over simplified since it does not take into account intradialytic urea generation and convective urea removal by ultrafiltration. Because the relative decrease in urea concentration during dialysis is the most significant determinant of Kt/V, direct measurement of URR is an accepted method for assessment of dialysis adequacy. The URR equation is as follows: URR = (BUNpre -BUNpost)/BUNpre where BUNpre is pre-dialysis urea concentration and BUNpost is post-dialysis urea concentration. By convention, the value is multiplied by 100 and expressed as a percentage. A minimum URR of 65% to 70% is recommended for adequate HD. Kt/V and URR are mathematically linked by the following equation: Kt/V= -ln(1-URR), where ln is the natural logarithm. (60) Accordingly, *Kt/V* equals 1.0 when URR equals 0.63 or 63% of whole-body urea has been removed. (60)

4.5 Limitations of UKM

One of the criticisms of UKM is the use of urea as the reference marker for measurement. We know that it's a very small solute. Clearance of a solute is multifactorial; it is dependent on the molecular weight, charge, volume of distribution, and protein binding. Furthermore, clearance of solutes with different molecular weights from urea or bound to proteins would be different. Thus, clearance of urea cannot be extrapolated to other substances such as "uremic toxin" because they act differently. In addition UKM does not take into account residual renal function (RRF), which has a significant impact on patient outcome. (57) Also, it has been shown that V calculated by anthropometric formulas systematically overestimates volume by about 15%. (58) Kt/V underestimate that body water has an independent effect on outcomes, it is now recognized that smaller patients require higher Kt/v compared to larger patients. (61) Also, Kt/V does not confer that time (t) has an independent effect on outcome. The National Cooperative Dialysis (NCDS) was the first multicenter, randomized controlled trial of hemodialysis adequacy in which UKM was used to analyse the effect of BUN and HD time. Longer time was associated with better outcomes, however the statistical relationship between treatment time and patient outcome in was considered not to be significant (*p* value of 0.056). (61-62) Kt/V does not account for QOL, BP and volume control, clinically stability or biochemical factors. We know from the analysis of Hurricane Katrina that patients who missed three HD sessions were associated with odds ratio for hospitalization of 2.15. (61,63) Thus, Kt/V only measure the adequacy of one dialysis session, it does not incorporate missed HD sessions or shorten dialysis time.

Some of these limitations are rectifiable. One can increase HD time for intradialytic hypotension, inability to control volume, or if dialysis dosage is inadequate. HD dose can be based on body surface area (BSA), thus, smaller patients can receive more dialysis.

4.6 Hemodialysis dose

Quantifying removal of toxic uremic solutes is important to assess the adequacy of HD. The delivered dialysis dose is a function of length of the session (*t*), dialysate and blood flow rates, volume of distribution (V) of the uremic toxin studied, and the dialyzer efficiency (K_oA). Volume of distribution is very different for urea (total body water volume), than other small-molecular-weight. The minimum frequency and dosage of dialysis is three times per week, for a minimum treatment time of 3 to 4 hours, a blood flow rate of at least 250 ml/min, and a dialysate flow rate of 500 to 800 ml/min. Patients that are initiated on HD, *V* is unknown and has to be estimated (men, 58% of body weight; women, 55% of body weight). After obtaining measured *Kt/V* the dialysis prescription can be adjusted to meet the *Kt/V* goals. For patients with severe and long-standing uremia, it's recommended to provide several sessions in achieving target dose to avoid the dialysis disequilibrium syndrome.

4.7 Recommendations for dialysis dose adequacy

Current recommendations in the United States are as follows (KDOQI) (64):

- A minimum *spKt/V* of at least 1.2 for both adult and pediatric HD patients. When URR is used, the delivered dose should be equivalent to a *Kt/V* of 1.2, that is, an average URR of 65%.
- To prevent the delivered dose of HD from falling below the recommended minimum dose, the prescribed dose of HD should be *spKt/V* of 1.3, which corresponds to an average URR of 70%.
- The delivered dose of HD should be measured at least once per month in all adult and pediatric HD patients.

4.8 Factors affecting delivered Kt/V

Factors that influences delivery of Kt/V is multifactorial: hematocrit, the effective dialyzer urea clearance *Kd* depends on blood and dialysate flow rates, dialyzer K_oA, effective dialyzer surface area, anticoagulation, and recirculation. (60) Dialysis session time (*t*) is critical for reaching the *Kt/V* goal. Prescribe treatment time (PTT) and effective treatment time (ETT) may not always correlate, EET may be significantly less secondary to patient demand, clotting of dialyser, or intermittent pump stops. *V* does not substantially change during a single HD session but may change over time. Dialysis dose needs to be adjusted for an increase in *V*. However, if there is a loss in body mass (weight loss, amputation of limb), is associated with a decrease in *V*, *Kt/V* should not be reduced but rather adjusted to the higher, ideal patient *V* or BSA.

If faced with an inadequate delivered *Kt/V*, first check if that session was representative of an average session and no unusual problems may have occurred (e.g., shortened time because of patient request, needle difficulty, leaks, alarm triggering). (60) The use of commercial technologies that measure ionic dialysance can be implemented to monitor each dialysis. A frequent cause of low *Kt/V* is fistula integrity that causes a vascular access problem leading to recirculation. Blood sampling errors should be considered because delayed post-HD sampling will reduce *Kt/V*. Standardized blood sampling procedures should be implemented in each center. If, despite these checks, a low *Kt/V* remains unexplained, treatment time should be increased to 4.5 or 5 hours. Prescription of a more efficient dialyzer and higher blood and dialysate flow rates should also be considered. However, increasing treatment time, rather than increasing dialysate flow, or using two dialysers, would be more beneficial and practical to improve adequacy. Muscle exercise before or during dialysis improves *Kt/V* by increasing blood supply to poorly perfused urea rich muscle tissue and thus facilitates urea equilibration. Delivered *Kt/V* should be checked whenever the dialysis prescription has been modified substantially. Online clearance monitoring allows assessment of *Kt/V* during each single session without blood sampling.

4.9 Should volume (V) be included in Kt/V to assess target clearance?

In an attempt to address the question of optimal dialysis dose, several clinical trial have proposed that patients with small urea *V*, such as women, do worst compared to larger people. This is secondary to the notion that muscle mass closely correlate to total body water than to body weight. Thus, small urea *V* is a good indicator for low muscle mass. The Hemodialysis Study (HEMO) was performed in which 1846 patients were randomly assigned to a standard or high dose of dialysis and a low- or high-flux dialyzer (based on clearance of beta-2-microglobulin) which revealed a beneficial effect of higher *Kt/V* for women but not for men. (65) This suggests that individuals with low muscle mass may require a higher clearance in relation to *V* and therefore raises the question of whether *V* is the appropriate denominator for dialysis dose. (60) Native renal clearances, in contrast, are commonly related to body surface area (BSA), not to total body water. (60) It has been suggested to relate BSA to dialysis clearances. The ratio of BSA to urea *V* is generally higher in women than in men and decreases with an increment in *V*. Prescribing dialysis dose in relation to BSA ($K \times t/\text{BSA}$) would result in more dialysis for smaller patients of either gender and for women of any size. (57,60) More work need to be done to validate this novel idea.

4.10 Other dialysis factors related to outcomes

There are many other factors that play a role in the outcome of dialysis adequacy. Such factor includes but is not restricted to middle molecule removal, hyperphosphatemia, preservation of RRF, vascular access, QOL and treatment time. In general, middle molecule removal is determined by the dialyser permeability, the presence of convection, protein binding, and dialysis duration. Given that daily dialysis results in more frequent solute level equilibration with less rebound, this technique provides higher middle molecule removal than with conventional hemodialysis. The retention of solutes of middle molecular size is proposed to play an important role in the pathogenesis of the uremic state and contribute significantly to the high mortality of dialysis patients. (60) High-flux dialyzers have the propensity to remove larger amounts of middle molecules than low-flux dialyzers due to higher membrane porosity, and this may even be further increased by the use of convective dialysis strategies, such as hemodiafiltration. Serum β_2-microglobulin, is a surrogate for other uremic middle molecules, is effectively removed by high-flux than by low-flux dialysis, and predialysis β_2-microglobulin levels were found to be related to mortality in patients treated randomly with high-flux or low-flux dialyzers. (70) Patient who has diabetes on HD, or on dialysis for longer than 3.7 years, and those with serum albumin levels below 40 g/l, may benefit most from high-flux dialysis. (69,71) The European Best Practice Guidelines have recommended maximizing the removal of middle molecules in all dialysis patients. (60,72)

Hyperphosphatemia is a major problem in HD and is managed by phosphate removal via dialysis, use of phosphate binder medication to prevent intestinal phosphate absorption from dietary phosphate and dietary restriction. With the use of larger dialyzer surface area, hemodiafiltration, high-flux HD, removal of phosphate is significantly removal. Must monitor for hypophosphatemia with long frequent dialysis

End stage renal patients initiated on dialysis initially posess considerable residual renal function (RRF). However, most of these patients lose their RRF by the end of the first year on dialysis. By year three only 10% to 20% of patients retain their RRF. RRF of 2 to 3 ml/min urea clearance contributes significantly to the elimination of uremic toxins. (73) The retention of RRF results in lower serum β_2-microglobulin, phosphate, potassium, urea, creatinine, and uric acid levels; higher hemoglobin concentration; enhanced nutritional status; better quality of life scores; and a reduced need for dietary and fluid restrictions. (60) Left ventricular hypertrophy is associated with loss of RRF. Patient with an estimated TBW of 40 liters, a residual urea clearance of 2 to 3 ml/min is equivalent to a *std-Kt/V* of 0.5 to 0.75/week. Dialysate water impurities, nephrotoxic agents such as radiocontrast, nonsteroidal anti-inflammatory drugs, aminoglycosides and activation of the immune system by bioincompatible membranes, intradialytic hypotension are risk factors for the loss of RRF. Patients who retain urine output may enhance survival augment with the regulation of fluid and electrolyte balance.

5. Frequency of dialysis

DePalma first reported in 1969 the successful use of short daily or "quotidian" hemodialysis. (35) Short daily dialysis (SDD) was based upon the premise that patient outcomes would improved, compared with conventional three times per week hemodialysis. SDD would occur with a dialysis schedule that consisted of the same number of hours of dialysis per week but delivered over twice as many sessions. More specifically, this schedule consists of daily hemodialysis (five to seven days per week) provided for a duration of 1.5 to 3 or more hours per session. Initial attempts to popularize daily dialysis in the United States were suppressed by financial and logistical issues. This led to a decline in its use both in the home and in-center settings. However, over the last decade there has been resurgence in the use of daily dialysis, with several studies emerging from the United States and Europe showing improvements in various intermediate outcomes. Most recently, in the wake of the HEMO study, attention has turned from increasing the per-session dialytic dose, to altering variables such as treatment frequency or duration to improve outcomes (75-76) Daily dialysis has also been proposed as a rescue therapy and in the intensive care unit setting.

The mortality rate of patients undergoing maintenance hemodialysis is unacceptably high. An extremely high morbidity, relatively low quality of life (due in part to a high level of dependence and unemployment), and high cost have also been observed. Contrast this with frequent dialysis which provides a more physiological renal replacement, because it allows more gentle volume removal, reduction of hemodynamic stress and better blood pressure control. More frequent dialysis and prolonged-duration HD have the greatest effect on middle molecule clearance. (74) In addition, phosphorus removal is increased secondarily to its predominant intracellular distribution. Protein bound solutes like p-cresol are not changed, because these solutes depend on RRF. The benefits of more frequent dialysis improve BP, thus decreasing anti-hypertensive medications, decreasing intradialytic hypotension, lowering serum phosphate, raising albumin and hemoglobin with lower requirements for erythropoiesis stimulating agents. HD patients switch to nocturnal dialysis improved sleep efficiency especially in stage 3 and 4 sleep with decreased in daytime fatigue after 6 months. (75) Nocturnal dialysis is also associated with beneficial effects on vascular smooth muscle which restore the proliferation of the apoptosis ratio, which directly associated to serum phosphorus. However, there are no published randomized trials of nocturnal hemodialysis compared to other modalities. Thus studies comparing nocturnal hemodialysis to conventional hemodialysis should be performed to better understand the benefits with nocturnal hemodialysis.

Due to the nightly schedule with nocturnal hemodialysis, the cost of consumables is higher than conventional hemodialysis and is similar to the cost of short daily hemodialysis. However, the personnel cost of nocturnal hemodialysis is lower than that with in-center hemodialysis regimens. (76)

Depending upon the consumable/personnel cost ratio in different countries, nocturnal hemodialysis can be less or more expensive than in-center conventional hemodialysis. In addition, the cost of medications, including EPO, antihypertensive agents, and phosphate binders, is lower with nocturnal hemodialysis as well as cost of hospitalization.

5.1 Vascular access

Performing hemodialysis requires the ability to access and return a patient's blood at a high rate. The optimal access would allow a high rate of blood flow, with no recirculation of dialyzed blood into the pre-dialysis blood, with maximal durability, minimal complications, and minimal gap from creation to use. Currently, no hemodialysis access approaches this goal; each available access has shortcomings.

The preferred access currently is the arteriovenous fistula (AVF). The AVF is created surgically by connecting an artery to a vein, with the subsequent increased flow and pressure causing the vein to "arterialize," with thickened wall and increased size. This arterialized vein can then be accessed for hemodialysis. The advantages to the AVF are a high rate of blood flow with minimal recirculation, minimal complications because of the absence of foreign material, and an extended functional life. The primary shortcoming of the AVF is the significant time from initial placement to maturation for use, which ranges from 25 to 98 days (81). Typically AVF is not used until 3 months after placement. However, a recent study of the practice patterns at dialysis facilities in DOPPS suggests that earlier cannulation of AVFs (even prior to 4 weeks) was not associated with increased risk of access failure (81). Other issues include a significant rate of primary failure of AVFs (82), vascular steal syndrome, inability to create AVFs because of lack of suitable vessels (82-84), and development of stenoses leading to AVF thrombosis and AVF failure (82-84).

Given the significant time for their maturation, AVFs must be placed well before initiation of hemodialysis to avoid use of other accesses, such as tunneled catheters. Currently, only 15 percent of patients starting on hemodialysis use an AVF, and only 24 percent have a maturing AVF (85). One cause is late referral to nephrologists, but even with a timely referral to nephrologists, 46% of the patients did not have a permanent access placed prior to starting HD (85). Some barriers leading to this problem include patient resistance to creation of AVFs, poor access to surgeons, and decreased rate of primary patency of AVFs (85). Possible solutions include improved patient education, often through patient support groups in CKD clinics and referral to nephrologist at earlier stage of chronic kidney disease (85).

Where creation of an AVF is impossible, insertion of an arteriovenous graft (AVG) may be feasible. The advantage of an AVG is the high primary patency rate and minimal gap between creation and first use (84,86). Because of the presence of foreign material, there is increased risk of access infection, although less than that with tunneled catheters, and there is an increased rate of stenosis, thrombosis, and graft failure compared with AVFs. One new technique in the creation of AVGs is the Hemodialysis Reliable Outflow (HeRO™) dialysis catheter, a new FDA approved device for catheter-dependent and significant vasculopathic patients. The HeRO device is an AVG that extends from the arm into the right ventricle. This may avoid problems with stenosis at the venous anastomosis leading to graft failure.

The third means of chronic hemodialysis access is the tunneled catheter. This catheter, like the standard non-tunneled dialysis catheter used for acute hemodialysis access and non-tunneled catheters used for venous access, is inserted into a central vein, usually the internal jugular vein, but the risk of infection is reduced by increasing the distance between the vein and skin entry by running the catheter through a subcutaneous tunnel. This access has the advantage of being usable immediately upon insertion, but it has the highest rate of infection, particularly catheter-related bacteremia, and is associated with higher costs, morbidity, and mortality, compared with other accesses (87-88). Other complications of the tunneled catheter include intraluminal thrombosis and fibrin sheath.

6. Management of access complications

6.1 Detection and treatment of stenosis and thrombosis of AVF and AVG

Stenosis of AVF and AVG commonly develop over time, generally resulting from response to endothelial damage. This can occur at the anastamosis between native vessels or between a graft and a native vessel, with endothelial damage caused by surgical trauma, or distal to the venous anastamosis, with endothelial damage from rapid turbulent flow. If these stenoses are not recognized and corrected, increased access pressures and decreased flow can result in thrombosis of the access. Once an access has thrombosed, even if it can be salvaged, the duration of secondary patency is relatively short, with 62% one year patency average (89). Therefore, monitoring and subsequent treatment of stenosis in AVFs and AVGs is critical to prolonging the life of these hemodialysis accesses. For an excellent review of the various methods of monitoring accesses, see reference 90. There are several ways to monitor for stenosis. Physical exam, looking for abnormalities such as change in thrill, bruit or pulse, presence of arm swelling, or prolonged bleeding after dialysis, can be quite helpful in detecting access problems (91). Another common way to detect stenosis is with dynamic venous pressure monitoring. With this technique, the pressure at the venous needle is measured with low dialysis pump rate. If the pressure is over 80, or if there is significant increase from prior pressures, there is a high likelihood of outflow stenosis (92). Measuring static access pressures (with blood pump off) is more accurate, and can also detect arterial stenoses, but this technique requires additional equipment, and is therefore not common (93). Another monitoring method growing in use is Doppler flow measurement. If the flow decreases to less than 650 mL/minute, or if there has been significant interval decrease in flow, there is a high likelihood of stenosis (94). Stenoses can be detected by Doppler ultrasound, but the gold standard for detection and treatment of access stenosis is fistulogram, or the injection of contrast into the access to demonstrate visually the stenosis. When a fistulogram demonstrates stenosis, the stenosis can be repaired with angioplasty or surgical revision. While angioplasty has a shorter secondary patency than surgical revision, angioplasty is generally the first line treatment of stenosis and thrombosis of AVF and AVG, since surgical revision can be performed after angioplasty in case of recurrent stenosis or

thrombosis (95). Treatment with anticoagulant or anti-platelet therapy, e.g. aspirin, ticlopidine or warfarin, has a modest effect on reducing stenosis and increasing patency of fistulas; however, this treatment is associated with increased risk of hemorrhage (96). Antiplatelet therapy should be a part of routine care in patient with graft but not AV fistula (97). Other pharmacological approaches for prevention of stenosis and patency of vascular access including calcium channel blocker, ACE-I and fish oil have been investigated, but further research is required to determine the role of these agents in maintaining fistula patency.
Another complication of AVF and AVG is vascular access induced ischemia and is related to significant amounts of blood flow via AV fistulas. This diversion of blood via the fistula could cause decrease of blood flow to the distal tissue and cause ischemia (known as steal syndrome). It could rarely cause exacerbation of heart failure in paints with underlying disease. Elderly patients, patients with diabetics, peripheral vascular disease or coronary artery disease are at increase risk of ischemia. Pain during hemodialysis is a characteristic symptom.
Another vascular access complication is central venous obstruction occurring in patients with previously inserted venous catheter or pacemaker placement. The rate of central venous obstruction is higher in patients who had their brachial venous accessed prior to dialysis access placement compare to patient who had internal jugular vein accessed. The most common clinical presentation is pain and swelling of the ipsilateral arm usually accompanied with the superficial collateral vein around the shoulder. Other clue for diagnosis of central venous obstruction is finger ulceration, pain and inadequate dialysis. The first option for treatment is percutaneous transluminal angioplasty and stent placement (angioplasty alone has a high rate of restenosis). The second option is surgical revision with bypass grafting and placement of HERO catheter (as discussed above).

6.2 Catheter thrombosis and fibrin sheath formation

One of the most common complications of hemodialysis catheters is decrease of flow or thrombosis. Catheter thrombosis prevention is generally achieved through instillation of heparin into the catheter ports after completion of dialysis; a recent study suggests that weekly instillation of recombinant tissue plasminogen activator (tPA) may prevent thrombosis more effectively (98). Catheter thrombosis can be treated effectively by instillation of tPA into the catheter lumens or with exchange of the catheter over a guidewire; however, thrombosis frequently recurs, necessitating further procedures. One cause of frequent catheter malfunction is the formation of a fibrin sheath around the tip of the catheter. This can be treated with a 3 hour infusion of low-dose tPA or with mechanical stripping, although secondary patency rates remain low (99).

6.3 Catheter related blood stream infection (CRBSI)

The prevalence of central venous catheters in the United States is about 20-30% despite recommendations from major societies to increase the use of AV fistulas known as fistula first initiative. There is an increased risk of mortality with the use of catheters compared with the use of AV fistulas (100). This increased rate of mortality is likely related to infection. The rate of catheter related blood stream infection is 0.5 to 6.6 episodes per 1,000 catheter days (101). The source of this infection is bacterial seeding from biofilms that form on the inside and outside of the blood stream catheter. The rate of CRBSI is directly related to the species and level of virulence of the seeding bacteria. Meticulous catheter care and reeducation of personnel responsible for insertion of the catheters are the key elements in lowering the rate of catheter related infection (101). The catheter care includes but is not limited to sterile technique of catheter placement, exit –site care, sterile technique during initiation and termination of dialysis (including the use of a sterile barrier, sterile gloves, and antiseptic to clean the tubes) and the replacement of malfunctioning catheters over a guidewire (empirical administration of antibiotics does not reduce the incidence of catheter associated bacteremia) (102). Using standard antiseptic precautions the incidence of catheter related infection could drop to one episode per 1,000 catheter days which could be used to assess the quality of catheter care.

The current guidelines indicate the use of tunneled cuffed catheter for long term use (more than 3 weeks duration) in patients in need of hemodialysis based on pathophysiological considerations as well as a generally lower rate of infection of tunneled, cuffed catheters compared to nontunneled catheters (103). The location of catheters influences the risk of infection. The femoral lines carry a higher rate of infection compare with the subclavian or jugular lines. Subsequent studies, however, only confirm an increase risk of femoral catheter infection in the patients with a higher BMI (87-88,102).

Although the prophylactic use of systemic antibiotics at the time of insertion of a catheter is not currently recommended, the antimicrobial lock solutions for prevention of catheter related infection and bactremia are recommended (101). The ideal lock solution has anticoagulant and antimicrobial activity, is safe, and does not induce bacterial resistance. The antimicrobial solutions most frequently used are antibiotics or chemicals, citrate (30% concentrated since the lower concentration has little antimicrobial affect) (104). Antimicrobial lock solutions substantially reduce the risk of catheter related infection (102). The potential disadvantage of usage of antibiotics for antimicrobial lock solution is bacterial resistance and predisposition to highly resistance bacterial infection. There is also a potential adverse effect of these antibiotics including aminoglycoside-related ototoxicity. The disadvantage of usage of citrate is hypocalcemia and adverse cardiac event if the locking solution is pushed to the patient blood (105).

Application of topical antibiotics to the exit site may reduce the incidence of catheter related infection in patients on hemodialysis. The most recent CDC guideline recommends use of povidone iodine antiseptic ointment or bacitracin/gramicidin/polymyxin B at the hemodialysis catheter exit site after each dialysis session (101). A recent Cochrane review on this subject concluded that the current data support only the topical application of mupirocin alone (among antibacterial agents) for prevention of catheter related infection (106). The use of antibiotic coated catheter in hemodialysis patients has not been shown to reduce the incidence of catheter related infection (101,107).

Staphylococcus species in general and S. aureus in particular are among the most common cause of bacterial related infection. Mortality rate is high among the patient infected with S. aureus (8%). Morbidity related to S. aureus is secondary to its high propensity to colonize prosthetic materials, heart valves, bones and joints. Nasal carriage of S. aureus is common among patients on dialysis, in whom it is associated with an increased risk of S. aureus infection. Successful elimination of S. aureus nasal carriage can be achieved by a short (5-day) course of mupirocin applied daily to the anterior nares (108).

Treatment of CRBSI requires systemic antibiotics and frequently discontinuation of the catheter and placement of temporary catheter. There are four possible options for treatment of CRBSI. Intravenous antibiotics alone, prompt catheter removal with delayed placement of a new long term catheter, exchange of the infected catheter with a new one over guidewire, or use of systemic antibiotics and an antibiotic lock in the existing catheter. Antibiotic therapy for catheter-related infection is often initiated empirically. The initial choice of antibiotics will depend on the severity of the patient's clinical disease, the risk factors for infection, and the likely pathogens associated with the specific intravascular device (109). Antibiotic therapy should be administered to patients with persistent fungemia or bacteremia after catheter removal (especially if the infection is caused by S. aureus). Long-term catheters should be removed from patients with CRBSI associated with any of the following conditions: severe sepsis; suppurative thrombophlebitis; endocarditis; bloodstream infection that continues despite antimicrobial therapy to which the infecting microbes are susceptible (110). In uncomplicated CRBSI involving long-term catheters due to pathogens other than S. aureus, P. aeruginosa, fungi, because of the limited access sites in many patients who require long-term intravascular access for survival in hemodialysis patients, treatment should be attempted without catheter removal, with use of both systemic and antimicrobial lock therapy for 14 days and cultures should be repeated one week after completion of antibiotics treatment. The rate of treatment failure, however, is higher for patient treated with antibiotics alone (111). If the symptoms resolve after 2–3 days of intravenous antibiotic therapy, guidewire exchange of the catheter is associated with cure rates that are comparable to those associated with immediate removal and delayed placement of a new catheter (110). Localized Cellulites (exit site infection) should be treated with systemic antibiotics and exit site care. Tunnel track infection, however, requires catheter removal since it involves space in an area with limited vascular supply (112).

6.4 Acute vascular access

A large diameter venous catheter (a dual lumen venous catheter) usually placed in the internal jugular or femoral vein, is needed for acute or urgent hemodialysis in the absence of permanent vascular access. This catheter is used in patients with acute kidney injury who need urgent hemodialysis, in patients who need removal of a toxic agent by means of dialysis, or with chronic dialysis patients with a temporary inability to use a permanent access, as with catheter-related bacteremia. Using this type of access, one lumen of the venous catheter is allocated to draw blood (arterial side) and the other lumen is allocated to return the blood. Separation of arterial from venous lumen minimized the recirculation of blood during hemodialysis. Because of high risk of infection, non-tunneled femoral catheter should be removed within a week, while non-tunneled internal jugular catheters can be used for about 2 weeks. Hemodialysis catheters placed in the subclavian veins have a significant risk of subclavian stenosis, which can cause the arm on that side to be unsuitable for AVF or AVG placement, and so catheters are generally not placed in the subclavian veins. An indwelling cuffed catheter is tunneled under the skin and placed in the internal jugular vein by an interventional nephrologist, interventional radiologist or surgeon. It is used when acute renal failure is expected to require hemodialysis for more than 2 weeks because of the decreased rate of infection (1034).

6.5 Extracorporeal therapies in the ICU setting - continuous renal replacement therapy

Critically ill, hemodynamically unstable intensive care unit (ICU) patients are typically the most challenging to treat with conventional dialytic modalities as described above. The intermittent volume and solute fluxes may cause significant morbidity, which includes worsening of hypotension and arrhythmias. Multiple modalities of renal replacement therapy are currently available. These include intermittent hemodialysis (IHD), continuous renal replacement therapies (CRRTs), and hybrid therapies, such as sustained low-efficiency dialysis (SLED).

INDICATIONS FOR AND TIMING OF INITIATION OF DIALYSIS – Accepted indications for renal replacement therapy (RRT) in patients with Acute Kidney Injury (AKI) generally include:
Refractory fluid overload
Hyperkalemia (plasma potassium concentration >6.5 meq/L) refractory to medical therapy
Signs of uremia, such as pericarditis, neuropathy, or an otherwise unexplained decline in mental status
Metabolic acidosis (pH less than 7.1) refractory to medical therapy.
Certain alcohol and drug intoxications

CRRTs involve either dialysis (diffusion-based solute removal) or filtration (convection-based solute and water removal) treatments that operate in a continuous mode (114-117). The major advantage of continuous therapy is the slower rate of solute or fluid removal per unit of time. Thus, CRRT is generally better tolerated than conventional therapy, since many of the complications of intermittent hemodialysis are related to the rapid rate of solute and fluid loss. It must be emphasized, however, that the protection afforded by CRRT is relative, not absolute.

7. Outcomes in CRRT

Outcomes of an increased dose of CRRT have been assessed in several randomized controlled trials and two meta-analyses (78-80,116-117). Conflicting results related to survival have been reported. To address the issue of optimal dose in CRRT and IHD, the United States VA/NIH Acute Renal Failure Trial Network study (ATN), the Randomized Evaluation of Normal versus Augmented Level of RRT study (RENAL) and two meta-analyses were performed. All studies found that, compared with standard intensity dialysis, higher intensity dialysis did not result in improved survival or clinical benefits:

In the United States VA/NIH Acute Renal Failure Trial Network study (ATN), all 1124 patients were treated with IHD, CRRT, or SLED based upon hemodynamic status. Patients were randomly assigned to one of two dosing arms:

- Intensive therapy: Hemodialysis and SLED were given six times per week and a target Kt/V of 1.2 to 1.4 per treatment, while CRRT was provided with an effluent flow rate of 35 mL/kg per hour.
- Less intensive therapy: Hemodialysis and SLED were given three times per week, while CRRT was provided with a flow rate of 20 mL/kg per hour.

The death rate at day 60 was the same for both groups (53.6 percent with intensive therapy and 51.5 percent with less intensive therapy). In addition, the duration of renal replacement therapy and the rate of recovery of kidney function or nonrenal organ failure were similar for both treatment arms. The group that received intensive therapy had an increased number of hypotensive episodes. Thus, more intensive renal support beyond that obtained with a standard thrice-weekly regimen (with a target Kt/V of 1.2 to 1.4 per treatment) or standard CRRT (with an effluent flow rate of 20 mL/kg per hour) does not improve clinical outcomes.

In the RENAL study (a trial in Australia and New Zealand), 1508 patients with AKI were randomly assigned to CVVHDF at an effluent flow of either 25 or 40 mL/kg per hour (119). At 90 days, mortality was the same in each group (44.7 percent, odds ratio 1.00, 95% CI 0.31 to 1.23). In addition, the incidence of patients who continued to receive renal replacement therapy at 90 days was similar with both dialysis doses (6.8 and 4.4 percent of higher and lower-intensity groups, odds ratio 1.59, 95% CI 0.86 to 2.92).

Two meta-analyses, one consisting of 3841 patients and 8 trials and the other 3999 patients and 12 trials, found that more intense therapy did not improve survival compared with less intensive regimens (118-119). There was significant trial heterogeneity.

8. References

Grassmann A, Gioberge S, Moeller S, Brown G. ESRD patients in 2004: global overview of patient numbers, treatment modalities and associated trends. Nephrol. Dial. Transplant. 2005, 20 (12): 2587-2593.

United States Renal Data System. USRDS 2010 Annual Data Report: Atlas of End-Stage Renal Disease in the United States 2010; Bethesda, MD, National Institute of Health, National Institutes of Diabetes and Digestive and Kidney Diseases.

Alper B, Shenava, R, Young, B, et. al. Uremia. Medscape. Batuman V. Mar 17, 2010. http://emedicine.medscape.com/article/245296-overview

Termorshuizen F, Dekker FW, van Manen JG et al., Relative contribution of residual renal function and different measures of adequacy to survival in hemodialysis patients: an analysis of the Netherlands Cooperative Study on the Adequacy of Dialysis (NECOSAD)-2, J Am Soc Nephrol 2004; 15:1061-70

Rosansky SJ, Clark WF, Eggers P, Glassock RJ. Initiation of dialysis at higher GFRs: is the apparent rising tide of early dialysis harmful or helpful? Kidney Int. 2009 Aug;76(3):257-61.

Schrier R. Manual of Nephrology: Diagnosis and Therapy. Philadelphia: Lippincott Williams & Wilkins, 2009.

Pendse, S, Singh, A, Zawada, E. Initiation of dialysis in Handbook of Dialysis, 4th ed, Daugirdas, JT, Blake, PG, Ing, TS (Eds). Lippincott Williams & Wilkins, Philadelphia 2007.

Rosansky SJ, Eggers P, Jackson K, Glassock R, Clark WF. Early Start of Hemodialysis May Be Harmful. Arch Intern Med. 2011; 171(5):396-403)

NKF-KDOQI Clinical Practice Guidelines. Am J Kidney Dis 1997; 30(3 Suppl 2): S67–S136.

Obrador RT, Auora P, Kausz AT et al. Level of renal function at the initiation of dialysis in the US end-stage renal disease population. Kidney Int 1999; 5: 2227– 2235.

National Kidney Foundation. KDOQI Clinical practice guidelines and clinical practice recommendations for 2006 updates: hemodialysis adequacy, peritoneal dialysis adequacy and vascular access. Am J Kidney Dis 2006; 48(Suppl 1): S1–S322.

Tang, SC, Ho, YW, Tang, AW, et al. Delaying initiation of dialysis till symptomatic uraemia--is it too late? Nephrol Dial Transplant 2007; 22:1926.

Cooper, BA, Branley, P, Bulfone, L, et al. A randomized, controlled trial of early versus late initiation of dialysis. N Engl J Med 2010; 363:609.

Clark, W., Na, Y., Rosansky, S., et.al. Association between estimated glomerular filtration rate at initiation of dialysis and mortality. CMAJ. 2011 Jan 11;183(1):47-53.

United States Renal Data System. Excerpts from the USRDS 2009 annual data report: Atlas of end-stage renal disease in the United States. Am J Kidney Dis 2010; 1(Suppl 1):S1.

USRDS: The United States Renal Data System: Overall hospitalization and mortality. Am J Kidney Dis 2010; 55(Suppl 1):S1.]

Van Biesen W, Vanholder R, Lameire N. The role of peritoneal dialysis as the first-line renal replacement modality. Perit Dial Int. 2000;20(4):375

Goldstein A, Kliger AS, Finkelstein FO. Recovery of renal function and the discontinuation of dialysis in patients treated with continuous peritoneal dialysis.Perit Dial Int. 2003;23(2):151

Teitelbaum I, Burkart J. Peritoneal dialysis. Am J Kidney Dis. 2003;42(5):1082

Wauters JP, Uehlinger D. Non-medical factors influencing peritoneal dialysis utilization: the Swiss experience. Nephrol Dial Transplant. 2004;19(6):1363

Mendelssohn DC, Langlois N, Blake PG. Peritoneal dialysis in Ontario: a natural experiment in physician reimbursement methodology. Perit Dial Int. 2004;24(6):531

Tonelli M, Hemmelgarn B, Culleton B, Klarenbach S, Gill JS, Wiebe N, Manns B, Alberta Kidney Disease Network. Mortality of Canadians treated by peritoneal dialysis in remote locations. Kidney Int. 2007;72(8):1023

Mehrotra R, Khawar O, Duong U, Fried L, Norris K, Nissenson A, Kalantar-Zadeh K. Ownership patterns of dialysis units and peritoneal dialysis in the United States: utilization and outcomes. Am J Kidney Dis. 2009;54(2):289.

Korevaar JC, Feith GW, Dekker FW, et al. Effect of starting with hemodialysis compared with peritoneal dialysis in patients new on dialysis treatment: a randomized controlled trial. Kidney Int 2003;64:2222-2228.

Ganesh SK, Hulbert-Shearon T, Port FK, et al. Mortality differences by dialysis modality among incident ESRD patients with and without coronary artery disease. J Am Soc Nephrol 2003;14:415-424

Stack AG, Molony DA, Rahman NS, et al. Impact of dialysis modality on survival of new ESRD patients with congestive heart failure in the United States. Kidney Int 2003;64:1071-1079

Vonesh EF, Snyder JJ, Foley RN, et al. The differential impact of risk factors on mortality in hemodialysis and peritoneal dialysis. Kidney Int 2004;66:2389-2401

Jaar BG, Coresh J, Plantinga LC, et al. Comparing the risk for death with peritoneal dialysis and hemodialysis in a national cohort of patients with chronic kidney disease. Ann Intern Med 2005;143:174-183.

Tattersall J, Martin-Malo A, Pedrini L, Basci A, Canaud B, Fouque D, Haage P, Konner K, Kooman J, Pizzarelli F, Tordoir J, Vennegoor M, Wanner C, ter Wee P, Vanholder R: EBPG guideline on dialysis strategies. Nephrol Dial Transplant 22[Suppl 2]: ii5–ii21, 2007.

Lowrie, E, Laird, NM. National Cooperative Dialysis Study. Kidney Int Suppl 1983; 23:19.

Eknoyan G, Beck GJ, Cheung AK, Daugirdas JT, Greene T, Kusek JW, Allon M, Bailey J, Delmez JA, Depner TA, Dwyer JT, Levey AS, Levin NW, Milford E, Ornt DB, Rocco MV, Schulman G, Schwab SJ, Teehan BP, Toto R, Hemodialysis (HEMO) Study Group. Effect of dialysis dose and membrane flux in maintenance hemodialysis. N Engl J Med. 2002;347(25):2010.

Paniagua R, Amato D, Vonesh E, Correa-Rotter R, Ramos A, Moran J, Mujais S, Mexican Nephrology Collaborative Study Group. Effects of increased peritoneal clearances on mortality rates in peritoneal dialysis: ADEMEX, a prospective, randomized, controlled trial. J Am Soc Nephrol. 2002;13(5):1307

Tattersall J, Martin-Malo A, Pedrini L, Basci A, Canaud B, Fouque D, Haage P, Konner K, Kooman J, Pizzarelli F, Tordoir J, Vennegoor M, Wanner C, ter Wee P, Vanholder R: EBPG guideline on dialysis strategies. Nephrol Dial Transplant 22[Suppl 2]: ii5–ii21, 2007

Kjellstrand CM, Buoncristiani U, Ting G, Traeger J, Piccoli GB, Sibai-Galland R, Young BA, Blagg CR: Short daily haemodialysis: Survival in 415 patients treated for 1006 patient-years. Nephrol Dial Transplant 23: 3283–3289, 2008.

DePalma, JR, Pecker, EA, Maxwell, MH. A new automatic coil dialyser system for 'daily' dialysis. Proc EDTA 1969; 6:26....DePalma, JR, Pecker, EA, Maxwell, MH. A new automatic coil dialyser system for 'daily' dialysis. Semin Dial 1999; 12:410.

Henderson LW, Leypoldt JK, Lysaght MJ, Cheung AK. Death on dialysis and the time/flux trade-off. Blood Purif. 1997;15(1):1.

FHN Trial Group, Chertow GM, Levin NW, Beck GJ, Depner TA, Eggers PW, Gassman JJ, Gorodetskaya I, Greene T, James S, Larive B, Lindsay RM, Mehta RL, Miller B, Ornt DB, Rajagopalan S, Rastogi A, Rocco MV, Schiller B, Sergeyeva O, Schulman G, Ting GO, Unruh ML, Star RA, Kliger AS. In-center hemodialysis six times per week versus three times per week. N Engl J Med. 2010;363(24):2287.

Kalirao P and Kaplan JM, Nocturnal Hemodialysis, Clin Exp Nephrol 2009; 13:257-62 Pierratos A, Ouwendyk M, Francoeur R, Vas S, Raj DS, Ecclestone AM, Langos V, Uldall R. Nocturnal hemodialysis: three-year experience. J Am Soc Nephrol. 1998;9(5):859.

Udall, PR, Francoeur, R, Ouwendyk, M. Simplified nocturnal home hemodialysis (SNHHD). A new approach to renal replacement therapy. J Am Soc Nephrol 1994; 5:428

Lindsay RM, Daily/Nocturnal Dialysis Study Group. The London, Ontario, Daily/Nocturnal Hemodialysis Study. Semin Dial. 2004;17(2):85

Lockridge RS Jr, Spencer M, Craft V, Pipkin M, Campbell D, McPhatter L, Albert J, Anderson H, Jennings F, Barger T. Nocturnal home hemodialysis in North America. Adv Ren Replace Ther. 2001;8(4):250.

Agar JW, Somerville CA, Dwyer KM, Simmonds RE, Boddington JM, Waldron CM. Nocturnal hemodialysis in australia. Hemodial Int. 2003;7(4):278.

Kooistra MP. Frequent prolonged home haemodialysis: three old concepts, one modern solution. Nephrol Dial Transplant. 2003;18(1):16.

Kjellstrand CM, Buoncristiani U, Ting G, et al. Short daily haemodialysis: survival in 415 patients treated for 1006 patient-years. Nephrol Dial Transplant 2008;23:3283-3289.

ERA-EDTA Registry: Annual Academic Medical Center. Amsterdam, The Netherlands, 2003.

Wizemann V, Külz M, Techert F, Nederlof B. Efficacy of haemodiafiltration. Nephrol Dial Transplant. 2001;16 Suppl 4:27.

Canaud B, Assounga A, Kerr P, Aznar R, Mion C. Failure of a daily haemofiltration programme using a highly permeable membrane to return beta 2-microglobulin concentrations to normal in haemodialysis patients. Nephrol Dial Transplant. 1992;7(9):924.

Jaber BL, Zimmerman DL, Teehan GS, Swedko P, Burns K, Meyer KB, Leypoldt JK. Daily hemofiltration for end-stage renal disease: a feasibility and efficacy trial. Blood Purif. 2004;22(6):481.

Zimmerman, DL, Swedko, P, Posen, G, Burns, K. Daily hemofiltration with a simplified method of delivery. J Am Soc Nephrol 2002; 13:61A.

Maduell F, Navarro V, Torregrosa E, Rius A, Dicenta F, Cruz MC, Ferrero JA. Change from three times a week on-line hemodiafiltration to short daily on-line hemodiafiltration. Kidney Int. 2003;64(1):305.

US Renal Data System: USRDS 2008 Annual Data Report: Atlas of Chronic Kidney Disease and End Stage Renal Disease in the United States, Bethesda, NIH, National Institute of Diabetes and Digestive and Kidney Disease, 2008

US Renal Data System: USRDS 2008 Annual Data Report: Atlas of Chronic Kidney Disease and End Stage Renal Disease in the United States, Bethesda, NIH, National Institute of Diabetes and Digestive and Kidney Disease, 2009

Vanholder R, Van Laecke S, Glorieux G: What is new in uremic toxicity?. Pediatr Nephrol 2008; 23:1211-1221.

Vanholder R, De Smet R, Glorieux G, et al: Review on uremic toxins: Classification, concentration, and interindividual variability. Kidney Int 2003; 63:1934-1943.

Ankit N. Mehta, MD; Andrew Z. Fenves, MD: Hemodialysis Adequacy: A Review; January 2010 Dialysis & Transplantation

Daugirdas JT. Simplifi ed equations for monitoring Kt/V, PCRn, eKt/V, and ePCRn. Adv Renal Replace Ther. 1995; 2:295-304.

Tattersall JE, DeTakats D, Chamney P, Greenwood RN, Farrington K. The post-hemodialysis rebound: predicting and quantifying its effect on Kt/V. Kidney Int. 1996; 50: 2094-2102.

Leypoldt JK, Jaber BL, Zimmerman DL. Predicting treatment dose for novel therapies using urea standard Kt/V. Semin Dial. 2004; 17:142-145.

Feehally, J, Floege, J, Johnson, R. The Comprehensive Clinical Nephrology. Chapter 90; Hemodialysis: Outcomes and Adequacy. Copyright © 2010 Elsevier

Agarwal, R, Mehrotra, R, Townsend RR, Goldfarb, S. NephSap, Vol9, No. 6, November 2010;pp 366-371

Powell JR, Oluwaseum O, Woo YM, Padmanabhan N, Narasingham E, Latta C, Tortolana J, Jardine AG, Geddes CC. Ten year experience of in-center thrice weekly long overnight hemodialysis. Clin J Am Soc Nephrol 4:1097-1101, 2009

Anderson AH, Cohen AJ, Kutner NG, Kopp JB, Kimmel PL, Mutner P; Missed dialysis sessions and hospitalization in hemodialysis patients after Hurricane Katrina. Kidney Int 75:1202-1208, 2009

National Kidney Foundation : KDOQI Clinical Practice Guidelines and Clinical Practice Recommendations for 2006 Updates: Hemodialysis Adequacy, Peritoneal

Dialysis Adequacy and Vascular Access. Am J Kidney Dis 2006; 48(Suppl 1):S1-S322

Eknoyan G, Beck GJ, Cheung AK, Daugirdas JT, Greene T, Kusek JW, Allon M, Bailey J, Delmez JA, Depner TA, Dwyer JT, Levey AS, Levin NW, Milford E, Ornt DB, Rocco MV, Schulman G, Schwab SJ, Teehan BP, Toto R, Effect of dialysis dose and membrane flux in maintenance hemodialysis. N Engl J Med. 2002; 347(25):2010. Hemodialysis (HEMO) Study Group

DePalma, JR, Pecker, EA, Maxwell, MH. A new automatic coil dialyser system for 'daily' dialysis. Proc EDTA 1969; 6:26.

DePalma, JR, Pecker, EA, Maxwell, MH. A new automatic coil dialyser system for 'daily' dialysis. Semin Dial 1999; 12:410.

Uldall, PR, Francoeur, R, Ouwendyk, M. Simplified nocturnal home hemodialysis (SNHHD). A new approach to renal replacement therapy. J Am Soc Nephrol 1994; 5:428.

Pierratos A, Ouwendyk M, Francoeur R, et al. Nocturnal hemodialysis: three-year experience. J Am Soc Nephrol 1998; 9:859.

Cheung AK, Rocco MV, Yan G, et al: Serum β2-microglobulin levels predict mortality in dialysis patients: Results of the HEMO study. J Am Soc Nephrol 2006; 17:546-555.

Locatelli F, Martin-Malo A, Hannedouche T, et al: Effect of membrane permeability on survival of hemodialysis patients. J Am Soc Nephrol 2009; 20:645-654.

European Best Practice Guidelines Expert Group on Hemodialysis, European Renal Association. Nephrol Dial Transplant 2002; 17(Suppl 7):16-31.

Bargman JM, Golper TA: The importance of residual renal function for patients on dialysis. Nephrol Dial Transplant 2005; 20:671-673.

Kliger AS, More Intensive hemodialysis. Clin J Am Soc Nephrol 4[suppll 1] S121-S124, 2009

Beecroft JM, Hoffstein V, Pierratos A, Chan Ct, McFarlane P, Hanly PJ, Nocturnal heamodialysis increases pharyngeal size in patients with sleep apnea and end stage renal disease. Nephrol Dialy Transplant 23: 673-679, 2008

McFarlane PA Reducing hemodialysis costs: conventional and quotidian home hemodialysis in Canada. Semin Dial. 2004: 17(2):118.

Manns M, Sigler MH, Teehan BP. Continuous renal replacement therapies: an update. Am J Kidney Dis. 1998;32(2):185.

Bouman CS, Oudemans-Van Straaten HM, Tijssen JG, Zandstra DF, Kesecioglu J. Effects of early high-volume continuous venovenous hemofiltration on survival and recovery of renal function in intensive care patients with acute renal failure: a prospective, randomized trial. Crit Care Med. 2002;30(10):2205.

Ronco C, Bellomo R, Homel P, Brendolan A, Dan M, Piccinni P, La Greca G. Effects of different doses in continuous veno-venous haemofiltration on outcomes of acute renal failure: a prospective randomised trial. Lancet. 2000;356(9223):26

Saudan P, Niederberger M, De Seigneux S, Romand J, Pugin J, Perneger T, Martin PY. Adding a dialysis dose to continuous hemofiltration increases survival in patients with acute renal failure. Kidney Int. 2006;70(7):1312.

Creation, cannulation and survival of arteriovenous fistulae: Data from the Dialysis Outcomes and Practice Patterns Study. Kidney International; Jan2003, Vol. 63 Issue 1, p323-330, 8p

Schild AF: Maintaining vascular access: the management of hemodialysis arteriovenous grafts. Vasc Access. 2010 Apr-Jun;11(2):92-9.

Robin M et al. Hemodialysis Arteriovenous Fistula Maturity: US Evaluation Radiology 2002, vol 221:1, 59-64

Biuckians A, Scott EC, Meier GH, et al: The natural history of autologous fistulas as first-time dialysis access in the KDOQI era. J Vasc Surg 2008; 47:415-421.

Ronald L Pisoni, Eric W Young, Dawn M Dykstra, Roger N Greenwood, Erwin Hecking, Brenda Gillespie, Robert A Wolfe, David A Goodkin and Philip J HeldVascular access use in Europe and the United States: Results from the DOPPS, Kidney International (2002) 61, 305–316

Lazarides MK, Georgiadis GS, Papasideris CP, et al: Transposed brachial-basilic arteriovenous fistulas versus prosthetic upper limb grafts: A meta-analysis. Eur J Vasc Endovasc Surg 2008; 36:597-601.

Parienti, J. J. et al. Femoral vs jugular venous catheterization and risk of nosocomial events in adults requiring acute renal replacement therapy: a randomized controlled trial. JAMA 299, 2413-2422 (2008).

Hamilton, H. C. & Foxcroft, D. R. Central venous access sites for the prevention of venous thrombosis, stenosis and infection in patients requiring long-term intravenous therapy. Cochrane Database of Systematic Reviews, Issue 3. Art. No.: CD004084. doi:10.1002/14651858.CD004084.pub2 (2007).

Kakkos SK, Haddad GK, Haddad JA et al., Secondary patency of thrombosed prosthethc vascular access grafts with aggressive surveillance, monitoring, and endovascular management, Eur J Endovasc Surg 2008; 36:356-65

Tessitore N, Bedogna V, Melilli E et al., In search of an optimal bedside screening program for arteriovenous fistula stenosis, Clin J Am Soc Nephrol 2011; 6:819-26

Beathard GA, An algorithm for the physical examination of early fistula failure, Semin Dial 2005; 18:331-335

Besarab A, Asif A, Roy-Chaudury P et al., The native arteriovenous fistula in 2007. Surveillance and monitoring. J Nephrol 2007; 20:656-667

Besarab A, Sullivan KL, Ross R et al., The utility of intra-access monitoring in detecting and correcting venous outlet stenoses prior to thrombosis, Kidney Int 1995; 1364- 1373

Tessitore N, Bedogna V, Gammaro L et al., Diagnostic accuracy of ultrasound dilution access blood flow measurement in detecting stenosis and predicting thrombosis in native forearm arteriovenous fistulae for hemodialysis, Am J Kidney Dis 2003; 42:331-341

Napoli M, Prudenzano R, Russo F et al., Juxta-anastomotic stenosis of native arteriovenous fistulas: surgical treatment versus percutaneous transluminal angioplasty, J Vasc Access 2010; 11:346-351

Dixon BS, Beck GJ, Vazquez MA, et al: Effect of dipyridamole plus aspirin on hemodialysis graft patency. N Engl J Med 2009; 360:2191-2201.

Dember LM, Besk GJ, Allon M, et al: Effect of clopidogrel on early failure of arteriovenous fistulas for hemodialysis: A randomized controlled trial. JAMA 2008; 299:2205-2207

Hemmelgarn BR, Moist LM, Lok CE et al., Prevention of dialysis catheter malfunction with recombinant tissue plasminogen activator, N Engl J Med 2011; 364:303-312

Kamper L, Piroth, W, and Haage P, Endovascular treatment of dysfunctional hemodialysis catheters, J Vasc Access 2010; 11:263-268
Allon M, Daugirdas J, Depner TA, et al: Effect of change in vascular access on patient mortality in hemodialysis patients. Am J Kidney Dis 2006; 47:469-477
2011 CDC Guidelines for the Prevention of Intravascular Catheter-Related Infections Rabindranath, K. S. et al. Systematic review of antimicrobials for the prevention of haemodialysis catheter-related infections. Nephrol. Dial. Transplant. 24, 3763-3774 (2009).
Vanholder, R. et al. Diagnosis, prevention and treatment of haemodialysis catheter-related bloodstream infections (CRBSI): a position statement of the European Renal Best Practice (ERBP). NDTPlus 3, 234-246 (2010).
Dogra GK, Herson H, Hutchison B, et al. Prevention of tunneled hemodialysis catheter-related infections using catheter-restricted filling with gentamicin and citrate: a randomized controlled study. J Am Soc Nephrol 2002; 13:2133–9
Punt, C. D. & Boer, W. E. Cardiac arrest following injection of concentrated trisodium citrate. Clin. Nephrol. 69, 317-318 (2008)
McCann, M. & Moore, Z. E. H. Interventions for preventing infectious complications in haemodialysis patients with central venous catheters. Cochrane Database of Systematic Reviews, Issue 1. Art. No.: CD006894. doi:10.1002/14651858. CD006894.pub2 (2010)
Chatzinikolaou, I. et al. Antibiotic-coated hemodialysis catheters for the prevention of vascular catheter-related infections: a prospective, randomized study. Am. J. Med. 115, 352-357 (2003).
von Eiff, C. et al. Nasal carriage as source of Stapylococcus aureus bacteremia. Study Group. N. Engl. J. Med. 344, 11-16 (2001)
Wilcox MH, Tack KJ, Bouza E, et al. Complicated skin and skin structure infections and catheter-related bloodstream infections: noninferiority of linezolid in a phase 3 study. Clin Infect Dis 2009; 48: 203–12.
Clinical practice guidelines for the diagnosis and management of intravascular catheter-related infection: 2009 Update by the Infectious Diseases Society of America
Mokrzycki MH, Zhang M, Cohen H, Golestaneh L, Laut JM, Rosenberg SO. Tunnelled haemodialysis catheter bacteraemia: risk factors for bacteraemia recurrence, infectious complications and mortality. Nephrol Dial Transplant 2006; 21:1024–31
NKF-K/DOQI Clinical Practice Guidelines for Vascular Access: update 2000. Am J Kidney Dis 2001; 37:S137-S181
McCarthy JT, Moran J, Posen G, Leypoldt JK, Hull AR, Jaber BL, Correa-Rotter R. A time for rediscovery: chronic hemofiltration for end-stage renal disease. Semin Dial. 2003;16(3):199.
Honore PM, Jamez J, Wauthier M, Lee PA, Dugernier T, Pirenne B, Hanique G, Matson JR. Prospective evaluation of short-term, high-volume isovolemic hemofiltration on the hemodynamic course and outcome in patients with intractable circulatory failure resulting from septic shock. Crit Care Med. 2000;28(11):3581.
Palevsky PM. Dialysis modality and dosing strategy in acute renal failure. Semin Dial. 2006;19(2):165.
Tolwani AJ, Campbell RC, Stofan BS, Lai KR, Oster RA, Wille KM. Standard versus

high-dose CVVHDF for ICU-related acute renal failure. J Am Soc Nephrol. 2008;19(6):1233.
Jun M, Heerspink HJ, Ninomiya T, Gallagher M, Bellomo R, Myburgh J, Finfer S, Palevsky PM, Kellum JA, Perkovic V, Cass A. Intensities of renal replacement therapy in acute kidney injury: a systematic review and meta-analysis. Clin J Am Soc Nephrol. 2010;5(6):956.
Van Wert R, Friedrich JO, Scales DC, Wald R, Adhikari NK, University of Toronto Acute Kidney Injury Research Group. High-dose renal replacement therapy for acute kidney injury: Systematic review and meta-analysis. Crit Care Med. 2010;38(5):1360.
RENAL Replacement Therapy Study Investigators, Bellomo R, Cass A, Cole L, Finfer S, Gallagher M, Lo S, McArthur C, McGuinness S, Myburgh J, Norton R, Scheinkestel C, Su S. Intensity of continuous renal-r

3

Management of Secondary Hyperparathyroidism in Hemodialysis Patients

Emanuel Zitt[1,2] and Ulrich Neyer[2]
[1]Department of Nephrology and Dialysis, Academic Teaching Hospital Feldkirch,
[2]Vorarlberg Institute for Vascular Investigation and Treatment (VIVIT), Feldkirch, Austria

1. Introduction

Secondary hyperparathyroidism (sHPT) represents the adaptive and very often finally maladaptive response of the organism to control the disturbed homeostasis of calcium, phosphorus and vitamin D metabolism caused by declining renal function. Dysregulation of calcium and phosphorus homeostasis leads to elevated levels of the phosphatonin fibroblast growth factor 23 (FGF23), decreased renal phosphorus excretion, increased serum phosphorus, and diminished synthesis of calcitriol ($1,25(OH)_2D_3$), the active form of vitamin D. These alterations result in increased secretion and synthesis of parathyroid hormone (PTH) and parathyroid cell hyperplasia (Cunningham et al., 2011).

Evidence is available that these disturbances in mineral metabolism lead to vascular (Goodman et al., 2000; Raggi et al., 2002) and valvular (Ribeiro et al., 1998) calcifications and are directly linked to an increased risk of cardiovascular morbidity and mortality as well as excess all-cause mortality (Covic et al., 2009). In accordance to a recent systematic review, the risk of cardiovascular and all-cause mortality is greatest with elevated serum phosphorus followed by increased serum calcium and PTH (Covic et al., 2009). Apart from extra-skeletal side effects, sHPT also leads to profound alterations in bone metabolism which become obvious in the different forms of renal osteodystrophy (Malluche & Faugere, 1990; Moe et al., 2006). This clinical syndrome encompassing mineral, bone and cardiovascular abnormalities has been termed CKD-related Mineral and Bone Disorder (CKD-MBD) (Moe et al., 2006). Furthermore, sHPT is thought to play a role in various other complications of end-stage renal disease as bone pain, bone fractures, muscle dysfunction, sexual dysfunction, disturbed hematopoiesis, immune dysfunction, pruritus and calcific uremic arteriolopathy (calciphylaxis) (Rodriguez & Lorenzo, 2009). An overview of the current understanding of the pathogenesis of sHPT is given in Figure 1.

In an attempt to improve clinical care, the National Kidney Foundation's Kidney Disease Outcomes Quality Initiative (NKF-K/DOQI™ [KDOQI]) has recommended target ranges for serum intact PTH, serum phosphorus and total corrected serum calcium (KDOQI, 2003). More recently, the Kidney Disease Improving Global Outcomes (KDIGO) guidelines for diagnosis, evaluation, prevention and treatment of CKD-MBD have been published (KDIGO, 2009) and endorsed by the US KDOQI (Uhlig et al., 2010) and European Renal Best Practice (Goldsmith et al., 2010) groups. These latter guidelines have tried to provide evidence-based recommendations, but due to the very limited availability of high quality

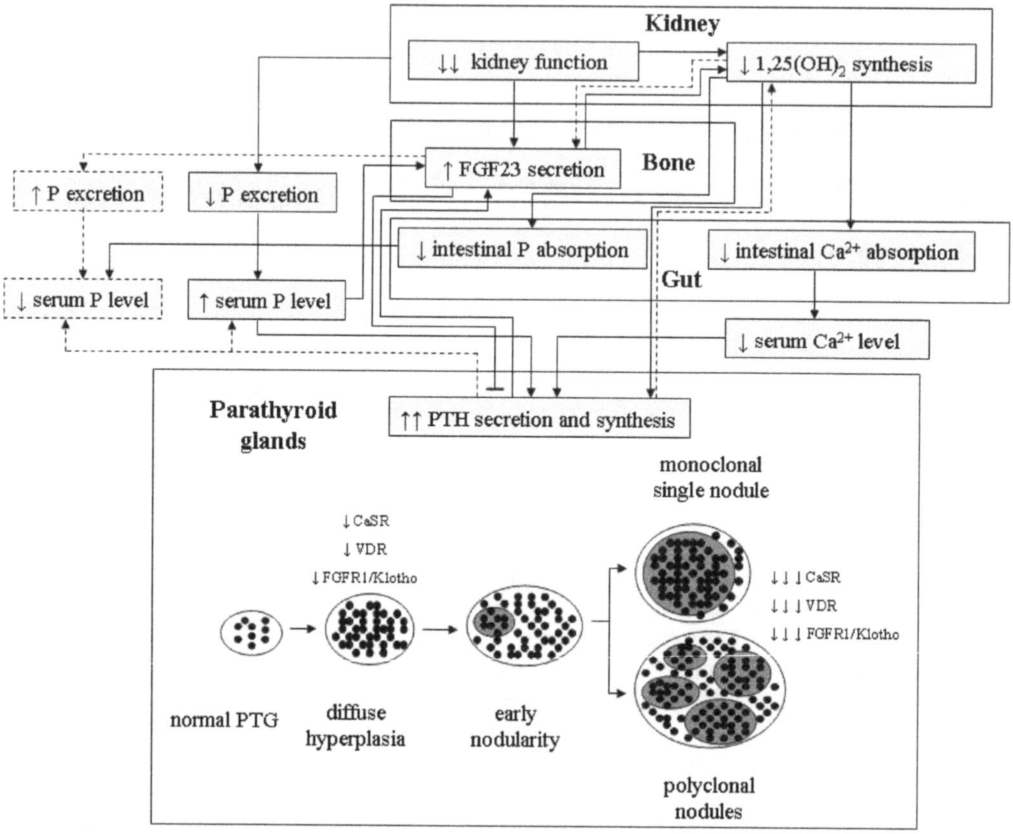

Fig. 1. Pathogenesis of secondary hyperparathyroidism. Declining kidney function causes reduced renal conversion of 25(OH)D to 1,25(OH)$_2$D by CYP27B1 (25(OH)D-1α-hydroxylase) and elevated serum phosphorus levels due to diminished phosphorus excretion. Increased phosphorus concentration, decreased calcium concentration and markedly reduced serum calcitriol levels lead to increased PTH synthesis and secretion in the parathyroid glands. Elevated FGF23 expression, to counteract the reduced phosphorus excretion, downregulates residual renal 25(OH)D-1α-hydroxylase, additionally promoting the development of sHPT. These metabolic changes are accompanied by a variable downregulation and underexpression of the calcium-sensing receptor and vitamin D receptor on parathyroidal cells, rendering the parathyroid gland unable to respond appropriately to calcium and calcitriol. Dashed lines indicate counter-regulatory pathways. Abbreviations: FGF23, fibroblast growth factor 23; P, phosphorus; Ca^{2+}, calcium; CaSR, calcium-sensing receptor; VDR, vitamin D receptor; FGFR1, fibroblast growth factor receptor 1, PTG, parathyroid gland.

clinical interventional trials with skeletal, cardiovascular or mortality end-points in this field, fewer and less mandatory recommendations are given compared to the older KDOQI guidelines.

The achievement of these target ranges set by the KDOQI or KDIGO guidelines is quite challenging (Young et al., 2004) and failure to reach these targets has been shown to be associated with increased risk for death compared to simultaneously achieving the targets for all three biochemical parameters PTH, calcium and phosphorus (Danese et al., 2008).

The 84-amino-acid peptide hormone PTH has a very short half-life of two to four minutes after parathyroid secretion. It is metabolized to shorter fragments in the liver which are then excreted by the kidneys. With increasing renal failure and progressive CKD the proportion of these fragments with a 5 to 10 times longer half-life raises due to decreased renal clearance. Although the exact composition and possible function of the various PTH fragments are not yet fully elucidated, experimental data clearly found a clinically relevant biological activity of some of these fragments. Routinely used second-generation PTH assays, globally called "intact" PTH assays because they were thought to measure the full-length PTH 1-84 molecule only, recognize with various cross-reactivities (from approximately 50 to 100%) a PTH fragment, which co-elutes in high-performance liquid chromatography with a synthetic PTH 7–84 fragment. With progressive renal failure the amount of this and related PTH fragments gradually increases from about 20% in healthy individuals to about 50% in hemodialysis patients (Brossard et al., 2000). Therefore, at least in part, the progressive increase in measured PTH with decreasing renal function is also linked to the decreased renal metabolism and clearance of PTH 1-84 and its fragments. The different commercially available second-generation PTH assays have variable cross-reactivity with the PTH 7-84 fragment, therefore PTH measurements with different assays are not fully comparable and due to lacking standardization of PTH measurement sHPT patients might be classified differently according to KDOQI or KDIGO guidelines, resulting in different and due to misclassification potentially disadvantageous therapeutic interventions (Koller et al., 2004). Newer third-generation PTH assays, which show no cross-reactivity with the PTH 7-84 and related fragments, have been developed. Unfortunately, in all bone biopsy studies, which were later used to establish the KDOQI and KDIGO PTH target ranges, the first available second-generation PTH assay was used, but this assay is no longer commercially available. In an attempt to provide some kind of comparability of PTH measurements and consistent classification, correcting factors for the different second-generation PTH assays were proposed (Souberbielle et al., 2010).

Current therapeutic strategies include the modification of calcium and phosphorus balance through restricted dietary calcium and phosphorus intake and removal during hemodialysis, administration of phosphate binders, vitamin D receptor activators (calcitriol and newer vitamin D analogues) and the calcimimetic cinacalcet, and ultimately parathyroidectomy in very severe sHPT. These interventions have been shown to improve the biochemical parameters (PTH, calcium, phosphorus), bone histology or histomorphometry and cardiovascular calcification, but still there is lacking evidence that improvements in these surrogate parameters translate into better patient outcomes. Traditionally interventions to treat sHPT primarily aimed at bone health, but over the years new experimental insights into cardiovascular calcification and epidemiological data about associated cardiovascular morbidity and mortality risk switched the emphasis from bone to cardiovascular health.

2. Treatment of hyperphosphatemia

Declining renal function inevitably causes phosphorus retention due to decreased renal phosphorus clearance. This mechanism starts early in chronic kidney disease. However, hyperphosphatemia is prevented until the late stages of chronic kidney disease by an increase in FGF23 and PTH which control phosphorus homeostasis for a definite time. Initially, phosphorus retention stimulates FGF23 and PTH secretion, which in turn suppress renal phosphorus reabsorption and increase renal phosphorus excretion. FGF23 also suppresses calcitriol ($1,25(OH)_2D_3$) production, which diminishes intestinal phosphorus absorption but allows increases in PTH levels. Whereas FGF23 suppresses PTH secretion in normal parathyroid glands, resistance to its effect occurs with further loss of kidney function because of decreased Klotho and FGF receptor 1 expression in the parathyroid glands and the kidney. Thus, as chronic kidney disease progresses to late stages, these homeostatic mechanisms are inevitably overwhelmed, hyperphosphatemia ensues, and the levels of PTH and FGF23 increase progressively (Cunningham et al., 2011).

Robust observational data show a clear association of higher serum phosphorus levels with cardiovascular events and mortality (Block et al., 1998, 2004). The exact threshold above which risk significantly increases is not definitely known and varies across the studies from 5.0 to 7.0 mg/dL (1.6 to 2.3 mmol/L) (Covic et al., 2009). However, it has never been determined in randomized placebo-controlled trials whether treating hyperphosphatemia to specific target ranges improves clinical patient outcomes. The KDIGO guidelines therefore suggest to decrease serum phosphorus levels toward the reference range in patients with chronic kidney disease 5D (KDIGO, 2009).

Therapeutic interventions to treat hyperphosphatemia include restriction of dietary phosphorus intake, administration of phosphate binders and increasing the frequency or length of dialysis sessions.

2.1 Dietary phosphorus restriction

Dietary phosphorus assessment and restriction is the cornerstone of the treatment of hyperphosphatemia. Educational support and dietary guidelines should be offered to the patients by a skilled dietician. Restriction of dietary phosphorus intake, however, requires a reduction in oral protein intake, as protein-rich foods are the main source of dietary phosphorus (Shinaberger et al., 2008). Lowering protein intake can lead to malnutrition and protein-energy wasting and thereby increasing mortality in dialysis patients (Lacson et al., 2007). It is very important to avoid concomitant malnutrition by forced dietary protein restriction, as protein restriction as means to lower dietary phosphorus intake may outweigh the benefit of controlled phosphorus and may lead to greater mortality (Shinaberger et al., 2008). One possibility for overcoming the problem of concordant overall protein restriction and the risk of malnutrition with reduced dietary phosphorus intake would be to avoid phosphorus-rich ingredients that are added to processed foods and beverages (Sherman & Mehta, 2009a, 2009b). Contrary to natural sources of organic phosphorus, such as meat or dairy products, such phosphorus sources are dissociated from protein intake. Reducing the consumption of such phosphorus additives might help to decrease phosphorus intake without the risk of protein-energy wasting (Sullivan et al., 2009). Additionally, the intake of protein sources with low phosphorus to protein ratios might further help to limit phosphorus intake (Noori et al., 2010). Nutritional guidelines recommend a maximum of 800 to 1000 mg (25 to 35 mmol) daily dietary phosphorus intake (Fouque et al., 2007). Nevertheless, dietary modifications alone are generally not sufficient to reduce phosphorus intake sufficiently in most patients, but help to save phosphate binders and probably reduce the high pill burden.

2.2 Phosphate binders

The use of oral phosphate binders to block intestinal phosphorus absorption has been shown to effectively reduce serum phosphorus levels irrespective of the phosphate binder class. Although no placebo-controlled randomized trial has been done so far to prove that reduction in serum phosphorus by the use of phosphate binders improves patient outcomes, a recent prospective observational study in a large number of incident dialysis patients has shown that the use of any phosphate binder (versus none) offers a clear survival benefit independent of absolute serum phosphorus concentration and co-medication (Isakova et al., 2009).

Available phosphate binders include the calcium salts calcium acetate and calcium carbonate, aluminium hydroxide, the polymeric anion-exchange resins sevelamer hydrochloride and sevelamer carbonate, lanthanum carbonate and the newer so far not well studied compounds ferric citrate, SBR759 (iron-based), magnesium/calcium carbonate and magnesium carbonate/calcium acetate. They differ in composition, phosphate-binding capacity, form and have specific potential advantages and disadvantages, which are summarized in Table 1.

Considering the different agents there are no data at present to favour one phosphate binder, because there is no proven superiority of any phosphate binder or binder class for relevant clinical outcomes. According to a recent systematic review and meta-analysis of available randomized controlled trials all phosphate binders decrease serum phosphorus levels compared with placebo. The newer drugs sevelamer hydrochloride and lanthanum carbonate do not result in superior control of biochemical parameters compared with calcium salts. In contrast, in head-to-head studies calcium salts enable a greater reduction of serum phosphorus than sevelamer hydrochloride. Whereas both calcium salts (calcium acetate and carbonate) do not differ with regard to serum calcium levels, sevelamer hydrochloride and lanthanum carbonate are associated with significantly lower rates of treatment-related hypercalcemia, which may result in decreased cardiovascular calcification. However, the finding of slower or less progression of cardiovascular calcification in sevelamer-treated patients is inconsistent across the studies. Studies revealed no difference in PTH suppression when comparing calcium acetate with calcium carbonate or lanthanum

Binder source	Form	Content (mineral/metal/element)	Phosphate-binding capacity	Daily dose	Advantages	Disadvantages
Calcium carbonate	tablet, capsule, chewable, gum, liquid	200 mg elemental Ca^{2+} per 500 mg carbonate (40% elemental Ca^{2+})	39 mg phosphate per 1 gramm calcium carbonate	1500 to 3500 mg (3–7 tablets)	effective phosphate-binding, inexpensive, readily available, long-term experience	potential for hypercalcemia and hypercalcemia-associated risks, gastrointestinal side effects
Calcium acetate	capsule, tablet	126.7 mg elemental Ca^{2+} per 500 mg tablet, 169 mg elemental Ca^{2+} per 667 mg capsule (25% elemental Ca^{2+})	45 mg phosphate per 1 gramm calcium acetate	3000 to 6000 mg (6 to 12 tablets)	effective phosphate-binding, potentially higher binding capacity and lower Ca^{2+} absorption than carbonate, inexpensive, long-term experience	potential for hypercalcemia and hypercalcemia-associated risks, gastrointestinal side effects, more costly than carbonate

Aluminium hydroxide	tablet, capsule, liquid	Varying with 100 to 600 mg aluminium per tablet	22.3 mg phosphate per 5 ml, 18.8 mg phosphate per 1000 mg	600 to 1800 mg (pill burden dependent on content per tablet)	very effective phosphate-binding capacity	potential for aluminium toxicity, gastrointestinal side effects
Sevelamer-HCl	tablet	none	64 mg phosphate per 800 mg sevelamer-HCl	2400 to 9600 mg (3 to 12 tablets)	effective phosphate-binding capacity, no Ca^{2+} and metal content, reduces LDL-cholesterol, possible potential for reduced calcification	costs, potential for decrease in bicarbonate levels, in presence of hypocalcemia need for Ca^{2+} supplement, higher risk of gastrointestinal side effects compared to Ca^{2+} salts
Sevelamer carbonate	tablet, powder	none	same as sevelamer-HCl	2400 to 9600 mg (3 to 12 tablets, 1 to 4 packets)	same as sevelamer-HCl, but lower risk of metabolic acidosis	assumed to have same disadvantages as sevelamer-HCl except decrease in bicarbonate levels, less well studied
Lanthanum carbonate	chewable tablet	250, 500, 750 or 1000 mg elemental lanthanum per tablet	NA	750 to 3750 mg (3 to 5 chewable tablets)	effective phosphate-binding capacity, no Ca^{2+}, chewable, reduced pill burden	costs, gastrointestinal side effects, potential for accumulation
Magnesium carbonate/calcium acetate	tablet	60 mg Mg per 235 mg $MgCO_3$, 110 mg elemental Ca^{2+} per 435 mg Ca^{2+} acetate	NA	705/1305 mg to 2820/5220 mg (3 to 12 tablets)	effective, potential for lower Ca^{2+} load than pure Ca^{2+}-based binders	potential for hypermagnesemia, gastrointestinal side effect, not well studied
Ferric citrate	capsule	176 mg elemental iron per 1g ferric citrate				potential for iron accumulation, not well studied, gastrointestinal side effects, less effective than Ca^{2+} salts
SBR759 (polymeric complex of starch with ferric iron)	powder	1.25 g per sachet			powder form	potential for iron accumulation, not well studied (1 phase I trial), gastrointestinal side effects, hypocalcemia

Table 1. Overview of available phosphate binders (adapted from KDOQI, 2003; KDIGO, 2009; Tonelli et al., 2010; Uhlig et al., 2010). Abbrevations: Ca^{2+}, calcium; HCl, hydrochloride; Mg, magnesium; CO_3, carbonate; NA, not available.

carbonate with calcium carbonate, but found a significantly lower PTH reduction with sevelamer hydrochloride in comparison to calcium salts. When all studies were pooled, gastrointestinal side effects occurred more often with sevelamer hydrochloride than with calcium salts. With the use of sevelamer hydrochloride significantly lower serum bicarbonate is found, aggravating already existing metabolic acidosis. The new formula of sevelamer carbonate does not negatively influence acid-base status. A possible advantage of sevelamer is its significant reduction of LDL-cholesterol. However, no difference in all-cause mortality could be found comparing calcium acetate and carbonate, or sevelamer with calcium salts. All-cause mortality as endpoint has not been studied with all other phosphate binders (Navaneethan et al., 2009).

Hypercalcemia is a known side effect of calcium salts, especially when combined with vitamin D receptor activators. Persistent hypercalcemia necessitates a dose reduction or cessation of calcium salts as phosphate binders. The KDOQI guidelines suggest limiting the daily calcium intake from calcium-containing phosphate binders to 1500 mg per day for elemental calcium and 2000 mg per day for total intake of elemental calcium including the dietary calcium content (KDOQI, 2003). Nevertheless, there is no data available to recommend a specific upper limit of a safe amount of calcium intake. Restrictive use of calcium-based phosphate binders may be considered in the following situations (Cozzolino et al., 2011; Goldsmith et al., 2010):

- presence of cardiovascular disease
- presence of vascular or valvular calcification
- older age (>65 years)
- diabetes mellitus
- evidence of adynamic bone disease
- hypercalcemia

Although very effective, a prolonged (>3 months continuously, or >6 months cumulative) use of aluminium hydroxide should be avoided because of the potential toxicity of accumulated aluminium leading to encephalopathy, osteomalacia and anemia (Goldsmith et al., 2010).

Irrespective of the phosphate binder class the successful practical management of hyperphosphatemia with phosphate binders includes:

- concomitant dietary phosphorus restriction (especially phosphorus-rich additives)
- administration of phosphate binders with the meal
- individual dosing with respect to eating habits and serum phosphorus level

A new and promising concept for the management of hyperphosphatemia was recently developed to enable patients to self-adjust the phosphate binder dose in relation to the phosphorus content of each individual meal: "Phosphate Education Program" (PEP) (Ahlenstiel et al., 2010). Patients are taught to eye-estimate the meal phosphorus content based on "phosphate units" (PU; 1 PU is defined per 100 mg of phosphorus per serving size of the meal) and then phosphate binders are prescribed dependent on an individual phosphate binder/PU ratio. This concept is similar to the individualized adjustments of insulin dose to carbohydrate intake in the treatment of diabetes mellitus.

Novel agents under development for the treatment of hyperphosphatemia are MCI-196 (colestilan) (Locatelli et al., 2010), a non-metallic anion-exchange resin, and niacin and nicotinamid, which probably directly inhibit the sodium-dependent phosphate cotransporter Na-Pi-2b in the gastrointestinal tract (Muller et al., 2007).

2.3 Dialytic methods for phosphorus removal

Dialytic methods to improve phosphorus removal include prolonged (nocturnal) hemodialysis (Culleton et al. 2007; Walsh et al., 2010) and convective strategies (Tonelli et al., 2009).

3. Vitamin D therapy

3.1 Correction of vitamin D deficiency and insufficiency

Neither the normal nor the desirable target ranges for 25-hydroxyvitamin D (25(OH)D) levels are known in patients on hemodialysis. In accordance with patients without chronic kidney disease, 25(OH)D levels <12.5 ng/mL (<30 nmol/L) are defined as vitamin D deficiency, values <30 ng/mL (<75 nmol/L) as vitamin D insufficiency. Observational studies have shown an association between low 25(OH)D levels and adverse clinical outcomes (Holick, 2005; Wolf et al., 2007; Giovannucci, 2008). Although data from clinical trials are missing to show a survival benefit after increasing 25(OH)D levels in insufficient or deficient hemodialysis patients, current guidelines suggest to replete 25(OH)D stores in these patients on grounds of low costs, relative safety of repletion and potential therapeutic impact (KDIGO, 2009). After initial measurement and diagnosis of vitamin D deficiency, a supplementation using cholecalciferol or ergocalciferol may be initiated with remeasurement after 3 months of supplementation. There are no data regarding the choice of vitamin D product or the administration route. Altogether, oral repletion seems to be more favourable compared to intramuscular route in hemodialysis patients. In accordance with the general population a daily dose of 1000 to 2000 IU of cholecalciferol or a corresponding weekly dose are given (KDOQI, 2003; KDIGO, 2009; Uhlig et al., 2010). In a recent study in 107 hemodialysis patients, 91% of the patients had a serum 25(OH)D level higher than the target level of 75 nmol/L (30 ng/mL) after 3 months of monthly oral substitution of 100,000 IU (at first dialysis session of the month) (Jean et al., 2009). This approach seems to be safe and guarantee patient compliance. If hypercalcemia or hyperphosphatemia occurs, vitamin D repletion should be temporarily discontinued or abandoned. Table 2 gives an overview of the key differences between 25(OH)D and its "active" form $1,25(OH)_2D$.

	25(OH)D	$1,25(OH)_2D$
Total plasma concentration (recommended normal values)	30 to 50 ng/mL (75 to 125 nmol/L)	30 to 50 pg/mL (75 to 125 pmol/L)
Total plasma concentration (relative values)	1000	1
Binding affinity to vitamin D-binding protein (relative values)	1000	1
Free concentration (relative values)	1	1
Half-life	25 to 30 days	4 to 8 hours
VDR affinity (relative values)	1	500 to 1000

Table 2. Characteristics and differences of 25(OH)D and $1,25(OH)_2D$. Abbrevations: VDR, vitamin D receptor.

3.2 Vitamin D receptor activators

Treatment of sHPT with active vitamin D receptor activators (VDRA) is a well established therapeutic modality, and current practice guidelines recommend to treat patients with elevated and/or increasing PTH levels with a VDRA (KDIGO, 2009). Observational studies are indicating a survival benefit of VDRA in hemodialysis patients in comparison with patients without VDRA treatment (Teng et al., 2003, 2005; Tentori et al., 2006; Naves-Diaz et al., 2008). Again, prospective controlled randomised clinical trials indicating a benefit on patient-level clinical outcomes with VDRA therapy are missing but strongly awaited. Calcitriol, the physiological VDRA, is the natural regulator of parathyroid gland function and growth and exerts its effect on PTH secretion by inhibiting mRNA synthesis through its action on the vitamin D receptor (VDR), a highly specific receptor that acts as a transcription factor. In addition, calcitriol is able to inhibit PTH secretion by increasing calcium absorption in the intestine, while also increasing bone resorption and, consequently, calcium release from bone. Moreover, calcitriol regulates the expression of its own receptor, stimulating its synthesis. The deficit of calcitriol observed in hemodialysis patients as well as a transformation into nodular hyperplasia with progressive sHPT is associated with a decrease in VDR levels in the parathyroid gland. Decreased VDR expression may than cause resistance to VDRA. VDRA generally control sHPT well in patients with moderately increased hypertrophic glands and less well in patients with enlarged hyperplastic glands and should therefore be started early in the development of sHPT (Cunningham et al., 2011). Beyond the classical endocrine effects on parathyroid gland, bone and intestine, the pleiotropic paracrine and autocrine effects of vitamin D have been associated with improvement of cardiovascular risk factors, including increased renin activity, hypertension, inflammation, insulin resistance, diabetes, albuminuria and an improved immune response.

Besides the native active hormone calcitriol ($1,25(OH)_2D_3$), the two prodrugs alfacalcidol ($1(OH)D_3$) and doxercalciferol ($1(OH)D_2$) and the two vitamin D analogues paricalcitol (19-nor-$1,25(OH)_2D_2$) and maxacalcitol (22-oxa-$1,25(OH)_2D_3$) can be used. Paricalcitol and maxacalcitol (oxacalcitriol) bind directly to the VDR, whereas doxercalciferol and alfacalcidol need an enzymatic 25-hydroxylation activation step in the liver. So far no prospective, placebo-controlled and blinded clinical trial involving 22-oxacalcitriol, paricalcitol, or doxercalciferol has yet demonstrated additional clinical benefits when compared with calcitriol, nor have any studies been published showing that either calcitriol or alfacalcidol has an advantage over the other with respect to biochemical or clinical end points (Cunningham & Zehnder, 2011). Therefore, low dose therapy with calcitriol (e.g. 0.25 µg/d orally or 0.25 µg thrice weekly orally or intravenously as a starting dose) is recommended with elevated or increasing PTH levels (KDIGO, 2009). Characteristics and oral calcitriol equivalent doses of various available VDRA are presented in Table 3.

According to current practice guidelines, the target range for PTH is now 2-9 times the upper limit of the normal range (KDIGO, 2009; Uhlig et al., 2010; Goldsmith et al., 2010). This wide range takes into account a significant interassay variability of values obtained with different commercial PTH assays (Koller et al., 2004; Souberbielle et al., 2010), inability to uniformly predict bone histologic and histomorphometric states by means of PTH within this range and the epidemiological observation of increased all-cause mortality starting from PTH values >400 to 600 pg/mL (Uhlig et al., 2010). If there is no successful response with PTH reduction into the suggested target range, or dose-limiting side effects occur, especially hypercalcemia and hyperphosphatemia, a calcimimetic can be initiated instead or combined with a low dose of VDRA.

VDRA	Chemical structure	Oral calcitriol equivalent dose (thrice weekly)
Calcitriol	$1,25(OH)_2D_3$; natural hormone	oral 0.25 μg intravenous 0.5 μg
Alfacalcidol	$1(OH)D_3$; synthetic prohormone	oral 0.5 μg intravenous 1 μg
Doxercalciferol	$1(OH)D_2$, synthetic prohormone	oral 2.5 μg intravenous 5 μg
Paricalcitol	19nor-$1,25(OH)_2D_2$; synthetic analogue	oral 1 μg intravenous 2 μg
Maxacalcitol (Oxacalcitriol)	22oxa-$1,25(OH)_2D_3$; synthetic analogue	NA

Table 3. Characteristics and oral calcitriol equivalent doses of vitamin D receptor activators (VDRA). Abbreviation: NA, not available.

4. Calcimimetics

Calcimimetics are allosteric modulators of the calcium sensing receptor that sensitize the receptor to extracellular calcium. This results in reduced PTH secretion and inhibited parathyroid cell proliferation (Nemeth et al., 1998; Chin et al., 2000). This decrease in serum PTH is accompanied by control of serum calcium and phosphorus levels in patients with sHPT as well as a halt or regression of parathyroid gland hyperplasia (Meola et al., 2009). Initial phase III trials and various observational studies have shown that cinacalcet enables more patients to reach the recommended biochemical targets (Block et al., 2004; Lindberg et al., 2005; Urena et al., 2009) and allows sustained biochemical control for long term up to 3 years (Sprague et al., 2009). At present cinacalcet hydrochloride is the only calcimimetic available for clinical use. In contrast to VDRA, cinacalcet decreases all three important biochemical parameters of CKD-MBD (PTH, phosphorus, calcium) (Urena et al., 2009). In addition to excellent results on laboratory parameters, cinacalcet has also shown favourable effects on cardiovascular hospitalization, bone fracture rate, parathyroidectomy rate and quality of life (Cunningham et al., 2005). In a prospectively designed observational study use of cinacalcet on top of standard sHPT therapy with VDRA and phosphate binders resulted in a 26% lower all-cause mortality and a 24% lower cardiovascular mortality than in patients without cinacalcet, with the largest survival benefit for patients with most severe sHPT (PTH >600 pg/mL) (Block et al., 2010). The ongoing double-blind, randomised placebo-controlled EVOLVE trial (Evaluation of cinacalcet HCl therapy to lower cardiovascular events) currently determines whether cinacalcet reduces all-cause mortality or non-fatal cardiovascular events (Chertow et al., 2007).

Generally, initial therapy starts with a daily dose of 30 mg followed by dose-titration every 2 to 4 weeks if necessary. Serum calcium levels must be monitored regularly because of its known hypocalcemic effect.

Whereas VDRA reduce PTH gene transcription and hormone synthesis over a period of several hours or even days, cinacalcet inhibits PTH secretion within minutes, with a maximal decrease occurring within 2 to 4 hours after administration. Besides gastrointestinal side effects, hypocalcemia is one of the most common adverse events seen with cinacalcet. It is thought to occur after decreased mobilization of calcium from bone caused by lowered PTH levels. In most patients, this hypocalcemia can be successfully managed with dose adjustments or a combination with low doses of VDRA in patients with moderate to severe sHPT. Clinical trials have demonstrated the superior suppression of PTH production and control of calcium and phosphorus in hemodialysis patients who use cinacalcet, both as adjunctive therapy to VDRA and as primary therapy with reduced doses of VDRA , compared with sHPT therapy with VDRA and phosphate binders only (Chertow et al., 2006; Block et al., 2008; Fishbane et al., 2008; Messa et al., 2008).

5. Parathyroidectomy

Persistently increased serum PTH levels >800 pg/mL (88.0 pmol/L) in presence of hypercalcemia or hyperphosphatemia refractory to medical therapy and calcific uremic arteriolopathy (calciphylaxis) with concomitantly elevated PTH levels are an indication for surgery (KDOQI, 2003; KDIGO, 2009). Subtotal and total parathyroidectomy (PTX) with or without forearm autograft arose as a treatment option in the 1990s (Tominaga et al., 1997) and PTX continues to be a primary therapeutic option for refractory sHPT in both Europe and the US. Rates of PTX increased for US patients on hemodialysis from 1998 to 2002 despite an increase in therapeutic options (Foley et al., 2005). The frequency of PTX across Europe has remained relatively stable since the mid-1980s (Malberti et al., 2001) and is lower in older patients (Pelletier et al., 2010).

PTX effectively decreases PTH, calcium and phosphorus and offers the highest percentage cure for sHPT, compared to all other medical and surgical treatments. However, recurrent hyperparathyroidism can be observed in 10 - 70% of patients dependent on follow-up time (Johnson et al., 1988; Gagne et al., 1992; Gasparri et al., 2001). For total parathyroidectomy with autotransplantation an intra-operative selection of parathyroid tissue with diffuse hyperplasia but low proliferative potential (and exclusion of nodular tissue) is feasible and minimizes the risk of graft-dependent recurrent hyperparathyroidism (Neyer et al., 2002). Alternatively to surgery, ultrasound-guided percutaneous fine-needle ethanol injection into nodular hyperplastic parathyroid glands is very common in Japan (Giangrande et al., 1992; Kitaoka et al., 1994; Fukagawa et al., 1999). Apart from ethanol, also calcitriol or novel VDRA can be directly placed into enlarged parathyroid glands using the same technique (Shiizaki et al., 2003).

To date no specific guidelines considering sHPT treatment in hemodialysis patients on kidney transplant waiting list have been established. After successful kidney transplantation persistent HPT can be observed in up to 25% of patients one year after transplantation despite adequate renal graft function. Severity of sHPT at time of transplantation was found to be a significant indicator of persistent HPT (Evenepoel et al., 2004). If indicated, therapy for persistent HPT should be initiated about three months after renal transplantation because further spontaneous improvement thereafter is rare. Because this special situation of persistent HPT after transplantation is usually accompanied by hypercalcemia and hypophosphatemia, conventional therapy with phosphate binders, VDRA or calcium supplements is not indicated in most patients. Therefore, PTX is the preferred treatment option in this situation and has been shown to be effective, safe, though associated with a mild deterioration of graft function in the early postoperative phase but similar graft survival in the long-term compared to kidney transplant patients without PTX and linked to a blood pressure and lipid lowering effect (Triponez et al., 2008). Recently, also cinacalcet has been proposed to offer an alternative therapeutic option to PTX, although not approved

for the use in this situation and cost-intensive if used for many years (Kruse et al., 2005; Serra et al., 2005; Srinivas et al., 2006; Zitt et al., 2007).
Therefore, we believe that a good and early control of sHPT prior to kidney transplantation is mandatory. This should be initially done using all medical options including cinacalcet, but if unsuccessful in control of severe sHPT proceeding straight to PTX for an optimal and cost-effective treatment. Randomized clinical trials directly comparing medical with surgical therapy of sHPT are lacking.
To avoid severe postoperative hypocalcemia ("hungry bone syndrome), pre-/peri- and postoperative calcium and calcitriol supplementation (e.g. 1 to 2 g elemental calcium thrice a day, 1 to 4 µg calcitriol per day; parenteral calcium substitution if symptomatic hypocalcemia is present with 1 to 2 mg elemental calcium/kg/h) must be guaranteed along with frequent controls of serum calcium levels. In case of recurrent or persistent hyperparathyroidism after parathyroidectomy, cinacalcet has been shown to be a viable and safe treatment option (Zitt et al., 2010).

6. Dialysate calcium concentration

A near-neutral calcium flux could be expected in patients with a dialysate calcium concentration of 1.25 mmol/L (2.5 mEq/L), although there is considerable interindividual variability among patients (Hou et al., 1991; Argiles et al., 1993). Based on calcium kinetic modelling even lower dialysate calcium concentrations of 1.0 mmol/L (2.0 mEq/L) might be needed to avoid net positive calcium balance (Gotch et al., 2010). The risks of hemodynamic instability and cardiac rhythm disturbances with a very low dialysate calcium concentration must be kept in mind (Drueke & Touam, 2009). Overall calcium balance is influenced by dietary calcium intake, vitamin D level, calcium-containing phosphate binders, use of VDRA and calcimimetics and dialysate calcium concentration. Therefore, selecting an individual dialysate calcium concentration is based on various parameters and must always be a compromise between the need to guarantee cardiovascular stability during the hemodialysis session and the goal to maintain normal bone turnover and mineralization in order to avoid bone pain and fractures but avoid extraskeletal calcification.

7. Summary

Whereas there are insufficient high-quality randomized controlled trials in the field, this shortcoming should not lead to a nihilistic approach to the relevant clinical problems of hemodialysis patients with sHPT. Nevertheless, because of insufficient clinical data, a single treatment modality, be it phosphorus binders, vitamin D substitution with inactive forms or vitamin D receptor activators, calcimimetics or parathyroidectomy may not claim to be uniformly superior to the others, and a wider therapeutic window often prompts the use of a combination of these options and individualization of sHPT management. The ultimate goal is to improve the very poor survival of hemodialysis patients, so any suggested approach for the management of sHPT should be tested.

8. References

Ahlenstiel, T., Pape, L., Ehrich, J. H., & Kuhlmann, M. K. (2010). Self-adjustment of phosphate binder dose to meal phosphorus content improves management of hyperphosphataemia in children with chronic kidney disease. *Nephrol Dial Transplant* 25(10): pp. 3241-3249

Argiles, A., Kerr, P. G., Canaud, B., Flavier, J. L., & Mion, C. (1993). Calcium kinetics and the long-term effects of lowering dialysate calcium concentration. *Kidney Int* 43(3): pp. 630-640

Block, G. A., Hulbert-Shearon, T. E., Levin, N. W., & Port, F. K. (1998). Association of serum phosphorus and calcium x phosphate product with mortality risk in chronic hemodialysis patients: a national study. *Am J Kidney Dis* 31(4): pp. 607-617

Block, G. A., Klassen, P. S., Lazarus, J. M., Ofsthun, N., Lowrie, E. G., & Chertow, G. M. (2004). Mineral metabolism, mortality, and morbidity in maintenance hemodialysis. *J Am Soc Nephrol* 15(8): pp. 2208-2218

Block, G. A., Martin, K. J., de Francisco, A. L., Turner, S. A., Avram, M. M., Suranyi, M. G., Hercz, G., Cunningham, J., Abu-Alfa, A. K., Messa, P., Coyne, D. W., Locatelli, F., Cohen, R. M., Evenepoel, P., Moe, S. M., Fournier, A., Braun, J., McCary, L. C., Zani, V. J., Olson, K. A., Drueke, T. B., & Goodman, W. G. (2004). Cinacalcet for secondary hyperparathyroidism in patients receiving hemodialysis. *N Engl J Med* 350(15): pp. 1516-1525

Block, G. A., Zaun, D. Smits, G., Persky, M., Brillhart, S., Nieman, K., Liu, J., & St Peter, W. L. (2010). Cinacalcet hydrochloride treatment significantly improves all-cause and cardiovascular survival in a large cohort of hemodialysis patients. *Kidney Int* 78(6): pp. 578-589

Block, G. A., Zeig, S., Sugihara, J., Chertow, G. M., Chi, E. M., Turner, S. A., & Bushinsky, D. A. (2008). Combined therapy with cinacalcet and low doses of vitamin D sterols in patients with moderate to severe secondary hyperparathyroidism. *Nephrol Dial Transplant* 23(7): pp. 2311-2318

Brossard, J.H., Lepage, R., Cardinal, H., Roy, L., Rousseau, L., Dorais, C., & D'Amour, P. (2000). Influence of glomerular filtration rate on non-(1-84) parathyroid hormone (PTH) detected by intact PTH assays. *Clin Chem* 46(5): pp. 697-703

Chertow, G. M., Blumenthal, S., Turner, S., Roppolo, M., Stern, L., Chi, E. M., & Reed, J. (2006). Cinacalcet hydrochloride (Sensipar) in hemodialysis patients on active vitamin D derivatives with controlled PTH and elevated calcium x phosphate. *Clin J Am Soc Nephrol* 1(2): pp. 305-312

Chertow, G. M., Pupim, L. B., Block, G. A., Correa-Rotter, R., Drueke, T. B., Floege, J., Goodman, W. G., London, G. M., Mahaffey, K. W., Moe, S. M., Wheeler, D. C., Albizem, M., Olson, K., Klassen, P., & Parfrey, P. (2007). Evaluation of Cinacalcet Therapy to Lower Cardiovascular Events (EVOLVE): rationale and design overview. *Clin J Am Soc Nephrol* 2(5): pp. 898-905

Chin, J., Miller, S. C., Wada, M., Nagano, N., Nemeth, E. F., & Fox, J. (2000). Activation of the calcium receptor by a calcimimetic compound halts the progression of secondary hyperparathyroidism in uremic rats. *J Am Soc Nephrol* 11(5): pp. 903-11

Covic, A., Kothawala, P., Bernal, M., Robbins, S., Chalian, A., & Goldsmith, D. (2009). Systematic review of the evidence underlying the association between mineral metabolism disturbances and risk of all-cause mortality, cardiovascular mortality and cardiovascular events in chronic kidney disease. *Nephrol Dial Transplant* 24(5): pp. 1506-1523

Cozzolino, M., Mazzaferro, S., & Brandenburg, V. (2011). The treatment of hyperphosphataemia in CKD: calcium-based or calcium-free phosphate binders? *Nephrol Dial Transplant* 26(2): pp. 402-407

Culleton, B. F., Walsh, M., Klarenbach, S. W., Mortis, G., Scott-Douglas, N., Quinn, R. R., Tonelli, M., Donnelly, S., Friedrich, M. G., Kumar, A., Mahallati, H., Hemmelgarn, B. R., & Manns, B. J. (2007). Effect of frequent nocturnal hemodialysis vs conventional hemodialysis on left ventricular mass and quality of life: a randomized controlled trial. *JAMA* 298(11): pp. 1291-1299

Cunningham, J., Danese, M., Olson, K., Klassen, P., & Chertow, G. M. (2005). Effects of the calcimimetic cinacalcet HCl on cardiovascular disease, fracture, and health-related quality of life in secondary hyperparathyroidism. *Kidney Int* 68(4): pp. 1793-1800

Cunningham, J., Locatelli, F., & Rodriguez, M. (2011). Secondary hyperparathyroidism: pathogenesis, disease progression, and therapeutic options. *Clin J Am Soc Nephrol* 6(4): pp. 913-921

Cunningham, J. & Zehnder D. (2011). New Vitamin D analogs and changing therapeutic paradigms. *Kidney Int* 79(7): 702-707

Danese, M. D., Belozeroff, V., Smirnakis, K., & Rothman, K. J. (2008). Consistent control of mineral and bone disorder in incident hemodialysis patients. *Clin J Am Soc Nephrol* 3(5): pp. 1423-9

Drueke, T. B. & Touam M. (2009). Calcium balance in haemodialysis--do not lower the dialysate calcium concentration too much (con part). *Nephrol Dial Transplant* 24(10): pp. 2990-2993

Evenepoel, P., Claes, K., Kuypers, D., Maes, B., Bammens, B., & Vanrenterghem Y. (2004). Natural history of parathyroid function and calcium metabolism after kidney transplantation: a single-centre study. *Nephrol Dial Transplant* 19: pp. 1281-1287

Fishbane, S., Shapiro, W. B., Corry, D. B., Vicks, S. L., Roppolo, M., Rappaport, K., Ling, X., Goodman, W. G., Turner, S., & Charytan, C. (2008). Cinacalcet HCl and concurrent low-dose vitamin D improves treatment of secondary hyperparathyroidism in dialysis patients compared with vitamin D alone: the ACHIEVE study results. *Clin J Am Soc Nephrol* 3(6): pp. 1718-1725

Foley, R. N., Li, S., Liu, J., Gilbertson, D. T., Chen, S. C., & Collins, A. J. (2005). The fall and rise of parathyroidectomy in U.S. hemodialysis patients, 1992 to 2002. *J Am Soc Nephrol* 16(1): pp. 210-218

Fouque, D., Vennegoor, M.,ter Wee, P., Wanner, C., Basci, A., Canaud, B., Haage, P., Konner, K., Kooman, J., Martin-Malo, A., Pedrini, L., Pizzarelli, F., Tattersall, J., Tordoir, J., & Vanholder, R. (2007). EBPG guideline on nutrition. *Nephrol Dial Transplant* 22 Suppl 2: pp. 45-87

Fukagawa, M., Tominaga, Y., Kitaoka, M., Kakuta, T., & Kurokawa, K. (1999). Medical and surgical aspects of parathyroidectomy. *Kidney Int Suppl* 73: pp. 65-69

Gagne, E. R., Urena, P., Leite-Silva, S., Zingraff, J., Chevalier, A., Sarfati, E., Dubost, C., & Drueke, T. B. (1992). Short- and long-term efficacy of total parathyroidectomy with immediate autografting compared with subtotal parathyroidectomy in hemodialysis patients. *J Am Soc Nephrol* 3(4): pp. 1008-1017

Gasparri, G., Camandona, M., & Dei Poli, M. (2001). Secondary and tertiary hyperparathyroidism: causes of recurrent disease after 446 parathyroidectomies. *Ann Surg* 233(1): pp. 65-69

Giangrande, A., Castiglioni, A., Solbiati, L., & Allaria, P. (1992). Ultrasound-guided percutaneous fine-needle ethanol injection into parathyroid glands in secondary hyperparathyroidism. *Nephrol Dial Transplant* 7(5): pp. 412-421

Giovannucci, E. (2008). Vitamin D status and cancer incidence and mortality. *Adv Exp Med Biol* 624: pp. 31-42

Goldsmith, D. J., Covic, A., Fouque, D., Locatelli, F., Olgaard, K., Rodriguez, M., Spasovski, G., Urena, P., Zoccali, C., London, G. M., & Vanholder, R. (2010). Endorsement of the Kidney Disease Improving Global Outcomes (KDIGO) Chronic Kidney Disease-Mineral and Bone Disorder (CKD-MBD) Guidelines: a European Renal Best Practice (ERBP) commentary statement. *Nephrol Dial Transplant* 25(12): pp. 3823-3831

Goodman, W. G., Goldin, J., Kuizon, B. D., Yoon, C., Gales, B., Sider, D., Wang, Y., Chung, J., Emerick, A., Greaser, L., Elashoff, R. M., & Salusky, I. B. (2000). Coronary-artery calcification in young adults with end-stage renal disease who are undergoing dialysis. *N Engl J Med* 342(20): pp. 1478-1483

Gotch, F. A., Kotanko, P., Thijssen, S., & Levin, N. W.. (2010). The KDIGO guideline for dialysate calcium will result in an increased incidence of calcium accumulation in hemodialysis patients. *Kidney Int* 78(4): pp. 343-350

Holick, M. F. (2005). Vitamin D for health and in chronic kidney disease. *Semin Dial* 18(4): pp. 266-275

Hou, S. H., Zhao, J., Ellman, C. F., Hu, J., Griffin, Z., Spiegel, D. M., & Bourdeau, J. E. (1991). Calcium and phosphorus fluxes during hemodialysis with low calcium dialysate. *Am J Kidney Dis* 18(2): pp. 217-224

Isakova, T., Gutierrez, O. M., Chang, Y., Shah, A., Tamez, H., Smith, K., Thadhani, R., & Wolf, M. (2009). Phosphorus binders and survival on hemodialysis. *J Am Soc Nephrol* 20(2): pp. 388-396

Jean, G., Souberbielle, J. C., & Chazot, C. (2009). Monthly cholecalciferol administration in haemodialysis patients: a simple and efficient strategy for vitamin D supplementation. *Nephrol Dial Transplant* 24(12): pp. 3799-3805

Johnson, W. J., McCarthy, J. T., van Heerden, J. A., Sterioff, S., Grant, C. S., & Kao, P. C. (1988). Results of subtotal parathyroidectomy in hemodialysis patients. *Am J Med* 84(1): pp. 23-32

K/DOQI (2003). K/DOQI clinical practice guidelines for bone metabolism and disease in chronic kidney disease. *Am J Kidney Dis* 42(4 Suppl 3): pp. S1-201

KDIGO (2009). KDIGO clinical practice guideline for the diagnosis, evaluation, prevention, and treatment of Chronic Kidney Disease-Mineral and Bone Disorder (CKD-MBD). *Kidney Int Suppl*(113): pp. S1-130

Kitaoka, M., Fukagawa, M., Ogata, E., & Kurokawa, K. (1994). Reduction of functioning parathyroid cell mass by ethanol injection in chronic dialysis patients. *Kidney Int* 46(4): pp. 1110-1117

Koller, H., Zitt, E., Staudacher, G., Neyer, U., Mayer, G.,& Rosenkranz, A. R. (2004). Variable parathyroid hormone(1-84)/carboxylterminal PTH ratios detected by 4 novel parathyroid hormone assays. *Clin Nephrol* 61(5): pp. 337-343

Kruse, A. E., Eisenberger, U., Frey, F. J., & Mohaupt, M. G. (2005). The calcimimetic cinacalcet normalizes serum calcium in renal transplant patients with persistent hyperparathyroidism. *Nephrol Dial Transplant* 20: pp. 1311-1314

Lacson, E., Jr., Ikizler, T. A., Lazarus, J. M., Teng, M., & Hakim, R. M. (2007). Potential impact of nutritional intervention on end-stage renal disease hospitalization, death, and treatment costs. *J Ren Nutr* 17(6): pp. 363-371

Lindberg, J. S., Culleton, B., Wong, G., Borah, M. F., Clark, R. V., Shapiro, W. B., Roger, S. D., Husserl, F. E., Klassen, P. S., Guo, M. D., Albizem, M. B., & Coburn, J. W. (2005). Cinacalcet HCl, an oral calcimimetic agent for the treatment of secondary hyperparathyroidism in hemodialysis and peritoneal dialysis: a randomized, double-blind, multicenter study. *J Am Soc Nephrol* 16(3): pp. 800-807

Locatelli, F., Dimkovic, N., Pontoriero, G., Spasovski, G., Pljesa, S., Kostic, S., Manning, A., Sano, H., & Nakajima, S. (2010). Effect of MCI-196 on serum phosphate and cholesterol levels in haemodialysis patients with hyperphosphataemia: a double-blind, randomized, placebo-controlled study. *Nephrol Dial Transplant* 25(2): pp. 574-581

Malberti, F., Marcelli, D., Conte, F., Limido, A., Spotti, D., & Locatelli, F. (2001). Parathyroidectomy in patients on renal replacement therapy: an epidemiologic study. *J Am Soc Nephrol* 12(6): pp. 1242-1248

Malluche, H. & Faugere M. C. (1990). Renal bone disease 1990: an unmet challenge for the nephrologist. *Kidney Int* 38(2): pp. 193-211

Meola, M., Petrucci, I., & Barsotti, G. (2009). Long-term treatment with cinacalcet and conventional therapy reduces parathyroid hyperplasia in severe secondary hyperparathyroidism. *Nephrol Dial Transplant* 24(3): pp. 982-989

Messa, P., Macario, F., Yaqoob, M., Bouman, K., Braun, J., von Albertini, B., Brink, H., Maduell, F., Graf, H., Frazao, J. M., Bos, W. J., Torregrosa, V., Saha, H., Reichel, H., Wilkie, M., Zani, V. J., Molemans, B., Carter, D., & Locatelli, F. (2008). The OPTIMA study: assessing a new cinacalcet (Sensipar/Mimpara) treatment algorithm for secondary hyperparathyroidism. *Clin J Am Soc Nephrol* 3(1): pp. 36-45

Moe, S., Drueke, T., Cunningham, J., Goodman, W., Martin, K., Olgaard, K., Ott, S., Sprague, S., Lameire, N., & Eknoyan, G. (2006). Definition, evaluation, and classification of renal osteodystrophy: a position statement from Kidney Disease: Improving Global Outcomes (KDIGO). *Kidney Int* 69(11): pp. 1945-1953

Muller, D., Mehling, H., Otto, B., Bergmann-Lips, R., Luft, F., Jordan, J., Kettritz, R. (2007). Niacin lowers serum phosphate and increases HDL cholesterol in dialysis patients. *Clin J Am Soc Nephrol* 2(6): pp. 1249-1254

Navaneethan, S. D., Palmer, S. C., Craig, J. C., Elder, G. J., & Strippoli, G. F. (2009). Benefits and harms of phosphate binders in CKD: a systematic review of randomized controlled trials. *Am J Kidney Dis* 54(4): pp. 619-637

Naves-Diaz, M., Alvarez-Hernandez, D., Passlick-Deetjen, J., Guinsburg, A., Marelli, C., Rodriguez-Puyol, D., & Cannata-Andia, J. B. (2008). Oral active vitamin D is associated with improved survival in hemodialysis patients. *Kidney Int* 74(8): pp. 1070-1078

Nemeth, E. F., Steffey, M. E., Hammerland, L. G., Hung, B. C., Van Wagenen, B. C., DelMar, E. G., & Balandrin, M. F. (1998). Calcimimetics with potent and selective activity on the parathyroid calcium receptor. *Proc Natl Acad Sci U S A* 95(7): pp. 4040-4045

Neyer, U., Hoerandner, H., Haid, A., Zimmermann, G., & Niederle, B. (2002). Total parathyroidectomy with autotransplantation in renal hyperparathyroidism: low recurrence after intra-operative tissue selection. *Nephrol Dial Transplant* 17(4): pp. 625-629

Noori, N., Kalantar-Zadeh, K., Kovesdy, C. P., Bross, R., Benner, D., & Kopple, J. D. (2010). Association of dietary phosphorus intake and phosphorus to protein ratio with mortality in hemodialysis patients. *Clin J Am Soc Nephrol* 5(4): pp. 683-692

Pelletier, S., Roth, H., Bouchet, J. L., Drueke, T., London, G., & Fouque, D. (2010). Mineral and bone disease pattern in elderly haemodialysis patients. *Nephrol Dial Transplant* 25(9): pp. 3062-3070

Raggi, P., Boulay, A., Chasan-Taber, S., Amin, N., Dillon, M., Burke, S. K., & Chertow, G. M. (2002). Cardiac calcification in adult hemodialysis patients. A link between end-stage renal disease and cardiovascular disease? *J Am Coll Cardiol* 39(4): pp. 695-701

Ribeiro, S., Ramos, A., Brandao, A., Rebelo, J. R., Guerra, A., Resina, C., Vila-Lobos, A., Carvalho, F., Remedio, F., & Ribeiro, F. (1998). Cardiac valve calcification in haemodialysis patients: role of calcium-phosphate metabolism. *Nephrol Dial Transplant* 13(8): pp. 2037-2040

Rodriguez, M. & Lorenzo V. (2009). Parathyroid hormone, a uremic toxin. *Semin Dial* 22(4): pp. 363-836

Serra, A. L., Schwarz, A. A., Wick, F. H., Marti, H.P., & Wuthrich, R. P. (2005). Successful treatment of hypercalcemia with cinacalcet in renal transplant recipients with persistent hyperparathyroidism. *Nephrol Dial Transplant* 20: pp. 1315-1319

Sherman, R. A. & Mehta O. (2009). Dietary phosphorus restriction in dialysis patients: potential impact of processed meat, poultry, and fish products as protein sources. *Am J Kidney Dis* 54(1): pp. 18-23

Sherman, R. A. & Mehta O. (2009). Phosphorus and potassium content of enhanced meat and poultry products: implications for patients who receive dialysis. *Clin J Am Soc Nephrol* 4(8): pp. 1370-1373

Shiizaki, K., Hatamura, I., Negi, S., Narukawa, N., Mizobuchi, M., Sakaguchi, T., Ooshima, A., & Akizawa, T. (2003). Percutaneous maxacalcitol injection therapy regresses hyperplasia of parathyroid and induces apoptosis in uremia. *Kidney Int* 64(3): pp. 992-1003

Shinaberger, C. S., Greenland, S., Kopple, J. D., Van Wyck, D., Mehrotra, R., Kovesdy, C. P., & Kalantar-Zadeh, K. (2008). Is controlling phosphorus by decreasing dietary protein intake beneficial or harmful in persons with chronic kidney disease? *Am J Clin Nutr* 88(6): pp. 1511-1518.

Souberbielle, J. C., Roth, H., & Fouque, D. P. (2010). Parathyroid hormone measurement in CKD. *Kidney Int* 77(2): pp. 93-100

Sprague, S. M., Evenepoel, P., Curzi, M. P., Gonzalez, M. T., Husserl, F. E., Kopyt, N., Sterling, L. R., Mix, C., & Wong, G. (2009). Simultaneous control of PTH and CaxP Is sustained over three years of treatment with cinacalcet HCl. *Clin J Am Soc Nephrol* 4(9): pp. 1465-1476

Srinivas, T. R., Schold, J. D., Womer, K.L., Kaplan, B., Howard, R. J., Bucci, C. M., & Meier-Kriesche, H. U. (2006). Improvement in hypercalcemia with cinacalcet after kidney transplantation. *Clin J Am Soc Nephro* 1: pp. 323-326.

Sullivan, C., Sayre, S. S., Leon, J. B., Machekano, R., Love, T. E., Porter, D., Marbury, M., & Sehgal, A. R. (2009). Effect of food additives on hyperphosphatemia among patients with end-stage renal disease: a randomized controlled trial. *JAMA* 301(6): pp. 629-635

Teng, M., Wolf, M., Lowrie, E., Ofsthun, N., Lazarus, J. M. ,& Thadhani, R. (2003). Survival of patients undergoing hemodialysis with paricalcitol or calcitriol therapy. *N Engl J Med* 349(5): pp. 446-456

Teng, M., Wolf, M., Ofsthun, M. N., Lazarus, J. M., Hernan, M. A., Camargo, C. A., Jr., & Thadhani, R. (2005). Activated injectable vitamin D and hemodialysis survival: a historical cohort study. *J Am Soc Nephrol* 16(4): pp. 1115-1125

Tentori, F., Hunt, W. C., Stidley, C. A., Rohrscheib, M. R., Bedrick, E. J., Meyer, K. B., Johnson, H. K., & Zager, P. G. (2006). Mortality risk among hemodialysis patients receiving different vitamin D analogs. *Kidney Int* 70(10): pp. 1858-1865

Tominaga, Y., Tanaka, Y., Sato, K., Nagasaka, T., & Takagi, H. (1997). Histopathology, pathophysiology, and indications for surgical treatment of renal hyperparathyroidism. *Semin Surg Oncol* 13(2): pp. 78-86

Tonelli, M., Pannu, N., & Manns, B. (2010). Oral phosphate binders in patients with kidney failure. *N Engl J Med* 362(14): pp. 1312-1324

Tonelli, M., Wang, W., Hemmelgarn, B., Lloyd, A., & Manns, B. (2009). Phosphate removal with several thrice-weekly dialysis methods in overweight hemodialysis patients. *Am J Kidney Dis* 54(6): pp. 1108-1115

Triponez, F., Clark, O.H., Vanrenterghem Y., & Evenepoel, P. (2008). Surgical Treatment of Persistent Hyperparathyroidism After Renal Transplantation. *Ann Surg* 248: pp. 18-30

Uhlig, K., Berns, J. S., Kestenbaum, B., Kumar, R., Leonard, M. B., Martin, K. J., Sprague, S. M., & Goldfarb, S. (2010). KDOQI US commentary on the 2009 KDIGO Clinical Practice Guideline for the Diagnosis, Evaluation, and Treatment of CKD-Mineral and Bone Disorder (CKD-MBD). *Am J Kidney Dis* 55(5): pp. 773-799

Urena, P., Jacobson, S. H., Zitt, E., Vervloet, M., Malberti, F., Ashman, N., Leavey, S., Rix, M., Os, I., Saha, H., Ryba, M., Bencova, V., Banos, A., Zani, V., & Fouque, D. (2009). Cinacalcet and achievement of the NKF/K-DOQI recommended target values for bone and mineral metabolism in real-world clinical practice--the ECHO observational study. *Nephrol Dial Transplant* 24(9): pp. 2852-2859

Walsh, M., B. J. Manns, et al. (2010). "The effects of nocturnal compared with conventional hemodialysis on mineral metabolism: A randomized-controlled trial." *Hemodial Int* 14(2): 174-81.

Wolf, M., Manns, B. J., Klarenbach, S., Tonelli, M., Hemmelgarn, B., & Culleton, B. (2007). Vitamin D levels and early mortality among incident hemodialysis patients. *Kidney Int* 72(8): pp. 1004-1013

Young, E. W., Young, E. W., Akiba, T., Albert, J. M., McCarthy, J. T., Kerr, P. G., Mendelssohn, D. C., & Jadoul, M. (2004). Magnitude and impact of abnormal mineral metabolism in hemodialysis patients in the Dialysis Outcomes and Practice Patterns Study (DOPPS). *Am J Kidney Dis* 44(5 Suppl 2): pp. 34-38

Zitt, E., Haid, A., Köberle-Wührer, R., Sprenger-Mähr, H., Hörandner, H., Zimmermann, G., & Neyer, U. (2007). Long-term observation after parathyroidectomy with autotransplantation of selected parathyroid tissue in chronic dialysis patients. *Nieren-Hochdruckkrkh* 36(3): pp. 87-95

Zitt, E., Rix, M., Urena Torres, P., Fouque, D., Jacobson, S. H., Petavy, F., Dehmel, B., & Ryba, M. (2010). Effectiveness of cinacalcet in patients with recurrent/persistent secondary hyperparathyroidism following parathyroidectomy: results of the ECHO study. *Nephrol Dial Transplant* Oct 28. [Epub ahead of print]

4

Sleep in Patients with ESRD Undergoing Hemodialysis

Mukadder Mollaoğlu
Cumhuriyet University
Turkey

1. Introduction

Sleep has been identified as an essential human need; this is partly because of the metabolic activities that occur while the individual is sleeping. Normal sleep is divided into non–rapid eye movement (NREM) and rapid eye movement (REM) sleep. NREM sleep comprises 75% to 80% of total sleep time (TST), and is characterized by relatively quiescent brain activity and decreased metabolic rate (Carskadon & Dement, 2000). NREM sleep consists of four stages (S1-S4), with each stage leading to a progressively deeper sleep. REM sleep follows slow wave sleep (SWS), or deep sleep, and increases over the night, comprising 20% to 25% of TST. REM sleep is characterized by an activated EEG pattern, muscle atonia, and episodic bursts of rapid eye movements. Normal sleep provides a period of physiologic and mental rest. During sleep, sympathetic tone decreases and parasympathetic tone increases, leading to a reduction in heart rate, arterial blood pressure, and cardiac output (Rosenthal, 1998). Deep sleep is theorized to be necessary for physiologic restoration. REM sleep is associated with dreaming, and is essential for maintaining emotional and cognitive well-being (Redline et al., 2004).

Waking and consciousness depend on the activity, of neurons in the ascending reticular activating system of the brainstem. These neurons project into the thalamus, hypothalamus and basal forebrain and eventually send projections to the cortex. There are particular neurotransmitters, such as the catecholamines, acetylcholine, histamine, glutamate and aspartate, that are localized within the reticular formation and have important roles in cortical activation and arousal (Jones, 1989). Sleep-promoting neurotransmitters include gamma aminobutyric acid (GABA), adenosine, and melatonin. Specific stages of sleep are regulated by the turning "on" and "off" of various neurons. REM "on" cells use GABA, acetylcholine, and glutamine, whereas REM "off" cells use norepinephrine and serotonin." REM On cells" are cholinergic cells in the lateral pontine and medial medullary reticular areas that innervate the thalamus, hippocampus and hypothalamus. These cells discharge at high rates during REM and show little or no activity during NREM."REM Off cells" are noradrenergic and serotonergic cells found in the locus coeruleus and raphe. These are cells which are slow or silent during REM sleep. Affecting levels of norepinephirne or serotonin can have an effect on REM sleep (Hoyt, 2005).

Sleep regulation is a balance between a homeostatic sleep need and an intrinsic body clock, or circadian pacemaker. Located in the suprachiasmic nucleus, the circadian pacemaker determines the onset and termination of sleep, and is partially regulated by environmental cues such as light and ambient temperature (Rosenthal, 1998). Melatonin, a physiologic sleep promoter, is inhibited by ambient light, and its circulation is decreased during daylight hours. The adrenal secretion of cortisol, which is associated with wakefulness, follows a circadian pattern. Regulated by the hypothalamic-pituitary axis, cortisol levels peak in the early morning hours in preparation for the increased metabolic demands during wakefulness (Mahowald, & Schenk, 1989).

Some medical illnesses, such as congestive heart failure (CHF), diabetes mellitus, chronic obstructive pulmonary disease and renal disease, can directly impair sleep physiology, leading to a cyclical interaction (Ballard, 2005). End-stage renal disease (ESRD) is one of these diseases. Approximately 50% of patients with chronic end-stage renal disease undergoing hemodialysis (HD) have insomnia and other sleep disorders (Hanly, 2007). Patients often complain of restless leg syndrome (RLS), periodic limb movement disorder (PLMD), bone pain, nausea, and pruritus (Merlino et al., 2006). The etiology of sleep disorders appears to be related to metabolic derangements associated with ESRD or from coexisting diabetes mellitus (Ballard, 2005).

2. Sleep problems in hemodialysis patients

Sleep complaints and sleep disorders are common in patients with end-stage renal disease. Although variable, their prevalence has been reported to be higher when compared to the general population (Merlino et al., 2006). The experiences of sleep alteration in ESRD patients have been studied. Interestingly, 80% of hemodialysis patients suffer from sleep abnormalities and the prevalence is higher than that in the general population (Gul et al., 2006). Holley et al. (1992) surveyed 70 dialysis patients, and reported sleep disturbance experienced mainly included trouble falling asleep (67%), nighttime waking (80%), early morning waking (72%), restless legs (83%), and jerking legs (28%). However, Walker et al. (1995) found daytime sleepiness was the most commonly reported problem (66.7%) followed by restless legs syndrome (57.4%). Generally, the most prominent sleep disorders among hemodialysis patients are sleep apnea syndrome, restless leg syndrome, periodic limb movement disorders, and insomnia (De Santo et al., 2005; Holley et al., 1992; Sabry et al., 2010).

2.1 Sleep apnea syndrome

The prevalence of sleep apnea syndrome in hemodialysis patients is at least 10 times higher (Kraus & Hamburger, 1997) than those values reported in the general population (Young et al., 1993). In another recent investigation, an apnea/hypopnea index higher than 5 was found in 31% of the (young) non-diabetic HD patients studied (Rodriquez et al, 2005).

Sleep apnea syndrome (SAS) is a major clinical disturbance defined as an intermittent interruption of air flow at the level of nose and mouth during sleep. These abnormalities cause frequent decreases in O_2 saturation and awakenings. Episodes of apnea are considered clinically significant if they persist for more than 10 s; however, apnea episodes may last up to 2 min. SAS is the clinical consequence of frequent (at least 10 events per hour) episodes of apnea during sleep (Tatomir et al., 2007). There are three major types of sleep apnea: obstructive sleep apnea (OSA), the central type (CSA), and the mixed type, which includes features of both obstructive and central apnea. OSA is characterized by obstruction of the air flow determined by the occlusion of the oropharyngeal tract (Zoccali et al., 2001).

OSA occurs when the patient no longer has airflow but there is respiratory effort. CSA is determined by the transient abolition of nerve conduction to the respiratory muscles. Central apnea is defined when the patient has both cessation of airflow and the lack of respiratory effort followed by spontaneous resumption of breathing. Mixed apnea is the combination of central and obstructive apneas. All of these conditions can cause arterial oxygen desaturation and they may even be present in the same person (Tatomir et al., 2007; Zoccali et al., 2001). Researchers have speculated that the chronic metabolic acidosis suffered by patients with hemodialysis causes these sleep disorders; as the body attempts to correct the acidosis, the patient exhales more carbon dioxide and the hypocapnia that results may be inadequate to fuel respiration (Kimmel, 1989). Another theory is that these patients frequently have peripheral neuropathy, either from the ESRD or diabetes mellitus, and if the neuropathy affects the nerves innervating the upper airway, then SAS will occur (Fletcher, 1993). There is also evidence that SAS is associated with increased morbidity, and mortality, as the patient with ESRD who suffers with SAS is looking at a future with probable pulmonary hypertension and right heart failure, as well as a shortened lifespan (Fletcher, 1993; Parker, 1997). While, there are no ready answers for the causes of these sleep disorders seen in patients with ESRD undergoing HD, it is crucial that the health care provider be aware of the syndrome.

The awareness of SAS as a potent cardiovascular risk factor in ESRD undergoing HD has generated new enthusiasm in examining novel therapeutic strategies to modify sleep apnea in the patient population. To date, conservative non-pharmacological treatments (e.g. weight loss and avoidance of potentiating medications) have yielded limited success. Nasal continuous positive airway pressure therapy remains a mainstay of treatment of SAS in the non-ESRD population. Continuous positive airway pressure involves a mask fitting over the nose or mouth in which positive pressure is administered to the airway keeping the upper airway patent during sleep. In the general population, the treatment of sleep apnea with continuous positive airway pressure improves quality of life (D'Ambrosio et al.,1999), vigilance, cognition, sexual performance, and normalizes nocturnal blood pressure profile (Faccenda et al., 2001). In the HD population, continuous positive airway pressure was used in a small study of eight patients with some improvement in nocturnal oxygenation, and five of six patients reporting improved daytime alertness (Pressman, 1993). Finally, given the contribution of uremia in the pathogenesis of SAS in ESRD, attempts in optimizing uremia control in the forms of nocturnal hemodialysis (NHD) and renal transplantation have shown early clinical success (Auckley et al, 1999;Hanly & Pierratos, 2001). It is tempting to speculate that similar to those with refractory hypertension, the treatment of sleep apnea in the HD population would improve their quality of life, augment rehabilitation, and perhaps impact on the poor survival of patients.

2.2 Restless Legs Syndrome

Restless Legs Syndrome (RLS) is a neurological movement disorder that is common, under-diagnosed, under-treated, and has a poorly understood etiology (Patrick,2007). Restless legs syndrome (RLS) is a sensorimotor movement disorder characterized by the irresistible need to move associated with feelings of discomfort and parasthesias (International Restless Legs Syndrome Study Group, 2003). The incidence of idiopathic RLS (iRLS) varies between 5–15% in the general population (Nicholas et al., 2003). In the HD population, the prevalence of secondary RLS may be greater, reported to be between 6–62% (Takaki et al., 2003;Unruh et al.,2004) with some geographic variability (Kavanagh et al., 2004). With employment of standardized criteria by IRLSSG, this decreased to 12–48% (Siddiqui et al.,2005; Takaki et al, 2003;Unruh et al., 2004). RLS is observed more commonly in women than men, more commonly with increasing age and with co-morbid diabetes. Other potential correlates of RLS include lower socio-economic status, worse somatic and mental health and diabetes (Berger et al., 2004; Siddiqui et al.,2005). A high correlation between RLS and PLMS has also been noted (Allen et al. 2003, Liao et al.,2008).

The pathophysiology of RLS in uremia remains unknown however, several theories have been proposed. Potential risk factors include anemia, iron deficiency, dialysis vintage, calcium/phosphate imbalance, and peripheral and central nervous system abnormalities(Berger et al., 2004;Unruh et al.,2004).

Evidence for a possible relationship of iron deficiency to RLS in this patient population has been explained by the universal occurrence of anemia, which is commonly acquired in patients with end-stage renal disease due to inadequate production of erythropoietin (Gigli et al.,2004). Anemia in ESRD is associated with several co-morbid conditions, including congestive heart failure, stroke, cognitive dysfunction, left ventricular hypertrophy,and worsening iron deficiency due to loss from hemodialysis (Allen,2004; Gigli et al.,2004) Ferritin levels under 100 ng/mL reflect depletion of iron stores and complicate the treatment of anemia in patients on dialysis (Easom, 2006; Patrick ,2007)

Multiple causes of secondary RLS including iron deficiency anemia, diabetes mellitus, Parkinsons disease, pregnancy, rheumatic disease, venous insufficiency and less commonly in association with peripheral neuropathies, vitamin deficiencies, lumbosacral radiculopathy, spinal stenosis, excess caffeine intake, administration of some tricyclic antidepressants, hypoglycemia and hypothyroidism (Nichols et al.,2003; Siddiqui et al.,2005;Unruh et al.,2004).

The revised IRLSSG criteria (Allen et al. 2003) for RLS included four essential diagnostic criteria additional supportive features. The criteria include unpleasant and uncomfortable sensations associated with an urge to move the limbs with symptoms worsened by rest, relieved by activity and typically worse toward the evening. Positive family history, initial therapeutic response to L-dopa or a dopamine-receptor agonist are supportive evidence. At least 85% of patients with RLS may also have concomitant periodic limb movements (PLMS) though this may be the result of other disorders such as obstructive sleep apnea.

Treatment of ESRD-associated anemia with erythropoietin has been shown to decrease arousal due to PLMS and produce trends toward higher sleep quality (Benz et al 2000). As will be reviewed later, intravenous (I.V.) iron in ESRD patients has been shown to be highly effective in causing remission of RLS symptoms (Sloand et al., 2004).

Given that alterations of the dopaminergic pathways may contribute to the development of RLS in ESRD, pharmacological treatment of RLS with Levodopa (L-DOPA) has been studied and was shown to improve sleep and reduce nocturnal limb movements in three prospective trials (Sandyk et al.1987; Trenkwalder et al., 1995; Walker, 1996). Recently, treatment with pergolide, a dopamine agonist was also examined in a double-blind placebo-controlled crossover study in ESRD patients (Pieta et al., 1998). In contrast to the use of L-DOPA, pergolide resulted in decreased symptoms without objective improvements in nocturnal limb movement or sleep architecture. Limited beneficial data regarding the use of other dopamine agonists have also been reported (Miranda et AL., 2004; Pellecchia et al., 2004). Folate is also involved in the production of dopamine in the CNS. Folate, as 5-methyltetrahydrofolate, increases production of CNS tetrahydrobiopterin, a cofactor in tyrosine hydroxylase production significant reduction in RLS symptoms and decreased leg movements during sleep ($p=0.018$). With the exception of this one trial, there is only limited information from case reports of significant symptom reduction in pediatric RLS using dopaminergic agents (Konofal et al.,2005)

2.3 Periodic Limb Movement Disorder

Periodic limb movement disorder (PLMD) is a condition characterized by periodic episodes of repetitive and highly stereotyped limb movements that occur either during sleep (PLMS) or in wakefulness (PLMW) (Walker et al., 1995). This syndrome is more often seen in the patient with ESRD than in the general population (Pressman et al., 1995). The presence of PLMS is responsible for sleep problems in up to 72% of patients with ESRD (Benz et al., 2000) and the presence of PLMS is a more accurate predictor of mortality than coexisting diseases, serum albumin, or urea reduction ratio (Winkelman et al., 1996). A high correlation between RLS and PLMS has also been noted (Allen et al. 2003).

Treatments with high-dose iron dextran and normalization of hematocrit with recombinant human erythropoietin have been demonstrated to improve RLPLMD in ESRD patients (Benz et al, 1999; Sloand et al., 2004). Alterations in dopamine and opioid synthesis may also play a role in the high prevalence of RLS and PLMD in uremia; however, data are limited. Indirect evidence stems from the notion that treatment with dopamine agonists, dopamine precursors in ESRD patients may improve RLS and PLMD symptoms (Sandyk et al.1987; Trenkwalder et al., 1995; Walker, 1996).

2.4 Insomnia

Insomnia is defined as a disorder of difficulty initiating sleep (DIS), difficulty maintaining sleep (DMS), and/or early morning awakening (EMA). Insomnia is commonly defined as the subjective sensation of short, unsatisfying sleep, despite the ability to sleep (Sabbatini et al., 2002). It may be secondary either to trouble falling asleep and/or to night-time waking, which must be persistently present (i.e. three to four times a week for several weeks) (Leger et al.,2002). The prevalence estimates of insomnia vary because of differences in definition, diagnosis, population characteristics, and research methodologies. Insomnia is a common sleep problem, however, and its prevalence in the general population ranges from 4% to 64% (Terzano et al., 2004; Chesson et al., 2000). The prevalence of insomnia is substantially greater in dialysis patients and has been reported to range from 45% to 59% (İliescu et al., 2003; İliescu et al., 2004; Sabbatini et al., 2002).

Insomnia is characterized by one or more of the following symptoms: difficulty falling asleep ("sleep onset insomnia"), difficulty staying asleep ("sleep maintenance insomnia"), early awakening or poor sleep quality ("non-restorative sleep") (Ohayon et al., 2002; Meyer, 1998). Insomnia is primarily a clinical diagnosis and it is most frequently diagnosed from data obtained from the history and from sleep diaries. PSG is not indicated in the initial evaluation of insomnia but may be necessary in chronic treatment-resistant cases and in patients in whom specific sleep disorders (SASRLSPLMS) are suspected (Bonner et al., 2008).

Insomnia may be caused by a variety of reasons, with the most frequent causes listed by researchers as: restless legs syndrome (RLS), periodic leg movements during sleep (PLMS), sleep apnea syndrome (SAS) and depression (Kimmel, 1989; Parker, 1997; Welch & Austin, 2001). The prevalence of insomnia due to RLS in dialysis patients ranges from 57% to 83% (Holley et al., 1992; Sabbatini et al., 2002; Walker et al., 1995). Elderly patients, those with longer dialysis durations, dialysis shift, and those with high levels of parathyroid hormone (PTH) or diabetes mellitus are at higher risk of insomnia; however, the dialysis type and biochemical parameters are not important determinants of insomnia (Han et al., 2002; Sabbatini et al., 2002).

Most studies assessing the effectiveness of different treatment modalities in insomniacs address short-term treatment of insomnia (Montgomery &Dennis., 2004; Morgan et al., 2003; Smith et al., 2002). Extra care and caution has to be exercised when treating insomnia in patients with renal impairment. Most hypnotics should be administered in appropriately reduced doses and interactions with the numerous medications used in the different HD populations should be considered carefully when prescribing a hypnotic to patients with renal failure (Novak et al., 2006). Surprisingly there is an almost complete lack of pharmacologic studies in renal patients suffering from insomnia. In a small randomized study using the PSQI Sabbatini et al. (2003). suggested that zaleplon improved sleep efficacy in maintenance hemodialysis patients.

Nonpharmacologic interventions include sleep hygiene measures relaxation therapy and biofeedback stimulus control therapy sleep restriction and cognitive behavioral therapy (Montgomery &Dennis., 2004; Morgan et al., 2003). These interventions have been shown to be beneficial in the long-term management of patients with chronic hypnotic use. Cognitive behavioral therapy for insomnia in the routine general practice setting improved sleep quality reduced hypnotic drug use and improved health-related quality of life at a favorable cost in chronic insomniacs.

3. Related factors with sleep problems in hemodialysis patients

A multitude of causes including anemia, blood urea levels, plasma creatinine levels, parathyroid hormone (PTH) concentrations, increased blood pressure, quality of life, and illness intrusiveness may contribute to sleep disturbances in patients on maintenance hemodialysis (Hanly et al., 2003; Iliescu et al., 2004; Sabbatini et al.,2003). Furthermore, there is a positive correlation between sleep disturbances and increased morbidity and mortality related to cardiovascular disease and infectious complications, the 2 major causes of death in hemodialysis patients (De Santo et al., 2005). Sleep disorders in hemodialysis patients is a multifactorial complaint, stemming from Uremic toxins and dialysis procedure, other medical problems, psychiatric or psychosocial background.

3.1 Uremic toxins

Several studies in the past 30 years have shown that uremic patients are at great risk for disordered sleep. A study by Millman et al. (1985) noticed a slight but significant relationship between sleep apnea syndrome and azotemia. In a recent prospective study of incident HD patients followed-up for 1 year, higher dialysis efficiency was associated with fewer sleep disturbances (Unruh et al., 2006). These latter data are further supported by the results of Hanly et al. (2001), who studied patients on conventional hemodialysis (4 h three times a week) who then switched to nocturnal (intensive) dialysis (8 h for 6 or 7 days/week). A spectacular correction of sleep apnea was recorded in this small-scale study (Hanly et al., 2001). Finally, the impact of uremic toxins is highlighted by the fact that sleep disorders are more frequent and more severe in dialyzed patients compared with subjects with pre-dialysis CKD (Merlino et al., 2006).

3.2 Interdialytic weight gain and hypertension

Excessive interdialytic weight gain has been associated with poor compliance and high blood pressure (Rahman et al., 2000). While the mechanism of the association between

interdialytic weight gain and sleep problems is unclear, we speculate that large interdialytic weight gains result in expanded intravascular volume, which has been associated with upper airway obstruction (Chiu et al., 2006).
The length of sleep during the night before a hemodialysis session after a long interdialytic interval (3 days, the "weekend interval") is significantly shorter compared to the usual sleep length following a short interdialytic interval. This led to some speculation regarding the possible effect of interdialytic weight gain (IWG) on sleep (Bertini et al., 1999). Furthermore, patients with uncontrolled pre-dialysis systolic pressure (usually a sign of hypervolemia in these patients) experience clinically overt insomnia more frequently (De Santo et al., 2001); in patients with chronic diseases, systolic hypertension appears to be a cause of sleep disturbances (Katz & McHorney 1998; Sabbatini et al., 2002; Thase, 2005).

3.3 Dialysis shift

The dialysis shift has several effects on patients with ESRD. Morning-shift HD patients experience more insomnia (Sabbatini et al., 2002), but also have longer survival times (Bliwise., 2001) than patients on other dialysis shifts. In according to another study (Merlino et al., 2006), for patients undergoing HD in the morning shift, the risk of subclinical insomnia is up to 18 times higher than for those who have their dialysis session in the afternoon. However, morning-shift HD patients have higher intradialytic sleepiness, which is associated with more decreased body temperature during HD, than patients on other dialysis shifts (Parker et al., 2003).

3.4 Dialysis vintage

The longer the dialysis vintage, the more significant is the prevalence of sleep quality disorders (Veiga et al., 1997). In a study by De Santo et al., (2005), patients with subclinical or clinical sleep disorders had double the dialysis vintage of those without sleep complaints; in patients with a medium dialytic age of 75 months, the prevalence of sleep disorders is close to 80%. These data are not surprising, taking into account the accumulation of comorbidites, including peripheral neuropathy and CVD, whilst on dialysis on long-term. In a polysomnographic study by Tatomir et al.,(2007) in patients hemodialyzed for more than 10 years, all patients has disturbed sleep with frequent awakening and reduced sleep efficiency. One-half of these patients had sleep-related breathing disorders, i.e. sleep apnea syndrome.

3.5 Restless legs syndrome

Restless legs syndrome (RLS) usually becomes apparent during resting and may significantly interfere with sleep. An association between RLS and insomnia in patients on maintenance hemodialysis has been suggested already by a few papers (Musci et al., 2005; Sabbatini et al., 2002; Walker et al., 1995). Moreover, RLS is associated with a low quality of sleep and lower quality of life.

3.6 Other medical factors

Other medical factors include the pain and discomfort caused by illnesses such as arthritis, cardiovascular disease, chronic obstructive pulmonary disease (COPD), cerebrovascular disease, neurological disorders, asthma, headaches, and more. The prognosis of patients with chronic uremia is influenced by the presence of comorbidities, mainly by cardiovascular disease (CVD), which causes roughly 50% of deaths (Covic et al., 2006). A study by Mucsi et al. (2004), demonstrated that comorbidities are independent predictors of sleep disturbances in patients on maintenance dialysis. According to another study, the average Charlson Comorbidity Index (CCI) in patients without sleep disorders was 4.10, while scores in patients with subclinical and clinically overt sleep disorders were 6.10 and 6.81, respectively (De Santo et al.,2005). This highly significant association in the Italian HD population was maintained regardless of age. To conclude so far, any in-depth research on the quality of sleep in renal patients must consider the magnitude of comorbidities.

3.7 Age

Sleep difficulties are closely correlated with older age in patients with chronic uremia (Iliescu et al., 2003). Yoshioka et al.(1993) found that advanced age and long-term dialysis therapy directly affected patients experiencing sleep problems. The disorders are similar to those described in the general population, where the prevalence and severity of sleep disorders are also associated with old age. Each decade of age increases the risk of insomnia by 239%, and the risk of overt clinical insomnia by 51% (De Santo et al., 2005). Mollaoğlu (2004) reported a negative correlation between age and sleep quality, with sleep quality decreasing with advanced age in their study of 105 HD patients. In addition, community-based studies have shown that sleep quality could be deteriorated in elderly patients due to increased frequency of physical diseases, multiple drug use, primary sleep disturbances, or lifestyle modifications (Brandenberger et al., 2003; Kamel & Gammack 2006).

3.8 Depression

The psychiatric condition most commonly causing sleep disorders is depression that may affect up to 50% of this patient population (Covic et al., 2006). The relationship between depression and sleep disorders is well known both in the general population and in patients undergoing hemodialysis (İliescu et al.,2003). Depression can be a cause, as well as a result, of insomnia. Dialysis patients with a Pittsburg Quality Index Sleep score of >5 (patients with a "difficult sleep") have a prevalence of overt depression of 20%, while among ESRD patients reporting a normal sleep, the prevalence of depression is almost nil (İliescu et al.,2003).

3.9 Medications and other substances

Medications and other substances which may cause insomnia include beta-blockers, bronchodilators, corticosteroids, CNS stimulants, Tagamet, cardiovascular drugs, neurological drugs, alcohol, caffeine and nicotine (Merlino et al., 2006; Rosenthal, 1998; Unruh et al., 2006). Most prescribed as well as over-the-counter medications produce side effects which are either sedating or stimulating. Drugs which cause daytime sleepiness include analgesics, benzodiazepines and antihistamines (Rosenthal, 1998; Unruh et al., 2006). According to recent investigations, the use of hypnotic medication in dialysis patients is rather modest: 8-10% (De Santo et al., 2005; De Santo et al., 2001). In a large study, the reported use of sleep-inducing medication was even lower—3.6% (Merlino et al., 2006). However, dialysis patients with severe sleep disorders use specific medication more frequently (24%) (De Santo et al., 2005). Improved hemodialysis techniques, socio-economical disparities in the studied populations, and reluctance by nephrologists to prescribe psychotropic medication may explain these disparities. However, we must be aware that chronic auto-administration of hypnotic medication may be more frequent in

ESRD patients compared to the general population. Moreover, according to recent data from the CHOICE incident dialysis population, use of benziodiazepines is associated with altered sleep quality during the first year of dialysis. Although this study was unable to distinguish between cause and effect, more effective dialysis and cognitive behavioral therapy have been suggested in patients with sleep disorders in need of sleep-inducing medication (Unruh et al., 2006). Moreover, many antidepressants actually cause paradoxical restlessness, therefore systematic administration of these drugs should be subjected to close clinical follow-up, which should be easy to accomplish in hemodialysis patients.

Alcohol is widely used as a sleep aid. Although it does shorten sleep latency, it also causes sleep fragmentation, decreased REM, REM rebound and early morning awakenings. The use of alcohol combined with hypnotics may exacerbate sleep difficulties even more (Rosenthal, 1998). Alcohol and (particularly) tobacco abuse is highly associated with increased prevalence of sleep disorders in ESRD (Merlino et al., 2006). Caffeine and other stimulants such as nicotine have been shown to increase sleep latency and sleep fragmentation, and to decrease total sleep time (Rosenthal, 1998). Current smoking is also related with decreases in sleep quality during the first year of dialysis therapy in incident patients (Unruh et al., 2006). Caffeine intake appears to have no significant impact on insomnia in ESRD (Sabbatini et al., 2002).

4. Sleep quality and evaluation of sleep in hemodialysis patients

Sleep quality is an important clinical construct for two major reasons. First, complaints about sleep quality are common; epidemiological surveys indicate that 15-35 % of the adult population complain of frequent sleep quality disturbance, such as difficulty falling asleep or difficulty maintaining sleep. Second, poor sleep quality can be an important symptom of many sleep and medical disorders (Buysse et al., 1989).

Sleep quality" is sometimes used to refer to a collection of sleep measures including total sleep time (TST), sleep onset latency (SOL), degree of fragmentation, total wake time, sleep efficiency, and sometimes sleep disruptive events such as spontaneous arousals or apnea. The widely employed Pittsburgh Sleep Quality Index (PSQI), for example, provides a measure of global sleep quality based on a respondent's retrospective appraisal (past month) of an array of sleep measures, including sleep latency, sleep duration, habitual sleep efficiency, sleep disturbances, use of sleeping medication, and daytime dysfunction (Krystal & Edinger, 2008). Sleep quality is also sometimes inferred from a collection of objective indices taken from polysomnography (PSG). PSG is the most valid and accurate way to assess sleep. Measures derived from PSG include: (a) total sleep time, (b) sleep efficiency (ratio of time spent asleep/time in bed), (c) sleep latency (time to fall asleep after lights out), (d) amount of wake time during sleep periods (waking after sleep onset, WASO), (e) number of awakenings, and (f) amount of each sleep stage (Landis al., 2002).

Among these objective indices are measures such as sleep onset latency, total sleep time, wake time after sleep onset, sleep efficiency, and number of awakenings that correspond to like measures taken from various available self-report instruments (e.g., sleep diaries, PSQI, etc.) (Buysse et al., 2006). However, PSG also provides a number of measures that reflect the architecture of sleep such as the percentage or temporal amounts of stage 1 sleep, stage 2 sleep, slow wave sleep or rapid eye movement (REM) sleep. Despite having no self-report analogues, these latter measures also have been employed by some as indices of sleep quality (Krystal & Edinger, 2008).

Most of the recent studies on quality of sleep use different questionnaires assessing various aspects of sleep. The Pittsburgh Sleep Quality Index, the Epworth Sleepiness Scale, and the Berlin Questionnaire are most frequently applied. Results derived from these questionnaires are limited by the subjective perception/sincerity of the patients, and thus are an imperfect substitute for more objective research methods on sleep in patients with chronic uremia (Chen et al, 2006; Iliescu et al., 2003; Mollaoglu & Mollaoglu, 2009; Sabbatini et al., 2003).

Researchers have documented that ESRD patients reported significantly poorer subjective quality of sleep in comparison to the general population (Holley et al., 1992; Parker, 2005). The reported prevalence of 'poor sleep', including sleep-wake complaints, sleep-disordered breathing and excessive sleepiness, in dialysis patients is in the range of 45–80% (Afshar et al., 2011; Parker, 1996; Walker et al., 1995; Wei et al., 2011). In a another study It was examined the quality of sleep in 89 subjects with ESRD on haemodialysis using the PSQI and found a prevalence of 'poor sleep' (global PSQI>5) of 71% (Iliescu et al., 2003). Also, decreased quality of sleep is common in dialysis patients and is associated with decreased health-related quality of life (Iliescu et al., 2003; Williams et al., 2002).

The complex evaluation of sleep in patients with renal disease may be accomplished only by means of polysomnography. Polysomnography includes the comprehensive evaluation of the patient during sleep by electroencephalography, electrooculography, myography, quantification of respiratory efforts (by plethysmography), pulseoxymetry and noninvasive evaluation of CO2 blood level, and heart rate measuring (Tatomir et al., 2007). Parker et al. (2003) examined by polysomnography 16 patients with HD and 8 patients with pre-dialysis CKD. Dialysis patients, in comparison with non-dialyzed CKD subjects, have a shorter sleep time. The REM phase is also shortened, time until falling asleep is longer, and respiratory events are more frequent. The sleep latency period was double in renal patients without dialysis compared to those with dialysis. Moreover, the prevalence and severity of periodical limb movement is higher in dialysis patients, as well as the number of short-term awakening periods (Parker et al., 2003). The authors suggest that sleep disturbances may have a different etiology in dialyzed patients compared to pre-dialysis CKD subjects. Functional and psychological factors may play a more prominent role in the pre-dialysis group, whereas intrinsic sleep disruption (arousals, apneas and limb movements) secondary to intermittent daytime HD sessions may play a more prominent role in patients with chronic uremia. Taken as a whole, renal patients experience a significant reduction in sleep length and efficiency compared to the general population (Parker et al., 2005).

The studies have shown poor the quality of sleep in HD patients to be associated with female sex, older age, caffeine intake, recombinant erythropoietin therapy, pain, cardiovascular disease, physical functioning, larger body mass index (BMI), exercise, dialysis adequacy, parathyroid hormone, serum creatinine and quality of life (QOL) (Benz et al., 1999; Sabatini et al., 2002; Walker et al., 1995). Hanly et al. (2003) examined daytime sleepiness with multiple sleep latency tests in 24 haemodialysis patients and found strong correlation between sleep latency and BUN. In addition, psychological problems do represent crucial factors in influencing the quality of sleep in hemodialysis patients, as emphasized by all the previous studies in prevalent patients with renal disease, with depression playing a prominent role, followed by anxiety, sexual problems, financial strains, and isolation (İliescu et al., 2003; İliescu et al., 2004; Markou et al.,2006; Novak et al.,2006).

Considering the strict linkage between some of these factors affecting sleep and hemodialysis, it is tempting to speculate that treating sleep problems, while improving the overall quality of life, might positively affect hemodialysis. In addition, with this point of

view, psychological, behavioural and pharmacologic interventions that promote sleep will represent a more than promising area for future research in hemodialysis patients.
The above studies results show that the sleep characteristics of hemodialysis patients need to be routinely evaluated. In addition to medical treatment to eliminate the sleep problems of hemodialysis patients and increase their sleep quality, the implementation of sleep hygiene interventions that can play a part in the regularity of patients' sleep could also be beneficial. These interventions would include an environment with a comfortable room temperature and ventilation, minimal noise, a comfortable bed, and proper lighting. These interventions should apply to each patient's personal routines (Mollaoglu & Mollaoglu, 2009).

5. Management of sleep problems in hemodialysis patients

Proper management of sleep problems in ESRD patients requires in the first instance a proper identification of sleep abnormalities (extensively discussed above). Although significant research has been done to characterize sleep abnormalities in hemodialysis patients (Holey et al., 1992; De Santo et al., 2005; Merlino et al., 2006), little has been published regarding proper treatment. In the absence of guidelines, nephrologists rely largely on some published data and on opinion-based medicine. Sleep problems lower quality of life and contribute to physical and mental health problems. Sleep disorders and lack of sleep are an under treated threat to the public health. Sleep professionals have recognized the behavioral components of sleep disorders for decades, yet most patients never get a proper diagnosis and treatment (Mollaoglu & Mollaoğlu, 2009).
Periodic clinical assessment of sleep complaints should become routine for dialysis staff. Early identification of sleep problems and interventions to improve sleep quality is essential, because sleep disturbance that persists for a long period of time could decrease general health and functioning (Sabbatini et al., 2003; Tatomir et al., 2007). Increasing evidence supports the effectiveness of both pharmacologic and nonpharmacologic therapies for sleep problems (Edinger et al., 2001; Montgomery & Dennis, 2004; Smith et al., 2002). Pharmacologic therapy are discussed in the sleep disorders section.
The most effective nonpharmacologic interventions tested to date include all or most of the following components: *sleep hygiene instruction, sleep restriction, stimulus control, relaxation training, and cognitive modification* (Edinger et al., 2001; Montgomery & Dennis, 2004).

5.1 Sleep hygiene

Sleep hygiene involves basic education on how the sleep environment, caffeine, alcohol, nicotine, food and exercise affect sleep (Smith et al., 2002). Sleep Hygiene is an educational approach designed to teach insomnia patients as well as the population at large how to maintain healthy behavioral habits which promote better sleep. It is important to understand that successful treatment is only possible if the patient complies with suggestions to improve sleep hygiene (*Edinger et al., 2001*). Below are summarized tips for sleep hygiene

Sleep hygiene tips

- Sleep only when sleepy. If you can't fall asleep within 20 min get up and do something boring until you feel sleepy,
- Don't take nap sunless your doctor advises so.

- Regular sleep-wake schedule is important. Get up and go to bed the same time every day even on weekends.
- Regular exercise improves sleep but most people should refrain from exercise at least 4 hr before bedtime.
- Develop sleep rituals (listening to musicetc.). It is important to give your body cues that it is time to slow down and sleep.
- Only use your bed for sleeping and intimacy. Refrain from using your bed to watch TV or work.
- Stay away from caffeine-containing beverages foods and medications nicotine and alcohol at least 4–6 hr before bedtime.
- Have a light snack before bed with a glass of milk which contains sleep-promoting tryptophan.
- Take a hot bath 90 min before bedtime. A hot bath will raise your body temperature but it is the drop in body temperature that may leave you feeling sleepy.
- Make sure your bed and bedroom are quiet and comfortable. Use appropriate curtains ear plugs or a white noise machine if necessary. A cooler room is recommended. Use a humidifier if the air is too dry.

These suggestions often combine several methods and may sound trivial. Compliance with such advice is still relatively poor however as it frequently requires changes in persistent "bad" habits which are ingrained (Morin et al., 1999). Building a regular sleep schedule and creating an appropriate sleeping environment as well as regular physical activity are very important in combating insomnia or insomnia-like presentations in RLS/PLMD (Montgomery & Dennis, 2004).

In terms of sleep hygiene for RLS/PLMD, there are a two main points that bear highlighting. First, the avoidance of alcohol, caffeine and nicotine may be underscored because of their potential contribution to RLS symptoms and/or PLMs. Second, other sleep hygiene practices may or may not have any utility for patients with RLS. Particularly when sleep hygiene is provided to patients as a handout or pamphlet, there is no indication that this helps promote sleep in any patient group. (Martin, 2000; Pigeon &Yurcheshen, 2009).

5.2 Relaxation and biofeedback techniques

Relaxation and biofeedback techniques for treating insomnia are based on the assumption that insomnia patients are overly aroused and anxious, and this interferes with their ability to initiate and/or maintain sleep (Lacks, 1993). Relaxation techniques are designed simply to teach patients to relax, and thus improve their ability to sleep. Of several relaxation methods, none has been shown to be more efficacious than the others. Progressive muscle relaxation, autogenic training and electromyographic biofeedback seek to reduce somatic arousal (e.g., muscle tension), whereas attention-focusing procedures such as imagery training and meditation are intended to lower presleep cognitive arousal (e.g., intrusive thoughts, racing mind) (Spielman et al., 1987).

In general, biofeedback training is an effective treatment for some insomnia patients, and is as effective as other non-pharmacologic interventions (Morin et al., 1999). If patients can train themselves to relax before sleep or at night after an awakening, they are more capable or falling asleep and staying asleep. It is believed that the beneficial effects of these methods extend beyond the sleep problems in that they facilitate better coping skills in general (Martin, 2000).

Structured exercise programs may also improve symptoms of insomnia (Montgomery & Dennis., 2004). Despite the promise of CBT the relative efficacy of these various nonpharmacologic approaches has not been well established. Data also suggest that CBTin contrast to medications may have a lasting effect beyond the termination of treatment. The extent to which the concomitant use of nonpharmacologic therapy augments the performance of pharmacologic treatments needs to be established in further studies (Novak et al., 2006).

5.3 Stimulus-control therapy

Stimulus-control therapy is a behavioral approach based on the premise that some sleep disturbances are behaviorally conditioned, so that the patient associates the bedroom environment with arousal. The main objective of stimulus control therapy is to reassociate the bed and bedroom with the rapid onset of sleep.
Below are summarized instructions for stimulus-control therapy (Martin, 2000).

Instructions for Stimulus-Control Therapy

- Patient goes to bed only when sleepy.
- If not asleep within about 10 minutes, patient gets out of bed, and does not return to bed until sleepy.
- When patient returns to bed, if not asleep within 15 minutes, gets out of bed.
- Pattern is repeated until patient can fall asleep within a few minutes.
- Must get up at the same time each morning (even if only slept 2 hours).
- Bed is used only for sleeping (not for watching television, reading exciting books, etc).
- All naps during the day must be avoided.

This method focuses primarily on shortening sleep onset, however, in the case of sleep maintenance insomnia, the instructions may be followed when the patient awakens and cannot fall back to sleep during the night. The patient should avoid lying awake in bed as much as possible and only go to bed when sleepy. No stimulating or distracting activities (e.g. reading exciting books or articles, watching television, looking at a clock) should be available. Although the patient cannot control sleep onset, wake up time should be fixed, so that a regular sleep/wake schedule will develop. Pro hibiting daytime naps is important to take advantage of the sleep deficit accumulated since the sleep period on the previous night, which in itself can shorten sleep onset. As with all psychological therapies, compliance is enhanced when the instructions and their rationales are explained to the patient.
Stimulus control therapy has been shown to be effective in shortening sleep latency compared with placebo intervention in insomnia patients (Lacks, Bertelson, Gans & Kunkel, 1996). Clinical trials have documented the efficacy of stimulus control therapy for both sleep onset and sleep-maintenance insomnia (Espie et al., 1989; Lacks et al., 1993)

5.4 Sleep restriction therapy

Sleep restriction therapy, is based on the observation that many insomnia patients spend an excessive amount of time in bed in futile attempts to achieve more sleep (Spielman, Saskin, & Thorpy, 1987).. Sleep restriction therapy consists of curtailing the amount of time spent in bed to increase the percentage of time spent asleep. This improves the patient's sleep efficiency (time asleep/time in bed). For example, a person who reports staying in bed for eight hours but sleeping an average of five hours per night would initially be told to decrease the time spent in bed to five hours. The allowable time in bed per night is increased 15 to 30 minutes as sleep efficiency improves. Adjustments are made over a period of weeks until an optimal sleep duration is achieved. Typically, it is best to alter the bedtime and to keep the rising time constant in order to maintain a regular sleep-wake rhythm. By creating a mild state of sleep deprivation, this therapy promotes more rapid sleep onset and more efficient sleep (Hauri, 2000). To minimize daytime sleepiness, time in bed should not be reduced to less than five hours per night. Sleep restriction therapy is modified in older adults by allowing a short afternoon nap.

Lichstein and Reidel (1994) concluded that sleep restriction therapy is actually the preferred technique for insomnia in older patients. In a later study they combined sleep restriction with sleep education for older insomnia patients, comparing a self-help technique (a guiding video) with therapist guidance (Riedel et al., 1995). While the self-help technique alone showed improvement on some sleep variables, therapist guidance was superior in that it improved sleep latency, wake time after sleep onset and sleep satisfaction.

Implementation of this technique requires a high level of motivation and compliance on the patient's part, and close follow up by the clinician. Below are listed the rules for sleep restriction therapy.

Instructions for Sleep Restriction Therapy

- Patient is only allowed to stay in bed for the amount of time they think they sleep each night, plus 15 minutes. For example, if patient reports sleeping only 5.75 hours, they are allowed to stayin bed for 6 hours.
- Patient must get up at the same time each day. If normal waking time is 6:30, patient is allowed to go to bed at 12:30.
- Napping is not allowed.
- When sleep efficiency has reached 85%, the patient can go to bed 15 minutes earlier.
- This procedure is repeated until the patient can sleep for the desired amount of time.

5.5 Weight loss

Upper-body obesity is a risk factor for OSA, and it is well documented that weight loss has a notable ameliorative impact on the occurrence of OSA (Ancoli-Israel et al., 1996; Smith et al., 1985). Since OSA results from closure of the airway, excess fatty tissue in theneck area may be a contributing factor. This supports the notion that weight plays a significant role in the presence and severity of sleep disordered breathing although no conclusive treatment trials have been published at this time.

5.6 Light therapy

The most influential treatment for circadian rhythm disturbances is increased exposure to bright light. This form of therapy, which directly targets the circadian system, is much preferred over hypnotics and other sedative medications. Since light is the most important synchronizer in our circadian system, increasing bright light exposure during certain times of the day can shift circadian rhythm phase and increase its amplitude. Specifically, bright light exposure in the evening causes a phase delay, while morning bright light exposure causes a phase advance in circadian rhythms, including rhythms of melatonin, core body temperature and sleepiness (Martin et al., 2000).

5.7 Cognitive-behavioral therapies

Many behavioral sleep medicine interventions are based on cognitive-behavioral therapies (CBT). The focus is on systematically introducing behavioral changes that have been proven to improve sleep. This could include changes in sleep schedule and changes in the contingencies and reinforcers that promote sleep. The cognitive approach focuses on looking internally to examine, manage, or modify sleep interfering thoughts and beliefs that can interfere with sleep. Cognitive behavioral therapy for insomnia in the routine general practice setting improved sleep quality reduced hypnotic drug use and improved health-related quality of life at a favorable cost in chronic insomniacs. Randomized controlled trials (RCTs) report somewhat conflicting results on the effectiveness of CBT in patients with insomnia but one systematic review including six RCTs (282 people) found that group or individual cognitive behavioral therapy (including sleep hygiene stimulus control sleep restriction muscle relaxation and sleep education) significantly improved PSQI scores compared with no treatment immediately after treatment and at 3 months (*Montgomery &Dennis, 2004*). Furthermore another meta-analysis involving 2102 patients in 59 trials found that sleep restriction and stimulus control therapies were more effective than relaxation techniques when used alone (*Edinger & Sampson., 2003*).

6. Conclusion

Considering that the most frequent sleep complaints, such as insomnia, OSAS and RLS, are related to a significant negative impact on functional health status in uraemic patients, the nephrologists should improve their recognition and treatment of these conditions to restore the quality of life of their patients. A good sleep history and, when indicated, a sleep recording, will help the clinician to make an accurate diagnosis and thus identify the best treatment. Nonpharmacologic methods such as behavioral techniques and cognitive therapyas well as pharmacologic approaches and combinations of these methods should be used for the treatment of sleep problems in hemodialysis patients.

7. References

Afshar, R., Emany, A. Saremi, A., Shavandi, N., & Sanavi, S. (2011). Effects of intradialytic aerobic training on sleep quality in hemodialysis patients. *Iranian Journal of Kidney Diseases,* Vol. 5, No. 2, Apr, pp. 119-23.

Allen, R. (2004). Dopamine and iron in the pathophysiology of restless legs syndrome (RLS). *Sleep Med,* Vol. 5, pp. 385-391.

Allen, R.P., Picchietti, D., Hening, W.A., Trenkwalder, C., Walters, A.S., & Montplaisi, J. (2003). Restless legs syndrome: Diagnostic criteria, special considerations, and epidemiology. A report from the restless legs syndrome diagnosis and epidemiology workshop at the National Institute of Health. *Sleep Med,* pp. 101–119

Ancoli-Israel, S., Kripke, D. F., Klauber, M. R., Fell, R., Stepnowsky, C., Estline, E., Khazeni, N. & Chinn, A.(1996). Morbidity, mortality and sleep disordered breathing in community dwelling elderly. *Sleep,* Vol. 19, pp. 277–282.

Auckley, D.H., Schmidt-Nowara, W., & Brown, L.K. (1999). Reversal of sleep apnea hypopnea syndrome in end-stage renal disease after kidney transplantation. *Am J Kidney Dis,* Vol. 34, pp. 739–744.

Ballard, R. D. (2005). Sleep and medical disorders. *Prim Care,* Vol. 35, pp. 511–533.

Benz, R.L., Pressman, M.R., Hovick, E.T. , & Peterson, D. D. (1999). A preliminary study of the effects of anemia with recombinant human erythropoietin therapy on sleep,

sleep disorders, and daytime sleepiness in hemodialysis patients (the SLEEPO study). *Am J Kidney Dis,* Vol. 34, pp. 1089–1095

Benz,R.L., Pressman, M.R., Hovik, E.H., & Peterson, D.D. (2000). Potential novel predictors of mortality in end-stage renal disease patients with sleep disorders. *American Journal of Kidney Disease,* Vol. 35, No. 6, pp. 1052-1060.

Berger, K., Luedemann, J., Trenkwalder, C., John, U. & Kessler, C. (2004). Sex and the risk of restless legs syndrome in the general population. *Arch Intern Med,* Vol. 164, pp. 196–202.

Bertini, M., Lucidi F, & De Santo RM (1999). Effeti dell' emodialisi sulla qualita del sonno, In: *Qualita della vita, etica ed economia in Nefrologia,* Bertini M, Di Iorio BR (eds). pp 79–90 Editoriale Bios, Cosenza.

Bliwise, D.L., Kutner, N.G, Zhang, R., & Parker, K.P. (2001). Survival by time of day of hemodialysis in an elderly cohort. *JAMA,* Vol. 286, pp.2690–4

Bonner, A., Wellard, S., & Caltabiano, M. (2008). Levels of fatigue in people with ESRD living in far North Queensland. *J Clin Nurs,* Vol. 17, No. 1, pp. 90-98.

Brandenberger, G., Viola, A.U., Ehrhart, J., Charloux, A., Geny, B. Piquard, F. & Simon C. (2003). Age-related changes in cardiac autonomic control during sleep. *J Sleep Res,* Vol. 12, No. 3, pp. 173–180.

Buysee, D.J., Reynolds, C.F., Monk, T.H., Berman, S.R., & Kupfer, D.J. (1989). The Pittsburgh Sleep Quality Index: A new ınstrument for psychiatric practice and research. *Psychiatry Research,* Vol. 28, pp. 93-213.

Buysse, D.J., Ancoli-Israel, S., Edinger, J.D., Lichstein, K.L., & Morin, C.M. (2006). Recommendations for a standard research assessment of insomnia. *Sleep,* Vol. 29, No. 9, pp. 1155–73.

Carskadon, M. A. and W. C. Dement (2000). Normal human sleep, In: *Principles and Practice of Sleep Medicine,* Kryger, M. H., Roth, T., Dementi, W. C., (editors), pp.15-16, W.B.Saunders,978-1416066453, Philadelphia.

Chen, W.C., Lim, P.S., Wu, W.C., Chiu, H.C., Chen, C.H., Kuo, H.Y., Tsai, T.W., Chien, P.I., Su, Y.J., Su, Y.L., Hung, S.H., & Woods, H.F. (2006). Sleep behavior disorders in a large cohort of chinese (Taiwanese) patients maintained by long-term hemodialysis. *Am J Kidney Dis.,* Vol.33 2, No. 48, pp. 277-284.

Chesson, A. J., Hartse, K., & Anderson, W.M. (2006). Practice parameters for evaluation of chronic insomnia. An American Academy of sleep medicine report. *Sleep,* Vol. 29, No. 11, pp. 1415-1419.

Chiu K-L, Ryan CM, Shiota S, Ruttanaumpawan P, Arzt M, Haight JS, Chan CT, Floras JS & Bradley TD (2006). Fluid shift by lower body positive pressure increases pharyngeal resistance in healthysubjects. *Am J Resp Crit Care Med,* Vol. 174, pp.1378–1383.

Covic, A., Gusbeth-Tatomir, P., & Goldsmith, D.J. (2006). The epidemics of cardiovascular disease in elderly patients with chronic kidney disease—two facets of the same problem. *Int Urol Nephrol,* Vol. 38, pp. 371–379.

D'Ambrosio, C., Bowman, T., & Mohsenin, V. (1999). Quality of life in patients with obstructive sleep apnea: effect of nasal continuous positive airway pressure – a prospective study. *Chest,* Vol. 115, pp. 123–129.

De Santo, R.M., Lucidi , F., Violani C, & Bertini, M. (2001). Insomnia is associated with systolic hypertension in uremic patients on hemodialysis. *Int J Artif Organs,* Vol. 24, pp. 853–862

De Santo, R.M., Lucidi, F., Violani, C., & Di Iorio, B.R. (2005). Sleep disorders in hemodialyzed patients—the role of comorbidities. *Int J Artif Organs,* Vol. 28, pp. 557–565.

Easom, A. (2006). The challenges of using serum ferritin to guide I.V. iron treatment practices in patients on hemodialysis with anemia. *Nephrol Nurs J,* Vol. 33, pp. 543-551.

Edinger, J.D., & Sampson, W.S. (2003). A primary care "friendly" cognitive behavioral insomnia therapy. *Sleep,* Vol. 26, pp. 177–182.

Edinger, J.D., Wohlgemuth, W.K., Radtke, R.A., Marsh, G.R., & Quillian, R.E. (2001). Cognitive behavioral therapy for treatment of chronic primary insomnia: a randomized controlled trial. *JAMA,* Vol. 285, pp. 1856–1864.

Espie, C.A., Lindsay, W.R., Brooks, D.N., Hood, E.M., & Turvey, T.A. (1989). Controlled comparative investigation of psychological treatments for chronic sleep-onset insomnia. *Behav Res Ther,* Vol. 27, pp. 79-88.

Faccenda, J.F., Mackay, T.W., Boon, N.A., & Douglas, N.J. (2001). Randomized placebo-controlled trial of continuous positive airway pressure on blood pressure in the sleep apnea-hypopnea syndrome. *Am J Respir Crit Care Med,* Vol. 163, pp. 344–348.

Fletcher, E.C. (1993). Obstructive sleep apnea and the kidney. *Journal of the American Society of Nephrology,* Vol. 4, No. 5, pp. 1111-1121.

Gigli, G.L., Adorati, M., Dolso, P., Piani, A., Brotini, S., & Budai, R. (2004). Restless legs syndrome in end-stage renal disease. *Sleep Med,* Vol. 5, pp. 309–315.

Gul, A., Aoun, N., & Trayner, E.M. (2006). Why do patients sleep on dialysis? *Semin Dial,* Vol. 19, No. 2, pp. 52-157.

Han, S.Y., Yoon, J.W., Jo, S.K., Shin, J.H., Shin, C., Lee, J.B., Cha, D.R., Cho, W.Y., Pyo, H.J.,Kim, H.K., Lee, K.B., Kim, H., Kim,. K.W., Kim, Y.S., Lee, J.H., Park, S.E., Kim, C.S., Wea, K.S., Oh, K.S.,Chung, T.S., & Suh, S.Y. (2002). Insomnia in diabetic hemodialysis patients. Prevalence and risk factors by a multicenter study. *Nephron,* Vol. 92, No. 1, pp. 127- 32.

Hanly, P.J., & Pierratos, A. (2001). Improvement of sleep apnea in patients with chronic renal failure who undergo nocturnal hemodialysis. *N Engl J Med,* Vol. 344, pp. 102–107.

Hanly, P.J., Gabor, J.Y., Chan, C., & Pierratos, A. (2003). Daytime sleepiness in patients with CRF: impact of nocturnal hemodialysis. *Am J Kidney Dis,* Vol. 41, pp. 403-410.

Hauri, P. J. (2000). The many faces of insomnia. In D. I. Mostofsky & D. H. Barlow (Eds.), The management of stress and anxiety in medical disorders (pp. 143-159). Needham Heights, MA: Allyn & Bacon.

Holley, J.L., Nespor, S., & Rault, R. (1992). A comparison of reported sleep disorders in patients on chronic dialysis and continuous peritoneal dialysis. *American Journal of Kidney Disease,* Vol. 14, No. 2, pp. 156–161.

Hoyt, B.D. (2005). Sleep in patients with neurologic and psychiatric disorders. *Prim Care.* Vol. 32, pp. 535–548.

Iliescu, E.A., Yeates, K.E., & Holland, D.C. (2004). Quality of sleep in patients with chronic kidney disease. *Nephrol Dial Transplant,* Vol. 19, pp. 95–99.

Iliescu, E.A., Coo, H., McMurray, M.H., Meers, C.L., Quinn, M.M., Singer, M.A., & Hopman, W.H.I. (2003). Quality of sleep and health-related quality of life in haemodialysis patients. *Nephrol Dial Transplant*, Vol. 18, No. 1, pp. 126–132.

International Restless Legs Syndrome Study Group (IRLSSG) (2003). Validation of the international restless legs syndrome study group rating scale for restless legs syndrome. *Sleep Med*, Vol. 4, pp. 121–132.

Jones, B.E., (1989). Basic mechanisms of sleep-wake states, In: *Principles and Practice of Sleep Medicine,* Kryger, M. H., Roth, T., Dementi, W. C., (editors), pp.121-140, W.B. Saunders , 978-1416066453, Philadelphia.

Kamel, N.S., & Gammack, J.K. (2006). Insomnia in the elderly: cause, approach, and treatment. *Am J Med*, Vol. 119, No. 6, pp. 463–469.

Katz, D.A., & McHorney, C.A. (1998). Clinical correlates of insomnia in patients with chronic illness. *Arch Intern Med*, Vol. 158, pp. 1099–1107.

Kavanagh, D., & Siddiqui, S. (2004). Restless legs syndrome in patients on dialysis. *Amer J Kidney Dis,* Vol. 43, No. 5, May, pp.763–771.

Kimmel, P.L. (1989). Sleep disorders in chronic renal disease. *Journal of Nephrology,* Vol. 1, pp. 59-65.

Konofal, E., Arnulf, I., Lecendreux, M., & Mouren, M.C. (2005). Ropinirole in a child with attention-deficit hyperactivity disorder and restless legs syndrome. *Pediatr Neurol,* Vol. 32, pp. 350-351.

Kraus, M.A., & Hamburger, R.J. (1997). Sleep apnea in renal failure. *Adv Perit Dial* Vol. 13, pp. 88–92.

Krystal, A.D.& Edinger, J.D. (2008). Measuring sleep quality. *Sleep Medicine,* Vol. 9, Suppl. 1, pp: 10–17.

Lacks, P, Morin, CM. (1993). Recent advances in the assessment and treatment of insomnia. *J Consult Clin Psychol.* Vol.60, pp.586.

Lacks, P., Bertelson, A.D., Sugerman, J., & Kunkel, J. (1996). The treatment of sleep maintenance insomnia with stimulus-control techniques. *Behav Res Ther,* Vol. 21, pp. 291-295.

Landis, C.A., Lentz, M.J., Tsuji, J., Buchwald, D., & Shaver J.L. (2004). Pain, psychological variables, sleep quality, and natural killer cell activity in midlife women with and without fibromyalgia, *Brain, Behavior, and Immunity,* Vol. 13, pp. 304–313.

Leger, D., Guillerminault, C., Dreyfus, J.P., Delahaye, C., & Paillard, M. (2000). Prevalence of insomnia in a survey of 12,778 adults in France. *J Sleep Res,* Vol. 9, pp. 35–42.

Liao, W.C., Ming-Jang Chiu, M.J., & Landis,C.A., (2008). A Warm Footbath before Bedtime and Sleep in Older Taiwanese with Sleep Disturbance. *Res Nurs Health.* Vol. 31, No. 5, pp. 514–528.

Lichstein, K. L. & Reidel, B. W. (1994). Behavioral assessment and treatment of insomnia: a review with anemphasis on clinical application. *Behavior Therapy,* Vol. 25, pp. 659-688.

Mahowald, M.W. and Schenk, C.H.(1989). "REM sleep behavior disorder" In: *Principles and Practice of Sleep Medicine,* Kryger, M. H., Roth, T., Dementi, W. C., (editors), pp.389-401, W.B. Saunders , 978-1416066453, Philadelphia.

Markou, N., Kanakaki, M., Myrianthefs, M., Hadjiyanakos, D., Vlassopoulos, D., Damianos, A., Siamopoulos, K., Vasiliou, M., & Konstantopoulos, S. (2006). Sleep-disordered breathing in nondialyzed patients with chronic renal failure. *Lung,* Vol. 184, pp. 43-49.

Martin, J. (2000). Assessment and treatment of sleep disturbances in older adults *Clinical Psychology Review,* Vol. 20, No. 6, pp. 783-805.

Merlino, G., Piani, A., Dolso, P.1, Adorati, M., Cancelli, I., Valentel, M., & Gigli, G.L. (2006). Sleep disorders in patients with end-stage renal disease undergoing dialysis therapy. *Nephrol Dial Transplant,* Vol. 21, pp. 184-190.

Meyer, T.J (1998). Evaluation and management of insomnia. *Hosp Pract (Minneap),* Vol. 33, No. 12, pp. 75-8, 83-6.

Millman, R.P., Kimmel, P.L., Shore, E.T., & Wasserstein, A.G. (1985). Sleep apnea in hemodialysis patients: the lack of testosterone effect on its pathogenesis. *Nephron,* Vol. 40, pp.407-410.

Miranda, M., Kagi, M., Fabres, L., Aguilers, L., Alvo, M., Elgueta, L., Erazo, S., & Venegas, P. (2004). Pramipexole for the treatment of uremic restless legs in patients undergoing hemodialysis. *Neurology,* Vol. 62, pp. 831-832.

Mollaoğlu, M. (2004). Depression and Health Related Quality of Life in Hemodialysis Patients. *Dialysis Transplant,* Vol 33, pp. 544-555

Mollaoğlu, M., & Mollaoğlu, M. (2009). Sleep Quality in Hemodialysis Patients. *Neurology Psychiatry &Brain Research,* Vol.15, pp.179-184.

Montgomery, P., & Dennis, J. (2004). A systematic review of non-pharmacological therapies for sleep problems in later life. *Sleep Med Rev,* Vol. 8, pp. 47-62.

Morgan, K., Dixon, S., Mathers, N., Thompson, J., & Tomeny, M (2003). Psychological treatment for insomnia in the management of long-term hypnotic drug use: a pragmatic randomised controlled trial. *Br J Gen Pract,* Vol. 53, pp. 923-928.

Morin, C.M., Colecchi, C., Stone, J., Sood, R., & Brink, D. (1999). Behavioral and pharmacological therapies for late-life insomnia: a randomized controlled trial. *JAMA,* Vol. 281, pp. 991-999.

Mucsi, I., Molnar, M.Z., Ambrus, C., Szeifert, L., Kovacs, A.Z., Zoller, R., Barotfi, S., Remport, A., & Novak, M. (2005). Restless legs syndrome, insomnia and quality of life in patients on maintenance dialysis. *Nephrol Dial Transplant,* Vol. 20, pp. 571-577

Mucsi, I., Molnar, M.Z., Rethelyi, J., Vamos, E., Csepanyi, C., Tompa, C., Barotfi, S., Marton, A., & Novak, M. (2004). Sleep disorders and illness intrusiveness in patients on chronic dialysis. *Nephrol Dial Transplant,* Vol. 19, pp. 1815-1822.

Nichols, D.A., Allen, R..P, Grauke, J.H., Brown,. J.B., Rice, M.L., Hyde, P.R., Dement, W.C., Kushida, C.A. (2003). Restless legs syndrome symptoms in primary care: a prevalence study. *Arch Intern Med,* Vol. 163, pp. 2323-2329.

Novak, M., Shapiro, C.M., Mendelssohn, D., & Mucsi, I. (2006). Diagnosis and management of insomnia in dialysis patients. Semin. Dial., Vol.19, pp.25-31.

Ohayon, M.M. (2002). Epidemiology of insomnia: what we know and what we still need to learn. *Sleep Med Rev* Vol. 6, No. 2. pp. 97-111.

Parker, K.P. (1997). Sleep and dialysis: A research-based review of the literature. *ANNA Journal,* Vol. 24, No. 6, pp. 626-641.

Parker, K.P., Bliwise, D.L., Bailey, J.L., & Rye, D.B. (2005). Polysomnographic measures of nocturnal sleep in patients on chronic, intermittent daytime haemodialysis vs those with chronic kidney disease. *Nephrol Dial Transplant,* Vol. 20, pp.1422-1428.

Parker, K.P., Kutner, N.G., Bliwise, D.L., Bailey, J.L., & Rye, D.B. (2003). Nocturnal sleep, daytime sleepiness, and quality of life in stable patients on hemodialysis. *Health Qual Life Outcomes,* Vol. 1, pp. 68.

Patrick, L. (2007). Restless Legs Syndrome: Pathophysiology and the Role of Iron and Folate. *Alternative Medicine Review,* Vol. 12, No. 2, pp. 101-112.

Pellecchia, M.T., Vitale, C., Sabatini, M., Longo, K., Amboni, M., Bonavita, V., & Barone, P. (2004). Ropinirole as a treatment of restless legs syndrome in patients on chronic hemodialysis: an open randomized crossover trial versus levodopa sustained release. *Clin Neuropharmacol,* Vol. 27, pp. 178–181.

Pieta, J., Millar, T., Zacharias, J., Fine, A., Kryger, M. (1998). Effect of pergolide on restless legs and leg movements in sleep in uremic patients. *Sleep,* Vol. 21, pp. 617–622.

Pigeon, W.R., & Yurcheshen, M. (2009). Behavioral Sleep Medicine Interventions for Restless Legs Syndrome and Periodic Limb Movement Disorder. *Sleep Med Clin,* Vol. 1, No. 4, December, pp. 487–494.

Pressman, M.R. Benz,.R.L., & Peterson, D.D. (1995). Periodic leg movements in sleep index(PLMSI) predicts mortality in end stage renal disease patients. *Sleep Research,* Vol. 24, pp. 416.

Rahman, M., Fu,P., Sehgal,A., & Smith, M.(2000). Interdialytic weight gain, compliance with dialysis regimen, and age are independent predictors of blood pressure in hemodialysis patients. *American Journal of Kidney Diseases,* Vol. 35, pp. 257-265

Redline, S., Kirchner, H.L., Quan, S.F., Gottlieb, D.J., Kapur, V., & Newman, A. (2004). The effects of age, sex, ethnicity, and sleep-disordered breathing on sleep architecture. *Arch Intern Med,* Vol. 164, pp. 406–418.

Riedel, B. W., Lichstein, K. L. & Dwyer, W. O. (1995). Sleep compression and sleep education for older insomniacs: Self-help versus therapist guidance. *Psychology and Aging,* Vol. 10, pp. 54–63.

Rodrigues, C.J.O., Marson, O., Tufic, S., Kohlmann, O., Guimar, S.M., Togeiro, P., Ribeiro, A.B., & Tavares, A. (2005). Relationship among end-stage renal disease, hypertension, and sleep apnea in nondiabetic dialysis patients. *Am J Hypertens,* Vol. 18, pp. 152–157.

Rosenthal, M.S. (1998). Physiology and Neurochemistry of Sleep. *American Journal of Pharmaceutical Education,* Vol. 62, pp. 204-208.

Sabbatini, M., Crispo, A., Pisani, A., Cesaro, A., Mirenghi, F., Cianciaruso, B., & Federico, S. (2003). Zaleplon improves sleep quality in maintenance hemodialysis patients. *Nephron Clin Pract,* Vol. 94, pp. 99–103.

Sabbatini, M., Minale, B., Crispo, A. Pisani, A., Ragosta, A., Esposito, R., Cesaro, A., Cianciaruso, B., & Andreucci, V.E. (2002). Insomnia in maintenance hemodialysis patients. *Nephrol Dial Transplant,* Vol. 17, pp. 852–856.

Sabry, A.A., Abo-Zenah, H., Wafa, E., Mahmoud, K., El-Dahshan, K., Hassan, A., Abbas, T.M., Saleh, A.M., & Okasha, K.. (2010). Sleep disorders in hemodialysis patients. *Saudi J Kidney Dis Transpl,* Vol. 21, pp. 300-305.

Sandyk, R., Bernick, C., Lee, S.M., Stern, L.Z., Lacono, R.P., & Bamford, C.R. (1987). L-dopa in uremic patients with the restless legs syndrome. *Int J Neurosci,* Vol. 35, pp. 233–235.

Siddiqui, S., & Kavanagh, D. (2005). Risk factors for restless legs syndrome in dialysis patients. *Nephro Clin Pract,* Vol. 101, pp. 155–60.

Sloand, J.A., Shelly, M.A., Feigin, A., Bernstein, P., & Monk, R.D. (2004). A double blind,placebo-controlled trial of intravenous iron dextran therapy in patients with ESRD and restless legs syndrome. *Am J Kidney Dis,* Vol. 43, pp. 663-670.

Smith, M.T., Perlis, M.L. Park, A., Smith, M.S., Pennington, J., Giles, D.E., & Buysse , D.J. (2002). Comparative meta-analysis of pharmacotherapy and behavior therapy for persistent insomnia. *Am J Psychiatry,* Vol. 159, pp. 5–11.

Smith, P.L., Gold, A.R., Meyers, D.A., Haponik, E.F., & Bleecker, E.R. (1985). Weight loss in mildly to moderately obese patients with obstructive sleep apnea. *Ann Intern Med,* Vol. 103, pp. 850-855.

Spielman, A.J., Saskin, P., & Thorpy, M.J. (1987). Treatment of chronic insomnia by restriction of time in bed. *Sleep,* Vol. 10, pp. 45-56.

Takaki, J., Nishi, T., Nangaku, M., Shimoyama, H., Inada, T., Matsuyama, N., Kumano, H., & Kuboki, T. (2003). Clinical and psychological aspects of restless legs syndrome in uremic patients on hemodialysis. *Am J Kidney Dis,* Vol. 41, pp. 833–839.

Tatomir, P., Seic, D.B. A., Buga, C., & Covic, A. (2007). Sleep disorders: a systematic review of an emerging major clinical issue in renal patients. *Int Urol Nephrol,* Vol.. 39, pp. 1217–1226

Terzano, M.G., Parrino, L., Cirignotta, F., Ferini-Strambi, L., Gigli, G., Rudelli, G., Sommacal, S., Studio Morfeo Committee (2004. Studio Morfeo: insomnia in primary care, a survey conducted on the Italian population. *Sleep Med,* Vol. 5, No. 1, pp. 67-75.

Thase, M.E. (2005). Correlates and consequences of chronic insomnia. *Gen Hosp Psychiatry,* Vol. 27, pp. 100–112.

Trenkwalder, C., Stiasny, K., Pollmacher, T., Wetter, T., Schwarz, J., Kohnen, R., & Kazenwadel, J. (1995). L-dopa therapy of uremic and idiopathic restless legs syndrome: a double-blind, crossover trial. *Sleep,* Vol. 18, pp. 681–688.

Unruh, M.L, Levey, A.S., D'Ambrosio, C. Fink, N.E., Powe, N., & Myer, B.K. (2004). Restless legs symptoms among incident dialysis patients: Association with Lower Quality of Liver and Shorter Survival (CHOICE). *Amer J Kidney Dis,* Vol. 43, No. 5, May, pp. 900–909.

Unruh, M.L., Sanders, M.H., Redline, S., Piraino, B.M., Umans, J.G., Hammond, T.C., Sharief, I., Punjabi, M., & Newman, B. (2006). Sleep apnea in patients on conventional thrice-weekly hemodialysis: comparison with matched controls from the sleep heart health study. *J Am Soc Nephrol,* Vol. 17, pp. 3503–3509

Veiga, J., Gonçalves, N., Gomes, F., Santos, N., Baptista, A., Paiva, T. (1997).Sleep disturbances in end-stage renal disease patients on hemodialysis. *Dial Transplant,* No.26, pp.380-384

Walker, S., Fine, A., & Kryger, M.H., (1995). Sleep complaints are common in a dialysis unit. *American Journal of Kidney Disease,* Vol. 5, No. 26, pp. 751–756.

Walker, S.L., Fine, A., & Kryger, M.H. (1996). L-DOPA/carbidopa for nocturnal movement disorders in uremia. *Sleep,* Vol. 19, pp. 214–218.

Wei, C.Y., Chung, T.C., Wu, S.C., Chung, C.F., & Wu, W.P. (2011). The Subjective sleep quality and heart rate variability in hemodialysis patients. *Ren Fail.* Vol. 5, No. 26, pp. 109-117.

Welch, J.L. & Austin, J.K. (2001). Stressors, coping and depression in haemodialysis patients. *Journal of Advanced Nursing,* Vol. 33, No. 2, pp. 200-207.

Williams, S.W., Tell, G.S., Zheng, B., Shumaker, S., Rocco, M.V., & Sevick, M.A. (2002). Correlates of sleep behavior among hemodialysis patients. *Am J Nephrol,* Vol. 22, pp. 18–28.

Winkelman, J.W., Chertow, G.M., & Lazarus, J.M. (1996). Restless legs syndrome in end-stage renal disease. *American Journal of Kidney Diseases,* Vol. 28, No. 3, pp. 372-378.

Yoshioka, M., Ishii ,T., & Fukunishi, I. (1993). Sleep disturbance of end-stage renal disease. *Jpn J Psychiatry Neurol.,* Vol. 47, pp.847-851.

Young , T., Palta, M., Dempsey, J., Skatrud, J., Weber, S., & Badr, S. (1993). The occurrence of sleep-disordered breathing among middle-aged adults. *N Engl J Med* Vol. 328, pp. 1230–1235.

Zoccali, C., Mallamaci, F., & Tripepi, G. (2001). Sleep Apnea in Renal Patients. *J Am Soc Nephrol,* Vol. 12, pp. 2854–2859.

5

Determinants of Cardiovascular Risk in Hemodialysis Patients without Significant Comorbidities

Aysegul Zumrutdal
Baskent University,
Adana Teaching and Research Hospital
Turkey

1. Introduction

Cardiovascular (CV) disease is a major cause of morbidity and mortality in patients with end-stage renal disease. Traditional risk factors for CV disease include hypertension, smoking, diabetes, dyslipidemia, left ventricular hypertrophy, advanced age and male sex in the general population. Although hemodialysis patients have a high prevalence of many of these factors, they also have nontraditional, or uremia-related, specific factors such as anemia, altered calcium-phosphorus metabolism, inflammation, oxidative stress, nitric oxide synthase inhibitors, hypoalbuminemia, carbamylation, abnormal lipoproteins and hyperhomocysteinemia (Parfrey, 2000; London&Drüeke 1997). So the risk markers that predict CV events in hemodialysis patients may differ from those in the general population.

This increased CV risk has often been attributed to 'accelerated atherosclerosis' in end-stage renal disease (Cheung, 2000; Kasiske et al., 2000). However, CV causes of death are most prominent in the first years of dialysis and are rare in patients who have been on long term dialysis - the reverse of what would be expected if dialysis itself caused 'accelerated atherosclerosis (Mailloux et al., 1991). Because many patients with end-stage renal disease already have one or more comorbidities and clinically evident vascular disease, it is difficult to determine from clinical or epidemiological studies whether traditional or non-traditional risk factors are more responsible for the high risk of CV events.

The presence of comorbid disease is an increasingly common problem, being much more prevelant in new patients started on dialysis today than previously (Godkin et al., 2003; Mailloux et al., 1996; Merkus et al., 2000; Miskulin et al., 2009; Wallen et al., 2001). Hemodialysis patients who are under 55 years of age and without diabetes, significant comorbid diseases and obesity are very rare in the general hemodialysis population. For this reason, fewer epidemiological studies which focus on the determinants of CV risk of a relatively 'healthy' hemodialysis population are available. However, it is increasingly appreciated that chronic kidney disease alone is an independent risk factor for the development of CV disease. In this topic review of available data, an overview is presented of CV risk factors in hemodialysis patients without significant comorbidities.

2. Markers of inflammation

Chronic inflammation is one of the well-known non-traditional cardiovascular risk factors in hemodialysis patients. Chronic kidney disease results in a chronic, low-grade inflammatory process that becomes evident even in the early stages of the disease. After the start of dialysis treatment, various factors associated with the dialysis procedure may also contribute to a stronger, more active inflammatory response. All available evidence suggests that chronic inflammation in hemodialysis patients may contribute significantly to the development and progression of CV disease (Filiopoulos&Vlassopoulos, 2009; Stenvinkel, 2006; Zimmermann et al., 1999).
Although few studies are available concerning the relationship between inflammatory status and CV risk in hemodialysis patients without co-morbid diseases, the studies that do exist in this area also support the role of inflammation.

2.1 C-reactive protein (CRP)

CRP is the best studied inflammation marker associated with CV events. It is the prototypical acute phase response protein produced by the liver under the control of various proinflammatory cytokines, namely interleukin-6, interleukin-1, and tumor necrosis factor-α. Its uniquiness is due to rapid (within 6 hours) and dramatic increases (up to 1000-fold) in circulating concentrations after a cytokine-mediated response to most forms of tissue injury, infection, and inflammation. Moreover, it was shown that plasma half-life (19 hours) and fractional clearance rates of CRP were nearly constant in normal subjects, as well as in patients with infectious, inflammatory, and neoplastic conditions. This marks CRP as a 'precise objective index' of overall inflammatory activity and a surrogate of underlying cytokine stimulus (Arici& Walls, 2001; Pepys&Baltz, 1983; Vigushin et al., 1993).
Several observations have demonstrated that in a significant proportion of hemodialysis patients CRP is elevated for no apparent reason. A wide variety of factors in hemodialysis patients may be responsible for this elevation. First, the uremic state is associated with an altered immune response and uremia per se may cause a proinflammatory status with ongoing acute phase response. Also, extracorporeal circulation of blood during each hemodialysis session may act as a fresh stimulus for acute phase response. Increased cytokine release, the role of dialysis membranes, the dialysate and the patient-specific processes, such as the type of vascular access or unrecognized infections, may also play a role in inciting an inflammatory response (Arici&Walls, 2001; Stenvinkel, 2002a, 2002b).
The predictive value of CRP in CV risk and mortality in hemodialysis patients was shown in numerous studies, and evidence from experimental and clinical studies showed that CRP may contribute directly to the pathogenesis of atherosclerosis and its complications through a variety of mechanisms (Arici&Walls, 2001; Yeun&Kaysen, 2000; Zimmermann et al., 1999). So it has been suggested that this hepatic–derived protein is not only a marker, but also a mediator, of vascular disease (Lagrand et al., 1997; Torzewski et al., 1998). Although a wide variety of potential sources may be associated with elevated CRP in this patient population, underlying silent CV disease may be one of the possible links for this elevation. So the clear association between CRP and CV disease in the hemodialysis population has added CRP as a new predictive CV risk factor which may actually be in a midway position between traditional and uremia-related CV risk factors (Arici&Walls, 2001).
One of the studies investigated the associations of different risk factors with carotid artery intima-media thickness in non-diabetic hemodialysis patients who had no clinical evidence

of atherosclerosis and no comorbidities (Zumrutdal et al., 2005). Seventy-two patients (43 men, 29 women; mean age 34.5 ± 10.6 years, mean time on hemodialysis 47.9 ± 40.0 months) were included in the study. Patients without history or evidence of myocardial, cerebrovascular or peripheral vascular disease, those without diabetes mellitus, and those who had been stabilized on hemodialysis therapy for more than six months and were less than 55 years old were enrolled. Patients were excluded whose chest radiograph showed calcified plaques in the aortic arch, or who had ischaemic findings on electrocardiography and/or ventricular wall motility disorders or valvular calcifications on echocardiography. Additionally, patients with conditions known to be associated with acute-phase responses were excluded. The control group consisted of 40 age-and sex-matched healthy subjects, who had been recruited from hospital staff. Body mass index, triglycerides, lipoprotein (a), fibrinogen, CRP, haematocrit-corrected erythrocyte sedimentation rate, serum cardiac troponin I, beta2 microglobulin, and homocysteine levels were found to be significantly different in patients on hemodialysis compared with control subjects. The mean value of the right and left carotid intima media thickness was 0.59 ± 0.06 mm for patients and 0.53 ± 0.07 mm for control subjects. The difference was significant (p=0.002). The carotid intima-media thickness of patients was correlated with age, body mass index, CRP, haematocrit-corrected erythrocyte sedimentation rate, beta2 microglobulin, serum cardiac troponin I, triglyceride, and fibrinogen. CRP, haematocrit-corrected erythrocyte sedimentation rate, serum cardiac troponin I, and fibrinogen were significantly correlated with each other, but not with beta2 microglobulin. The only parameter correlated with beta2 microglobulin was time on hemodialysis. The mean carotid intima-media thickness was significantly greater in patients with both left ventricular hypertrophy and a CRP level > 6.0 mg/L than it was in those with a CRP level ≤ 6.0 mg/L. In that study, multivariate regression analysis showed that age, CRP, beta2 microglobulin, and left ventricular hypertrophy were independent predictors of carotid artery intima-media thickness. The results of that study supported the hypothesis of an 'accelerated atherogenesis' in the hemodialysis population, even if those patients do not have clinical evidence of atherosclerosis. And CRP was found to be one of the independent predictors of early-onset atherosclerosis.

Most investigations of CV risk in patients on hemodialysis have been cross-sectional in nature and representative of the general hemodialysis population. In the previous study, the same subgroup of hemodialysis patients was followed up over the course of one year and the determinants of the progression of carotid artery intima-media thickness were assessed again (Zumrutdal et al., 2006). Fifty-four of the 72 patients completed the study and re-tested under the same standardized conditions after 12 months. The findings at 12 months showed that carotid artery intima-media thickness had progressed in 75.9 % patients. Age, CRP, beta2 microglobulin and left ventricular hypertrophy were independently related with baseline carotid artery intima-media thickness. At 12 months, age and CRP were found to be independent variables related with carotid artery intima-media thickness. The independent risk factors related with the change in carotid artery intima-media thickness from baseline to 12-month stage were age and male sex.

According to those results, age and male sex were related to progression of carotid artery intima-media thickness as unavoidable risk factors in this subgroup of the hemodialysis population. That agreed with the results of major clinical and epidemiological studies of the general population. The independent relation between CRP and carotid artery intima-media thickness both at baseline and 12 months supports the additional role of non-specific inflammation in hemodialysis patients without comorbidities.

2.2 Hematocrit-corrected erythrocyte sedimentation rate (Hct-corrected ESR)

Although ESR is widely used in the general population as an inflammation marker, it was judged to be of no clinical utility in chronic hemodialysis patients in the mid-1980s. So ESR has seldom been studied in patients on hemodialysis. However, in 2001, it was proposed that after correction of ESR values according to Hct levels in hemodialysis patients, Hct-corrected ESR could serve to select the inflammation-afflicted hemodialysis patients from those without this comorbid state (Borawski& Mysliwic, 2001). Supporting that study, while no relationship between ESR and carotid artery intima-media thickness was found, a relationship in hemodialysis patients without comorbidities was found between Hct-corrected ESR and carotid artery intima-media thickness, beyond other inflammatory markers, CRP, and fibrinogen. Although larger additional studies are needed to determine the potential value of Hct-corrected ESR as an inflammatory marker for early-onset atherosclerosis, this relationship may again reflect the role of non-specific inflammation in CV risk of the 'healthy' hemodialysis patients (Zumrutdal et al., 2005).

2.3 Fibrinogene

In the normal population, increased activity of procoagulant proteins including factor VII and fibrinogen is associated with coronary risk. Factor VII coagulant activity and markers of thrombin activation are elevated in patients with chronic renal failure and correlate positively with serum triglycerides and the acute phase reactants interleukin 6 and fibrinogen and negatively with serum albumin (Tomson, 2000). The presence of generalized endothelial dysfunction in uraemic patients is also suggested by higher plasma levels of fibrinogen, endothelin and other factors. The relationship between carotid artery intima-media thickness and fibrinogene in hemodialysis patients without comorbidities may reflect the role of fibrinogene in early-onset atherosclerosis as one of the best-studied inflammation markers (Zumrutdal et al., 2005).

3. Cardiac markers

3.1 Left ventricular hypertrophy

Left ventricular hypertrophy is a well-known potent predictor of CV mortality in patients on renal replacement therapy (Ma et al., 1992). This may result either from pressure overload, causing increased tensile stress, or from volume overload, causing increased shear stres (Tomson, 2000). Recently published results demonstrated that even with good control of hypertension and anaemia, conventional hemodialysis is associated with significant left ventricular hypertrophy. And high prevalence of CV disease was positively associated with left ventricular hypertrophy in hemodialysis population.

In the study assessing the predictive markers of CV risk in asymptomatic hemodialysis patients, in total, 113 hemodialysis patients were included. Demographic, anthropometric, clinical, and laboratory data were collected. Silent myocardial damage was defined by elevated cardiac troponin I values above cutoff values. Cardiac troponin I concentrations were below cutoff value in 103 (91.2%) patients (group 1), whereas 10 (8.8%) patients (group 2) had elevated concentrations. Group 1 patients had higher levels of hemoglobin and high-density lipoprotein cholesterol and lower C-reactive protein and tumor necrosis factor-alpha levels, as well as less incidence of left ventricular hypertrophy, when compared to group 2 patients. Diabetes mellitus, left ventricular hypertrophy, uncontrolled blood pressure, normalized protein equivalent of total nitrogen appearence, hemoglobin and tumor necrosis factor-alpha were found to be independently associated with silent myocardial damage (Afsar et al., 2009).

In hemodialysis patients without comorbidities, mean carotid intima-media thickness, which reflects generalized atherosclerosis and CV risk, was significantly greater in patients with left ventricular hypertrophy, than it was in patients without left ventricular hypertrophy. Mean carotid intima-media thickness in subjects in the heathy control group was significantly lower than it was in hemodialysis patients both with and without left ventricular hypertrophy. The mean serum cardiac troponin I level in the control group was significantly lower than it was in patients both with and without left ventricular hypertrophy. The mean serum cardiac troponin I level was significantly higher in patients with left ventricular hypertrophy than it was in those without left ventricular hypertrophy (Zumrutdal et al., 2005). The relationship between carotid artery intima-media thickness, serum cardiac troponin I levels and left ventricular hypertrophy may demonstrate that subclinical atherosclerotic changes and/or adaptation may occur along with cardiac alterations. So it may be reasonable to apply early strategies for prevention and treatment of left ventricular hypertrophy in hemodialysis patients before clinically evident CV disease.

3.2 Cardiac troponins

Cardiac troponins are the most specific biomarkers for myocardial damage, although they may be elevated in situations other than acute coronary syndrome. Hemodialysis patients often have raised cardiac troponin I and T levels in the absence of acute ischaemic symptoms. The source of this increase has been a point of confusion over the past decade. At the beginning, some authors suggested that this might be related to the cardiac expression of troponins, while others argued for the skeletal muscle as a possible extracardiac source of abnormally elevated cardiac troponins in hemodialysis patients (Bodor et al., 1997; Kals et al., 2011; McLaurin et al., 1997).

In initial experience with two troponin subunits, serum troponin T was elevated more frequently than troponin I in patients with renal failure, and that led the clinicians to question its specificity for the diagnosis of myocardial infarction. Additionally, the poorer specificity of troponin T was attributed to subclinical myocardial injury in the setting of left ventricular hypertrophy or to uremia-induced skeletal muscle expression of the cardiac isoform of troponin T, while cardiac troponin I has been exclusively of cardiac origin and does not express in the skeletal muscle at any developmental stage. Thus, troponin I was proposed to be a better marker of myocardial injury in renal failure than T (Yeun&Kaysen, 2000). However, subsequent studies reported the absence of extracardiac cardiac troponin T expression in truncal skeletal muscle biopsy specimens from patients with end-stage renal failure at the RNA and protein levels (Haller et al., 1998). Another study, based on the electromyographic evaluation of 50 chronic hemodialysis patients, investigated the relationship between increased cardiac troponin T levels and uremic myopathy. Proximal-extremity muscles-deltoid, biceps, vastus laterali-, which were the most common targets of uremic myopathy, were studied. Five of 50 patients (10%) had a positive troponin T test, but only 1 of those patients had characteristic electromyographic findings. Totally, 4 of 50 patients (8%) had electromyographic findings characteristic of uremic myopathy. Positive troponin test results were not associated with calcium, phosphate, parathormone levels. There was no association between serum cardiac troponin T levels and uremic myopathy (Zumrutdal AO et al., 2000).

Subsequent studies showed that frequently positive T test results in hemodialysis patients were likely due to use of the older and less specific troponin T assay with some cross-reactivity to skeletal muscle (Yeun&Kaysen, 2000). And with the use of the latest generation assays, accumulated data from groups of renal failure patients have suggested that elevated levels of both troponin T and I in asymptomatic hemodialysis patients could be associated with added CV risk, including general mortality. Most of the recent studies supported the troponin tests as predictive markers of asymptomatic atherosclerosis and silent myocardial damage in hemodialysis patients (Kanderian& Francis, 2006; Kanwar et al., 2006).

The carotid artery intima-media thickness measurement has been proposed as a method for establishing risk stratification for CV events. To the best of our knowledge, we were the first to examine the relationship between serum cardiac troponin I level and early onset atherosclerosis in a selected subgroup of hemodialysis patients without any clinical evidence of either atherosclerosis or comorbidities. Based on those results, the increased serum cardiac troponin I level was positively correlated with the carotid intima-media thickness and seemed to be a valuable predictive marker for the assessment of CV risk in asymptomatic hemodialysis patients (Zumrutdal et al., 2005). Also, a possible association was found between elevated serum cardiac troponins and inflammatory markers such as CRP, fibrinogen and Hct-corrected ESR. The association between carotid intima-media thickness, serum cardiac troponin I levels and inflammatory parameters needs to be clarified with further studies. Although the underlying pathophysiology of elevated cardiac troponins is still not clearly understood, it may reflect ongoing, often subclinical, myocardial damage or microinfarctions that are partially independent of acute ischaemic injury. So serum cardiac troponin elevations might be very effective in elucidating cardiac risks of hemodialysis patients without any clinical evidence of atherosclerosis and comorbidities.

In conclusion, in addition to traditional risk factors such as age and male sex, non-specific inflammation may play a key role in the progression of atherosclerosis in patients on hemodialysis without comorbidities. Although it is well-established that end-stage renal failure is a state of chronic systemic inflammation, both nondialysis-related factors and the dialysis procedure per se may be responsible for this high risk. Beta2 microglobulin and serum cardiac troponins may be the potential new additions for CV risk in this group of patients. Further studies are needed to determine whether there is a causal relationship.

4. Metabolic markers

4.1 Beta 2 microglobulin

Elevated plasma beta2 microglobulin is a well-known characteristic of chronic renal failure, and among uremic toxins in the middle molecule range, it is certainly one of the most studied compounds. Beta 2 microglobulin is a key component in the genesis of dialysis-associated amyloidosis. The source of the elevated serum beta2 microglobulin has not been explained absolutely in hemodialysis patients. There is controversy as to whether elevated levels are caused predominantly by increased synthesis of beta2 microglobulin, the use of membranes in hemodialysis with different clearance capacities, or diminished renal elimination (Drüeke et al., 2009). Use of middle and high-flux biocompatible membranes was shown to be associated with a notable reduction in beta2 microglobulin and, in some other studies, the systemic inflammatory response, in the general hemodialysis population. However, the role of proinflammatory monocytic cytokines, such as interleukin-1 and

interleukin-6, in the pathogenesis of elevated beta2 microglobulin, and its role as a potential initiator of the inflammatory response were discussed (Vraetz et al., 1999; Xie & Yi, 2003).
Recently, a study comparatively evaluated the effect of hemodialysis and peritoneal dialysis on oxidative stress and inflammatory biomarkers and the associated factors. It found similar degrees of inflammaton and oxidative stress activation in both groups. In that study, beta2 microglobulin was one of the parameters which correlated to oxidative stress and inflammatory biomarkers. It was negatively correlated both with total antioxidant capacity in hemodialysis patients and with superoxide dismutase in peritoneal dialysis patients (Filiopoulos et al., 2009).
Previously, for what was probably the first time in the available literature, we provided data about the association between beta2 microglobulin and early-onset atherosclerosis in hemodialysis patients without comorbidities (Zumrutdal et al., 2005). In our study, the only parameter correlated with beta2 microglobulin was time on hemodialysis therapy. At that time, we speculated that the relationship we found might be casual (inflammatory) or just an epiphenomenon, and added that further follow up studies were needed to elucidate the importance of beta2 microglobulin as a new nontraditional cardiovascular risk factor in hemodialysis patients. Subsequently, few studies have evaluated the association of beta 2 microglobulin levels with clinical outcome in dialyzed patients. The patients were divided into two groups according to their serum beta2 microglobulin levels (lower beta2 microglobulin group, n=245 and higher beta2 microglobulin group, n=245) and followed-up. During the follow-up period of 40±15 months, there were 91 all-cause deaths, and out of them, 36 were from CV disease. All cause mortality in the higher beta2 microglobulin group was significantly higher compared to that in the lower beta2 microglobulin group. And serum beta2 microglobulin level was a significant predictor of mortality in hemodialysis patients, independent of hemodialysis duration, diabetes, malnutrition and chronic inflammation (Okuno et al., 2009).
A few studies also supported the correlation between serum beta2 microglobulin levels and various cardiovascular risk factors, including CRP, in hemodialysis patients (Kuragano et al., 2010). And recently, beta2 microglobulin has been suggested to be a novel biomarker of peripheral arterial disease and an independent predictor of aortic stiffness in atherosclerosis, in the general population (Wilson et al., 2007). Additionally, higher serum beta2 microglobulin levels were proposed to be a novel marker to distinguish levels of risk in acute heart failure patients with creatinine ≤ 3mg/dl (Kawai et al., 2010).
All of those findings strongly support the role of beta2 microglobulin in CV risk of hemodialysis patients, and it seems it will be a potential new CV risk marker in the future. Further studies are needed to clarify the importance of beta2 microglobulin as a CV risk factor in hemodialysis patients without comorbidities.

5. Determinants of cardiovascular risk in nondiabetic hemodialysis patients

Diabetes is not only a traditional risk factor for CV disease, but also one of the most common causes of end-stage renal disease. While a decline in CV deaths has occurred in the general population, a similar trend has not been observed in dialysis patients. This discrepancy is in part due to the demographics of patients about to be started on dialysis: about 40 percent are diabetic. Also, the average age of hemodialysis patients is approximately 60 years and about 20 percent are over 75 years, and many patients have underlying cardiac disease

(Mailloux, 2010). Thus, epidemiologic studies concerning the predictive factors of CV disease in nondiabetic hemodialysis patients are less available.

5.1 Association with traditional and nontraditional risk factors

In a study of the CV assessment of 75 nondiabetic hemodialysis patients, the main cause of renal failure was hypertension. Compared with normal controls, the patients were found to have increased inflammatory cytokines such as interleukin- 6, tumor necrosis factor alpha, and intercelluler adhesion molecule, as well as a high frequency of carotid intima media thickening, left ventricular hypertrophy, and aortic calcifications (Kunstmann et al., 2009). Mortality predictors among 84 diabetic and 161 nondiabetic patients undergoing hemodialysis were investigated for two years. Forty-three diabetic patients and 30 nondiabetic patients died. Among diabetic patients, oliguria, elevated CRP, and elevated D-dimer levels predicted all-cause mortality. Oliguria was the most important predictor, particularly for infectious disease-related death. Among nondiabetic patients elevated cardiac troponin T levels, elevated D-dimer levels, and low cholesterol levels predicted all-cause mortality rates. Subdivision of the causes of death among nondiabetic patients revealed that cardiac troponin T levels predicted CV mortality rates. According to those results, mortality predictors among hemodialysis patients differed between diabetic and nondiabetic patients (Hocher et al., 2003). In one comparison, two groups of nondiabetic hemodialysis patients (both groups n=30) matched for age and sex, were selected according to the absence or presence of symptomatic atherothrombotic vascular disease affecting the coronary, cerebral, or peripheral arteries. The two groups were identical regarding primary renal disease, duration of hemodialysis, and Epo treatment. The presence of hypertension, lipoprotein (a), and fibronectin levels were independent predictors for the presence of atherothrombotic CV disease which may contribute to the high prevalence of CV risk. Smoking was not a predictor. (Tzanatos et al., 2009).

Left ventricular hypertrophy: Left ventricular hypertrophy is one of the strongest predictors of CV mortality in the general dialysis population. It is an independent predictor of survival in patients with chronic renal failure and it is present in a large number of patients on hemodialysis. In 30 nondiabetic hemodialysis patients, predictive factors associated with left ventricular hypertrophy at baseline and in the follow-up period (at 0, 12, and 24 months) were studied. Systolic blood pressure, residual glomerular filtration rate and serum albumin levels were the predictive factors for left ventricular mass index at initiation of hemodialysis. Systolic blood pressure, human atrial natriuretic peptide, and hemoglobin levels were independent risk factors for left ventricular mass index, after 24 months. Systolic blood pressure, human atrial natriuretic peptide, and hemoglobin levels were also predictive factors for left ventricular mass index after initiation of hemodialysis (Io et al., 2010). Better management of hypertension and anaemia may be priorities for preventing or improving CV risk in these patients.

Carotid intima-media thickness: Carotid intima-media thickness is a strong predictor of CV events in the general population. The predictive value of carotid intima-media thickness in 99 nondiabetic hemodialysis patients was investigated. During a follow-up of 42.4±19.5 months, 33 patients died, 19 (57.6%) of them of CV causes. In those 19 patients carotid thickness was significantly higher than in those who survived. So carotid intima-media thickness was an independent predictor of CV death in nondiabetic hemodialysis patients (Ekart et al., 2005). Asymptomatic atherosclerosis and major risk factors in 104 nondiabetic patients with different stages of chronic kidney disease (stage 1-5) were also investigated. Carotid intima-media thickness and plaque occurrence were compared with 40 healthy control subjects. Nondiabetic patients with chronic kidney disease showed advanced atherosclerosis, intima-media thickness, and plaque occurrence, and their numbers increased directly with the level of renal dysfunction. Another important risk factor was hypertension (Ekart et al., 2008).

Vascular calcification: The uremic state is associated with numeous metabolic abnormalities and endocrine disturbances primarily involving calcium and phosphorus metabolism. Vascular calcification is highly prevelant in dialysis patients and increases CV mortality. The presence and progression of vascular calcification in hemodialysis patients have been significantly associated with chronic inflammation, malnutrition, and disorders of mineral metabolism. Through a review of the literature examining vascular calcification in end stage renal failure patients, hyperphosphatemia is significantly associated with vascular calcification in nondiabetic patients, while it may not be a significant risk factor for vascular calcification in diabetic patients. In diabetic patients vascular calcification occurs long before the initiation of dialysis therapy and and the factors associated with vascular calcification in non-uremic diabetics appear to be hyperglycemia and related metabolic disorders, such as increased glycation and oxidative stress. In diabetic end stage renal failure patients, hyperglycemia is also suggested to be a significant factor associated with the progression of vascular calcification. Thus, the importance of glycemic control in diabetic and phosphate control in nondiabetic end stage renal failure patients is suggested (Ishimura et al., 2008).

The accumulating data demonstrate the role of abnormalities of calcium, phosphorus, vitamin D, and parathyroid hormone in CV disease and the importance of phosphate control is suggested for preventing vascular calcification and CV risk (Andress, 2008; London et al., 2000).

Diabetes mellitus and ethnicity are known factors that affect the extent of CV calcifications. The extent of CV calcifications was assessed in non-diabetic Caucasian hemodialysis patients by a novel composite calcification score. Body mass index, cholesterol, triglycerides, intact PTH, and serum levels of fetuin-A and uncarboxylated matrix Gla protein were not associated with CV calcifications. Age, male gender, dialysis vintage, smoking, calcium-phosphate product, CRP, and lower Kt/V were independent risk factors for CV calcifications (Schlieper et al., 2009). Increasing dialysis efficiency and lowering calcium-phosphate product can reduce CV calcifications. Generally, a calcium X phosphate product of less than 55 is the therapeutic optimum and it is possible that even lower levels offer further survival advantage. However, no prospective randomized studies have demonstrated a CV benefit and/or a survival advantage with any of the current therapeutic options. But observational studies have shown improved survival in hemodialysis patients treated with active vitamin D analogues (Levin&Li, 2005).

Metabolic abnormalities: Chronic kidney disease is associated with complex metabolic changes including insulin resistance, and insulin resistance is associated with increased CV risk (O'Sullivian&Kelly, 2007). In contrast to the general population, a higher body mass index is associated with better survival among hemodialysis patients. Theoretically, high energy supplementation in nondiabetic hemodialysis patients might adversely affect insulin resistance, and with this goal in mind, the effects of high energy supplementation on nondiabetic hemodialysis patients was investigated. According to the results, body fat mass and CRP were the primary determinants of insulin resistance in nondiabetic hemodialysis patients. High energy supplementation, increased adiposity, and inflammation exacerbated insulin resistance. However, long term metabolic effects of this strategy were unclear (Hung & Tang, 2009).

Another study on nondiabetic hemodialysis patients showed that liver fat, visceral adiposity, and sleep disturbances contributed to the development of insulin resistance and glucose intolerance. However, further studies in the long term are still needed to clarify whether interventions that improve insulin sensitivity improve clinical outcomes and CV risk in nondiabetic hemodialysis patients (Sakkas et al., 2008). The study comparing fasting glucose levels and impaired fasting glucose levels with malnutrition and inflammatory parameters in nondiabetic hemodialysis patients demonstrated that fasting glucose levels predict one-year all-cause mortality in non-diabetic hemodialysis patients. And they also showed that basal fasting glucose levels, or the presence of impaired fasting glucose, plays an important role in inflammation, malnutrition and short term mortality (Lin-Tan, 2007).
Diabetes mellitus and deficiency in n-3 long-chain polyunsaturated fatty acids are known to increase the incidence of CV disease. The study investigated the relationship between n-3 long-chain polyunsaturated fatty acids and the pulse wave velocity from the brachium to the ankle, which was measured as a marker of atherosclerosis in 54 diabetic and 93 nondiabetic hemodialysis patients. The mean pulse wave velocity in diabetic patients was significantly higher than that of nondiabetic patients. There was a significant inverse association between pulse wave velocity and docasahexaenoic acid levels and docasahexaenoic acid/aracidonic acid ratios in nondiabetic patients. It was concluded that n-3 long-chain polyunsaturated fatty acids may be a negative risk factor for CV disease in nondiabetic hemodialysis patients (Hamazaki et al., 2009).
Numerous abnormalities of lipid and lipoprotein metabolism are described in renal disease. These abnormalities are caused by complex alterations in several pathways of lipoprotein metabolism. In addition, nonenzymatic modification of lipoprotein particles enhances their atherogenicity without affecting the measured levels of cholesterol, triglycerides, or the HDL, LDL and very-low-density lipoprotein fractions (Tomson, 2000). Dyslipidemia may be present in more than 90 % of hemodialysis patients and has been reported to correlate with CV disease in some, but not all, cross sectional studies of nondiabetic patients on hemodialysis. Among other lipid parameters, low HDL cholesterol was one of the independent determinants of coronary artery disease in nondiabetic hemodialysis patients (Zumrutdal et al., 2007). However there are limited data concerning the effectiveness of lipid lowering with statins in decreasing CV outcomes in patients on hemodialysis.
Coagulation defects: In 68 nondiabetic hemodialysis patients, the probable association of circulating levels of plasminogen activator inhibitor type-1 and the expression of plasminogen activator inhibitor type-1 in internal iliac artery walls with atherosclerotic disease was investigated. Fifty age- and sex-matched healthy normotensive controls participated in the study. Atherosclerotic disease in both groups was assessed by measuring carotid intima-media thickness. Compared with control subjects, hemodialysis patients had significantly increased carotid thickness. Atherosclerotic plaques were detected in 61.7% of hemodialysis patients and 4% of controls. Carotid intima-media thickness was correlated with age, systolic blood pressure, low-density lipoprotein, CRP, and interleukin-6. In hemodialysis patients, a close correlation was found between serum plasminogen activator inhibitor type-1 level, CRP, and interleukin-6 level. Also, carotid intima-media thickness and plaque score were correlated with circulating levels of plasminogen activator inhibitor type-1 and with the expression of it in internal iliac artery walls. The circulating levels of plasminogen activator inhibitor type-1 and the expression of plasminogen activator inhibitor type-1 in internal iliac rtery walls were statistically associated with CRP, interleukin-6, and low density lipoprotein cholesterol. With all of those correlations, authors have suggested that increased circulating plasminogen

activator inhibitor type-1 and an upregulated expression of plasminogen activator inhibitor type- 1 in the vasculature could indicate a chronic endothelium activated state and that may identify the risk of atherothrombosis related with inflammation in nondiabetic hemodialysis patients (Peng et al., 2008). Among nondiabetic patients, generalized endothelial dysfunction is associated with an increase in CV risk.

Gene polymorphisms: Cytokine gene polymorphisms have been implicated as potential genetic risk factors for CV disease. The study assessed the role of cytokine gene polymorphisms in carotid intima-media thickness and left ventricular mass index, as surrogate markers for CV risk, in nondiabetic hemodialysis patents. Carotid intima-media thickness and left ventricular mass index progression for 2 years were detected at higher levels in patients with high-producer genotypes than in the patients with the low-producer genotype during the study period. The TNF-alpha-308 G/A polymorphism was closely associated with CRP. So polymorphisms in inflammatory genes could be additional factors affecting inflammation and CV risk in non diabetic hemodialysis patients (Yilmaz et al., 2010).

Synthesis of nitric oxide by endothelial nitric oxide synthase plays a key role in the atherosclerotic process. Several polymorphisms of the gene encoding endothelial nitric oxide synthase are known and have been investigated with respect to their influence on CV disease risk in the general population. The association between endothelial nitric oxide synthase gene polymorphism and CV events in nondiabetic Japanese hemodialysis patients was also investigated. Three endothelial nitric oxide synthase polymorphisms were genotyped for the patients and two endothelial nitric oxide synthase polymorphisms were found to be associated with major cardiac, cerebrovascular, or peripheral vascular events (Asakimori et al., 2004).

5.2 Coronary artery disease in nondiabetic hemodialysis patients

It is increasingly appreciated that chronic renal failure alone is an independent risk factor for the development of coronary artery disease. For evaluating the determinants of coronary artery disease in nondiabetic hemodialysis patients, among 312 consecutive patients on regular hemodialysis, 26 nondiabetic patients with angiographically defined coronary artery disease were compared with a subject group of nondiabetic hemodialysis patients of the same gender, smoking status, and hypertension with similar ages and body mass indexes, who had normal electrocardiography and myocardial perfusion scintigraphy. Demographics, CRP, ESR, Hct-corrected ESR, beta 2 microglobulin, cardiac troponin I, parathyroid hormone, albumin, calcium X phosphorus, and lipid profiles were compared between the groups. The nondiabetic patients with coronary artery disease had higher CRP, higher cardiac troponin I, and lower HDL-cholesterol levels than the patients without coronary artery disease. Backwards stepwise logistic regression analysis revealed that high CRP and troponin I levels and low HDL cholesterol levels were independently related with coronary artery disease in nondiabetic hemodialysis patients (Zumrutdal et al., 2007).

The predictive value of CRP in CV risk and mortality in hemodialysis patients was previously shown in numerious studies, and underlying coronary artery disease may be one of the possible links for this elevation. Additionally, even small elevations of serum cardiac troponin I concentration, at levels lower than those traditionally used for the diagnosis of acute events, were independently associated with the presence of coronary artery disease in asymptomatic hemodialysis patients. Thus, small and non-specific increases in cardiac troponin I levels may reflect underlying coronary artery disease in nondiabetic hemodialysis patients.

6. Conclusion

All hemodialysis patients, diabetic or nondiabetic, are at markedly increased CV risk, with chronic renal disease alone currently considered a coronary heart disease risk equivalent. A large number of risk factors for CV disease and decreased survival that are related or unrelated to the dialysis procedure have been identified. Since no data are available about the outcome comparing hemodialysis patients with comorbidities with those without, it is not possible to suggest increased benefits for survival for hemodialysis patients without comorbidities. Cardiovascular risk factor modification should be undertaken for all dialysis patients with or without comorbidities, given that they are considered a coronary heart disease equivalent.

7. References

Afsar, B., Elsurer, R., Akgul, A., Sezer, S., & Ozdemir, FN. (2009). Factors related to silent myocardial damage in hemodialysis patients. *Renal Failure*. Vol.31, No:10, pp.933-941, ISSN 0886-022X

Andress, DL. (2008). Bone and mineral guidelines for patients with kidney disease: a call for revision. *Clinical Journal of the American Society of Nephrology*. Vol.3, No:1, pp.179-183, ISSN1555-9041

Arici, M., Walls, J. (2001). End stage renal disease, atherosclerosis, and cardiovascular mortality: Is C- reactive protein the missing link? *Kidney International*. Vol.59, No:2, pp. 407-414, ISSN0085-2538

Asakimori, Y., Yorioka, N., Tanaka, J., Takasugi, N., Harada, S., Shigemoto, K., Yamashita, K. et al. (2004). Association between ENOS gene polymorphism and cardiovascular events in nondiabetic hemodialysis patients: a prospective study. *American Journal of Kidney Disease*. Vol.44, No:1, pp.112-120,0272-6386.

Bodor, GS., Survant, L., Voss, EM., Smith, S., Porterfield, D., & Apple, FS. (1997). Cardiac troponin T composition in normal and regenerating human skeletal muscle. *Clinical Chemistry*. Vol. 43, No:3, pp.476-484, ISSN0009-9147

Borawski, J., Mysliwic, M. The hematocrit corrected erythrocyte sedimentation rate can be useful in diagnosing inflammation in hemodialysis patients. (2001). *Nephron*. Vol.89, No:4, pp.381-383, 0028-2766

Cheung, AK.,Sarnak, MJ., Yan, G., Dwyer, JT., Heyka, RJ., Rocco, MV., Teehan, BP. et al.(2000). Atherosclerotic cardiovascular disease risks in chronic hemodialysis patients. *Kidney International*. Vol.58, No:1, pp.353-362, ISSN0085-2538

Cianciolo, G., Cli, L., La Mana, G., Donati, G., D'Addio, F. Comai, G., Ricci, D., et al. (2007). Is beta 2 microglobulin- related amyloidosis of hemodialysis patients a multifactorial disease? A new pathogenetic approach. *The Internal Journal of Artificial Organs*. Vol 30, No: 10, pp. 864-878, ISSN0391-3988

Drüeke, TB., Massy, ZA. (2009). Beta 2 microglobulin. *Seminars in Dialysis*. Vol.22, No: 4, pp. 378-380, 0894-0959

Ekart, R., Hojs, R., Hojs-Fabjan, T., & Balon, BP.(2005). Predictive value of carotid intima media thickness in hemodialysis patients. *Artificial Organs*. Vol. 29, No: 8, pp. 615-619, ISSN0160-564X

Ekart, R., Hojs, R., Bevc, S., & Balon, BP. (2008). Asymptomatic atherosclerosis and hypertension in nondiabetic patients with chronic kidney disease. *Artificial Organs*. Vol. 32, No: 3, pp.220-225, ISSN0160-564X

Filiopoulos, V., Hadjiyannakos, D., Takouli, L., Metaxaki, P., Sideris, V., & Vlassopoulos, D. (2009). Inflammation and oxidative stres in end stage renal disease patients treated with hemodialysis or peritoneal dialysis. *The International Journal of Artificial Organs.* Vol. 32, No: 12, pp. 872-882, ISSN 0391-3988

Filiopoulos, V., Vlassopoulos, D. (2009). İnflammatory syndrome in chronic kidney disease: pathogenesis and influence on outcomes. *İnflammation& Allergy Drug Targets.* Vol. 8, No:5, pp. 369-382. ISSN 1871-5281

Goodkin, Da., Bragg-Gresham, JL., Koenig, KG., Wolfe, RA., Akiba, T., Andreucci, VE., & Saito, A et al. (2003). Association of comorbid conditions and mortality in hemodialysis patients in Europe, Japan, and the United States: the dialysis Outcomes and Practice Patterns Study (DOPPS). *Journal of American Society of Nephrology.* Vol.14, No:12, pp. 3270-3277, ISSN 1046-6673

Haller, C., Zehelein, J., Remppis, A., Müler-Bardorff, M., & Katus, HA. (1998). Cardiac Troponin T in patients with end stage renal disease. Absence of expression in truncal skeletal muscle. *Clinical Chemistry.* Vol.44, No:5, pp. 930-938, ISSN0009-9147

Hamazaki, K., Terashima, Y., Itomura, M., Sawazaki, S., Inagaki, H., Kuroda, M., Tomita, S. et al. (2009). The relationship between n-3 long-chain polyunsaturated fatty acids and pulse wave velocity in diabetic and non-diabetic patients under long-term hemodialysis. *Clinical Nephrology.* Vol.71, No: 5, pp. 508-513, ISSN0301-0430

Hocher, B., Ziebig, R., Altermann, C., Krause, R., Asmus, G., Richter, CM., Slowinski, et al. Different impact of biomarkers as mortality predictors among diabetic and nondiabetic patients undergoing hemodialysis. (2003). *Journal of American Society of Nephrology.* Vol.14, No: 9, pp. 2329-2337, ISSN1046-6673

Hung, SC., Tarng, DC. (2009). Adiposity and insulin resistance in nondiabetic hemodialysis patients: effects of high energy supplementation. *The American Journal of the Clinical Nutrition.* Vol.90, No:1, pp.64-69,0002-9165

Io, H., Matsumoto, M., Okumura, K., Sato, M., Masuda, A., Furukawa, M., Nohara N, et al. (2010). Predictive factors associated with left ventricular hypertrophy at baseline and in the follow-up period in non-diabetic hemodialysis patients. *Seminars in Dialysis.* Epub ahead of print.Augst.13., ISSN0894-0959

Ishimura, E., Okuno, S., Taniwaki, H., Kizu, A., Tsuchida, T., Shioi A, Shoji T, et al. (2008). Different risk factors for vascular calcification in end-stage renal disease between diabetics and non-diabetics: the respective importance of glycemic and phosphate control. *Kidney Blood Pressure Research.* Vol. 31, No: 1, pp.10-15, ISSN1420-4096

Kals, J., Zagura, M., Serg, M., Kampus, P., Zilmer, K., Unt, E., Lieberg, et al. (2011). Beta 2 microglobulin, a novel biomarker of peripheral arterial disease, idependently predicts aortic stifness in these patients. *Scandinavian Journal of Clinical and Laboratory Investigation.* Epub ahead of print. 2011 Feb.14. ISSN 0085-591X

Kanderian, AS., Francis, GS. (2006). Cardiac troponins and chronic kidney disease. *Kidney International.* Vol. 69, No:7, pp.1112-1114, ISSN0085-2538

Kanwar, M., Hashem, M., Romsan, H., Kamalakannan, D., Cheema, A., Ali, A., Gadrin, J., & Maciejko, JJ. (2006). Usefulness of clinical evaluation, troponins, and C-reactive protein in predicting mortality among stable hemodialysis patients. *American Journal of Cardiology.* Vol.98, No: 9, pp.1283-1287, ISSN 0002-9149

Kasiske, BL.,Chakkera, HA., Roel, J. (2000). Explained and unexplained ischemic herat disease risk after renal transplantation. *Journal of the American Society of Nephrology.* Vol.11, No:9, pp. 1735-1743, ISSN1046-6673

Kawai, K., Kawashima, S., Miyazaki, T., Tajiri, E., Mori, M., Kitazaki, K., Shirotani, T. et al. (2010). Serum Beta 2 microglobulin concentration as a novel marker to distinguish levels of risk in acute heart failure patients. *Journal of Cardiology*. Vol.55, No:1, pp.99-107, ISSN0914-5087

Kaysen, GA., Eiserich, JP. (2004). The role of oxidative stres-altered lipoprotein structure and function and microinflammation on cardiovascular risk in patients with minor renal dysfunction. *Journal of American Society of Nephrology*. Vol:15, No:3, pp. 538-548,ISSN 1046-6673

Kumar, J., Shah, SV. (2005). Kidney disease as an independent risk factor for cardiovascular events. *Journal of Renal Nutrition*. Vol. 15, No:1, pp. 99-104. ISSN 1051-2276

Kunstmann, S., Vukusich, A., Michea, L., Varela, C., Allende, I., Bravo S, Gainza D, et al. (2009). Cardiovascular assessment of non diabetic patients on hemodialysis. *Revista Medica de Chile*. Vol. 137, No:3, pp: 351-360, ISSN0034-9887

Kuragano, T., Kida, A., Furuta, M., Nanami, M., Otaki, Y., Hasuike, Y., Nonoguchi, H., & Nakanishi, T. (2010). The impact of beta 2microglobulin clearence on the risk factors of cardiovascular disease in hemodialysis patients. *American Society for Artificial Internal Organs*. Vol. 56, No:4, pp. 326-332, ISSN1058-2916

Lagrand, WK., Niessen, HWM., Wolbink, GJ., Jaspars, LH., Visser, CA., Verheugt, FW., Meijer, CJ,. et al. (1997). C-reactive protein colocalizes with complement in human hearts during acute myocardial infarction. *Circulation*. Vol.95, No:1, pp. 97-103, ISSN0009-7322

Levin, A., Li, YC. (2005). Vitamin D and its analogues: do they protect against cardiovascular disease in patients with kidney disease? *Kidney International*. Vol.68, No: 5, pp.1973-1981, ISSN0085-2538

Lin-Tan, DT., Lin, JL., Wang, LH., Wang, LM., Huang, LM., Liu, L., Huang, JY., & Huang, YL. (2007). Fasting glucose levels in predicting 1-year mortality in patients who do not have diabetes and are on maintenance hemodialysis. *Journal of the American Society of Nephrology*. Vol. 18, No: 8, pp. 2385-2391, ISSN1046-6673

London, GM; Drüeke, TB. (1997). Atherosclerosis and arteriosclerosis in chronic renal failure. *Kidney International*. Vol.51, No. 6, pp. 1678-1695, ISSN0085-2538

London, GM., Marchais, SJ., Metivier, F., & Guerin, AP. (2000). Cardiovascular risk in end stage renal disease: vascular aspects. *Nephrology Dialysis Transplantation*. Vol.15, Suppl 5, pp.97-101, ISSN0931-0509

Ma, KW., Grene, EL., Raij, L. Cardiovascular risk factors in chronic renal failure and hemodialysis populations. (1992). *American Journal of Kidney Disease*. Vol. 19, No:6, pp.505-513, 0272-6386

Mailloux, LU., Bellluci, AG., Wilkes, BM.,Napolitano, B., Mosset, RT., Lesser, M., & Bluestone, PA. (1991). Mortality in dialysis patients: analyses of the causes of death. *American Journal of Kidney Diseases*. Vol.18, No:3, pp. 326-335, ISSN0272-6386

Mailloux, LU., Napolitano, B., Bellucci, AG., Mossey, RT., Vernace, MA., & Wilkes, BM. (1996). The impact of co-morbid risk factors at the start of dialysis upon the survival of ESRD patients. *American Society for Artificial Internal Organs*. Vol 42, No:3, pp.164-169, ISSN 1058-2916

Mailloux, LU., Henrich, WL. (2010). Patient survival and maintenence dialysis. wwwUpToDatecom, Editors; Berns JS& Post WT, pp.1-27

McLaurin, MD., Apple, FS., Voss, EM., Herzog, CA., & Sharkey, SW. (1997). Cardiac troponin I, cardiac troponin T, and creatinine kinase MB in dialysis patients without ischemic heart disease: Evidence of cardiac troponin T expression in skeletal muscle. *Clinical Chemistry*. Vol.43, No:6, pp.976-982, ISSN 0009-9147

Merkus, MP., Jager, KJ., Dekker, FW., de Haan, RJ., Boeschoten, EW., & Kredit, RT. (2000). Predictors of poor outcome in chronic dialysis patients: The Netherlands Cooperative Study on the Adequacy of Dialysis. The NECOSAD Study Group. *American Journal Of Kidney Disease*. Vol.35, No:1, pp. 69-79, ISSN 0272-6386

Miskulin, D., Bragg-Gresham, J., Gillespie, BW., Tentori, F., Pisoni, RL., Tiqhiouart, H., Levey, AS. et al. (2009). Key comorbid conditions that are predictive of survival among hemodialysis patients. *Clinical Journal of the American Society of Nephrology*. Vol. 4, no:11, pp.1818-1826, 1555-9041

O' Sullivan, AJ., Kelly, JJ. (2007). Insulin resistance and protein catabolism in non diabetic hemodialysis patients. *Kidney International*. Vol.71, No:2, pp.98-100, ISSN0085-2538

Okuno, S., Ishimura, E., Kohno, K., Fujino-Katoh, Y., Maeno, Y., Yamakawa, T., Inaba, M., & Nishizawa, Y. (2009). *Nephrology Dialysis Transplantation*. Vol.24, No: 2, pp.571-577, ISSN0931-0509

Parfrey, PS. (2000). Cardiac disease in dialysis patients: diagnosis, burden of disease, prognosis, risk factors and management. *Nephrology Dialysis and Transplantation*, Vol.15, Suppl.5, pp. L58-68, ISSN0931-0509

Peng, Y., Liu, H., Liu, F., Ouyang, L., Cheng M, Gao L, Pan F. et al. (2008). Atherosclerosis is associated with plasminogen activator inhibitor type-1 in chronic hemodialysis patients. *Nephrology (Carlton)*. Vol.13, No: 7, pp. 579-586, ISSN1320-5358

Pepys, MB., Baltz, ML.(1983). Acute phase proteins with special reference to C-reactive protein and related proteins (pentaxins) and serum amyloid a protein. *Advances in Immunology*. Vol: 34, pp. 141-212, ISSN 0065-2776

Sakkas, GK., Karatzaferi, C., Zintzaras, E., Giannaki, CD., Liakopoulos, V., Lavdas, E., Damani, E. et al. (2008). Liver fat, visceral adiposity, and sleep disturbances contribute to the development of insulin resistance and glucose intolerance in nondiabetic dialysis patients. *American Journal of Physiology: Regulatory, Integrative and Comparative Physiology*. Vol. 295, No: 6, pp.1721-1729, ISSN0363-6119

Sarnak, MJ., Levey, AS., Scoolwerth, AC., Coresh, J., Culleton B, Hamm, LL., McCullough, PA. et al. (2003). Kidney disease as a risk factor for development of cardiovascular disease: a statement from the American Heart Association Councils on Kidney in Cardiovascular Disease, High Blood Pressure Research, Clinical Cardiology, and Epidemiology and Prevention. *Circulation*. Vol. 108, No:17, pp. 2154-2169, ISSN 0009-7322

Schlieper, G., Brandenburg, V., Djuric, Z., Damjanovic, T., Markovic, N., Schurgers, L., Kruger, T. et al. (2009). Risk factors for cardiovascular calcifications in-diabetic Caucasian Hemodialysis patients. *Kidney Blood Pressure Research.*. Vol.32, No: 3, pp161-168, ISSN1420-4096

Stenvinkel, P. (2002). İnflammation in end-stage renal failure: could it be treated? *Nephrology Dialysis Transplantation*. Vol.17, suppl.8, pp. 33-38, ISSN0931-0509

Stenvinkel, P., Alvestrand, A. (2002). Inflammation in end-stage renal disease: sources, consequences, and therapy. *Seminars in Dialysis*. Vol.15, No:5, pp. 329-337, ISSN 0894-0959

Stenvinkel, P. (2006). İnflammation in end-stage renal disease: the hidden enemy. *Nephrology* (Carlton). Vol. 11, No:1, pp.36-41, ISSN 1320-5358

Tomson, CRV. (2000). Cardiovascular disease in chronic renal failure. In: *Comprehensive Clinical Nephrology (2nd edition)*. Johnson RJ & Feehally J, pp. 887-904, Mosby-Elsevier, ISBN 07234 32589, Philadelphia

Torzewski, J., Torzewski, M., Bowyer, DE., Fröhlich, M., Koenig, W., Waltenberger, J., Fitzsimmons, C. et al. (1998). C-reactive protein frequently colocalizes with the terminal complement complex in the intima of early atherosclerotic lesions of human coronary arteries. *Arteriosclerosis, Thrombosis, and Vascular Biology*. Vol. 18, No:9, pp.1386-1392,ISSN 1079-5642

Tzanatos, HA., Tseke, PP., Pipili, C., Retsa, K., Skoutelis, G., & Grapsa, E. (2009). Cardiovascular risk factors in non-diabetic hemodialysis patients: a comparative study. *Renal Failure*. Vol. 31, No:2, pp.91-97, ISSN0886-022X

Vigushin, DM., Pepys, MB., Hawkins, PN.(1993). Metabolic and scintigraphic studies of radioiodinated human C- reactive protein in health and disease. *The Journal of Clinical Investigation*. Vol. 91, No:4, pp. 1351-1357, ISSN 0021-9738

Vraetz, T., Ittel, TH., Mackelenbergh, MG., Heinrich, PC., Sieberth, HG., & Graeve, L. (1999). Regulation of beta 2 microglobulin expression in different human cell lines by proinflammatory cytokines. *Nephrology Dialysis and Transplantation*. Vol.14, no:9, pp.2137-2143, 0931-0509

Wallen, MD., Radhakrishnan, J., Appel, G., Hodgson, ME., & Pablos-Mendez, A. (2001). An analysis of cardiac mortality in patients with new-onset end stage renal disease in New York state. *Clinical Nephrology*. Vol. 55, No.2, pp.101-108, ISSN0301-0430

Wilson, AM., Kimura, E., Harada, RK., Nair, N., Narasimhan, B, Meng, XY., Zhang, F., et al. (2007). Beta 2 microglobulin as a biomarker in peripheral arterial disease: proteomic profiling and clinical studies. *Circulation*. Vol.116, No: 12, pp.1396-1403, ISSN0009-7322

Xie, J., Yi Q. (2003). Beta 2 microglobulin as a potential initiator of inflammatory responses. *Trends in Immunology*. Vol. 24, No:5, pp. 228-229, ISSN1471-4906

Yeun, JY., Kaysen GA. (2000). C-reactive protein, oxidative stres, homocysteine, and troponin as inflammatory and metabolic predictors of atherosclerosis in ESRD. *Current Opinion in Nephrology and Hypertension*. Vol. 9, No:6, pp.621-630, ISSN1062-4821

Yılmaz, R. Altun, B., Ozer, N., Hazirolan, T.,& Turgan, C. (2010). Impact of cytokine genotype on cardiovascular surrogate markers in hemodialysis patients. *Renal Failure*. Vol.32, No:7, pp.806-816, ISSN0886-022X.

Zimmermann, J., Herrlinger, S., Pruy, A., Metzger, T., & Wanner, C. (1999). İnflammation enhances cardiovascular risk and mortality in hemodialysis patients. *Kidney International Suppl*. Vol. 55, No:2, pp. 648-658, ISSN 0098-6577

Zumrutdal, AO., Bakıner, O., Ucan, H., Atalay, HV., & Bodur, H. (2000). Relationship between uremic myopathy and false-positive cardiac troponin T test. *Nephron*. Vol. 86, No:4, pp. 522-523, ISSN0028-2766

Zumrutdal, A., Sezer, S., Demircan. S., Seydaoglu. G., Ozdemir, FN, & Haberal, M. (2005). Cardiac troponin I and beta 2 microglobulin as risk factors for early- onset atherosclerosis in patients on haemodialysis. *Nephrology*. Vol. 10, No:5, pp. 453-458, ISSN 1320-5358

Zumrutdal, A., Demircan, S., Seydaoglu, G., Singan, M., Sezer, S., Ozdemir, FN., & Haberal, M. (2006). Atherosclerosis in haemodialysis patients without significant comorbidities: Determinants of progression. *Nephrology*. Vol. 11, No:6, pp 489-493, ISSN 1320-5358

Zumrutdal, A., Baltali, M., Micozkadioglu, H., Torun, D., Sezer, S., Ozdemir, FN. & Haberal M. (2007). Determinants of coronary artery disease in nondiabetic hemodialysis patients: A matched case-control study. *Renal Failure*. Vol. 29, No:1, pp.67-71, ISSN0886-022X

6

Complications and Management of Hyperphosphatemia in Dialysis

Eiji Takeda, Hironori Yamamoto, Hisami Yamanaka-Okumura and Yutaka Taketani
University of Tokushima Graduate School
Japan

1. Introduction

1.1 High mortality in dialysis patients

Dialysis patients have extraordinarily high mortality rates. Cardiac disease is the major cause of death accounting for 43% of all-cause mortality among patients receiving hemodialysis and peritoneal dialysis [Henry et al., 2002; US Renal Data System Annual Data Report Bethesta, 2005]. In previous report, patients with end-stage kidney disease (chronic kidney disease (CKD) stage 5) on dialysis, in comparison with the general population, also have a 3- to 30-fold increase in mortality, depending on the age group examined, and cardiovascular disease accounts for more than half of all deaths, with myocardial infarction, ischaemic cardiomyopathy, stroke and peripheral vascular disease making up the bulk of deaths (Foley et al., 1998). The marked excess in cardiovascular mortality in CKD, compared with the general population, is not explained by the presence of traditional Framingham risk factors, such as diabetes, smoking, hypertension and elevated cholesterol levels (Zoccali, 2000; Longenecker et al., 2002). With vascular calcification and arterial stiffness being observed in young and middle-aged dialysis patients without conventional cardiovascular risk factors (London et al., 2003), the search for non-traditional risk factors has led to increasing evidence of a multitude of factors that contribute to ectopic calcification in CKD.

1.2 High mortality rate and hyperphosphatemia

Inorganic phosphate (phosphate) retention, or hyperphosphatemia, has been identified as playing a major role in the progression of renal failure and in the generation of secondary hyperparathyroidism and uremic bone disease (Slatopolsky et al., 2002). Further observational data have also shown a significant association of hyperphosphatemia with increased mortality among patients who have end-stage kidney disease and are on hemodialysis (Block et al., 1998; Owen & Lowrie, 1998; Ganesh et al., 2001). Moreover, elevated serum phosphorus has been associated with an increased risk for cardiovascular mortality and hospitalization (all-cause, cardiovascular, and fracture) among dialysis patients (Block et al., 2004). Elevated phosphorus and Ca × P are also independent risk factors for all-cause and cardiovascular mortality in CKD stage 5, and increased levels of parathyroid hormone may be associated with both cardiovascular disease and increased vascular calcification (Braun et al., 1996; Block et al., 1998; Ganesh et al., 2001; Wang et al., 2003; Young et al., 2005). Thus, phosphorus has the potential to induce vascular calcification and may be cardiotoxic (Achinger & Ayus, 2006). Hyperphosphatemia is sometimes regarded as a distinct syndrome (Hruska et al., 2008), and its treatment should be considered preferentially and even independently of other laboratory values (Fig. 1).

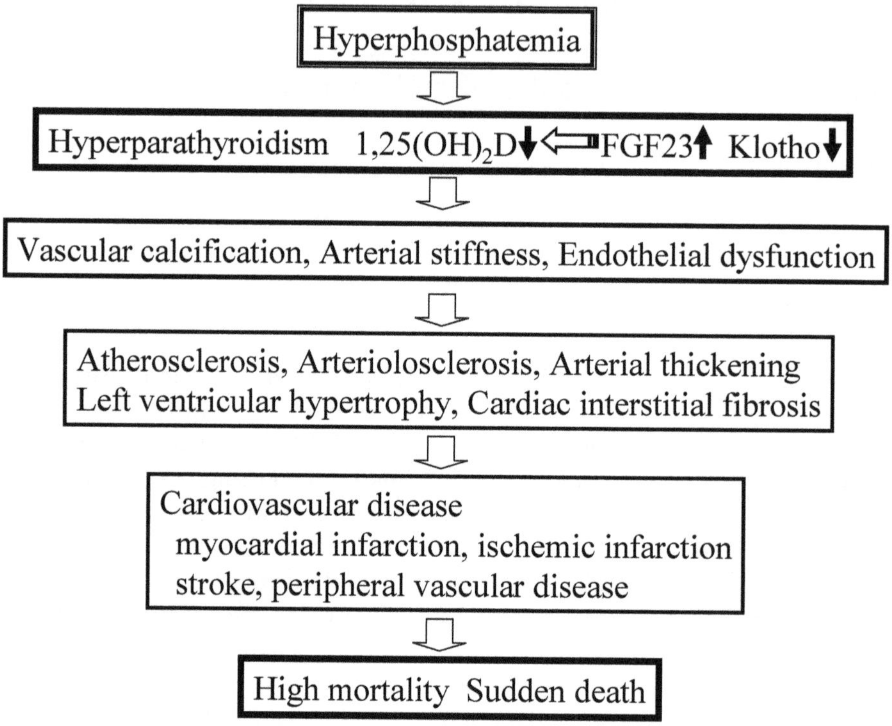

Fig. 1. Hyperphosphatemia in hemodialysis

2. Phosphate metabolism in human

2.1 Phosphate metabolism in normal physiology

Phosphorus is essential for multiple and diverse biological functions, including cellular signal transduction, mineral metabolism, and energy exchange. Although more than 80% of total body phosphorus is stored in bone and teeth, intracellular phosphorus exists in the form of organic compounds such as adenosine triphosphate and as free anions like $H_2PO_4^-$, which are commonly referred to as phosphate. Serum phosphorus primarily occurs in the form of inorganic phosphate, which is maintained within the physiological range by regulation of dietary absorption, bone formation, and renal excretion, as well as equilibration with intracellular stores (Takeda et al., 2000; Bringhurst et al., 2004; Fukagawa et al., 2004; Blumsohn, 2004).

Phosphate absorption in the renal proximal tubule and the small intestine is important for phosphate homeostasis. This is a major regulator of phosphate homeostasis and has the phosphate reabsorptive capacity to accommodate physiologic phosphate requirement. Up to 70% of filtered phosphate is reabsorbed in the proximal tubule where sodium-dependent phosphate transport systems in the brush-border membrane mediate the rate limiting step in the overall phosphate reabsorptive process (Murer et al, 2000; Takeda et al, 2000; Miyamoto et al, 2007; Tenenhouse, 2005; Biber et al, 2009). Three different types of sodium-dependent phosphate transporters have been identified till now, types I, II and III. The sodium-dependent phosphate transport system includes the type IIa and type IIc Na-dependent phosphate cotransporters, which are localized in the apical membrane of the renal proximal tubular cells, and the type IIb Na-dependent phosphate cotransporter, which is localized in the apical membrane of the intestinal epithelial cells. The type IIa Na-dependent phosphate transporter is the major determinant of plasma phosphate level and urinary phosphate excretion (Murer et al, 2000; Takeda et al, 2000; Miyamoto et al, 2007; Tenenhouse, 2005; Biber et al, 2009). This transporter is regulated by physiological stimuli, for example, type IIa transporter levels in the apical membrane are increased in response to dietary restriction of phosphate and 1,25-dihydroxy-vitamin D_3 [1,25$(OH)_2D_3$] and decreased in response to parathyroid hormone, or a high- phosphate diet. In addition, intestinal phosphate transport activity and type IIb Na-dependent phosphate transporter levels are upregulated by 1,25$(OH)_2D_3$ (Xu et al., 2002; Segawa et al., 2004).

In addition, fibroblast growth factor 23 (FGF23), a recently identified member of the FGF family, is involved in renal phosphate homeostasis (Yu X & White, 2005; Yu & White, 2005). FGF23 induces urinary phosphate excretion by suppressing the expression of type IIa and IIc Na-dependent phosphate cotransporters in the brush border of renal proximal tubules (Shimada et al., 2004; Shimada et al., 2005). It also suppresses 1,25$(OH)_2D$ production by inhibiting 1a-hydroxylase (CYP27B1), which converts 25-hydroxyvitamin D [25(OH)D] to 1,25$(OH)_2D$, and by stimulating 24-hydroxylase (CYP24), which converts 1,25$(OH)_2D$ to inactive metabolites in the proximal tubule of the kidney (Shimada et al., 2004; Shimada et al., 2005). Given the fact that FGF23 promotes renal phosphaturia, its secretion should be regulated by serum phosphate levels. Experimental and clinical studies showed that several days of dietary phosphate loading lead to an increase in serum FGF23 in humans (Ferrari et al, 2005; Perwad et al., 2005; Nishida et al., 2006).

2.2 Phosphate metabolism in hemodialysis patients

Several studies have measured circulating FGF23 levels in predialysis and dialysis patients and reported progressively elevated FGF23 levels as serum creatinine or phosphate levels increase (Larsson et al., 2003; Imanishi et al., 2004). Thus, it appears that in patients with CKD, FGF23 production increases to counteract chronic phosphate retention by promoting urinary phosphate excretion in the face of reduced nephron mass. Notably, in this setting, a previous study showed that FGF23 was a strong independent predictor of diminished 1,25$(OH)_2D$ levels, even after adjustment for renal function, serum phosphorus levels and 25(OH)D levels (Gutierrez et al., 2005). This finding suggests that in patients with CKD, increases in FGF23 intended to maintain neutral phosphate balance result in suppression of renal 1,25$(OH)_2D$ production, thereby triggering the early development of secondary hyperparathyroidism (Fig. 1).

3. Cardiovascular disease in hemodyalysis

3.1 Hyperphosphatemia and cardiovascular disease

Cardiomyopathy and ischemic heart disease including acute myocardial infarctions, which are both common conditions in dialysis patients, likely play a role in the development of sudden death. After percutaneous and surgical coronary revascularization, dialysis patients are still remaining at a high risk for sudden cardiac death (Furgeson, 2008). Hyperphosphatemia is a known factor contributing to the increased risk of cardiac death both in patients with end-stage renal disease and in those under renal replacement treatment with dialysis (Goodman et al., 2000). In patients with renal disease, in fact, the well-known relationship between hyperphosphataemia, secondary hyperparathyroidism, bone turnover and extra osseous calcifications has recently been followed by the recognition of a major role played by elevated serum phosphorus levels in the induction of vascular calcification, cardiac interstitial fibrosis and arterial thickening which highly increase the risk of cardiac death (Goodman et al., 2000; Block & Port, 2000; Amann et al., 2003; Goldsmith et al., 2004; Floege & Ketteler, 2004).

3.2 Vascular calcification

Phosphate is probably the predominant inducer of vascular calcification, and elevated serum levels are strongly associated with increased vascular calcification and mortality (Goodman et al., 2000). Elevated phosphate triggers a concentration-dependent precipitation of calcium in vascular smooth muscle cells, and phosphate is also a potent stimulus for the differentiation of vascular smooth muscle cells. In vitro studies demonstrate that high phosphate levels in incubation media enhance calcification with associated extracellular matrix synthesis(Jono et al., 2000). Phosphate and sodium dependent phosphate transporter seem to play a very important role in vascular smooth muscle cells mineralization. Type III sodium-dependent phosphate transporter presents two discrete subtypes, Pit-1 and Pit-2. In human vascular smooth muscle cells, Pit-1 is mainly expressed (London et al., 2000). Apatite formation by smooth muscle cells, as a response to increased phosphate levels, is fully inhibited by phosphonoformic acid (PFA), a sodium dependent phosphate transporter inhibitor, a finding supporting the notion that vascular calcification is an active rather than passive cellular process (Giachelli et al., 2001; Ketteler et al., 2003).

Hyperphosphataemia induces osteocalcin and Cbfa-1 in vascular smooth muscle cells and promotes vascular calcification. Animals deficient in Cbfa-1 fail to mineralize bone(Komori et al., 1997), and there is also increased expression of Cbfa-1 when vascular smooth muscle cells are incubated in uremic serum compared with pooled human serum (Moe et al., 2003). There is now considerable evidence that hyperphosphataemia regulates several signalling pathways of cell functions. Of great interest is the recent identification of a novel phosphate-regulating gene, klotho (Kuro-o et al., 1997; Yoshida et al., 2002), which in mice is involved in the development of a syndrome resembling human ageing. The klotho mutant mice show abnormal calcium phosphate vitamin D metabolism and develop hyperphosphataemia and vascular calcification (Kuro-o et al., 1997; Yoshida et al., 2002). Hyperphosphataemia also down-regulates klotho gene expression (Fig. 1).

3.3 Endothelial dysfunction

Endothelial dysfunction is the principal cause of atherosclerosis resulting in cardio vascular disease (Ross, 1999). High phosphate loading on endothelial cells inhibited nitrogen oxide (NO) production through increased reactive oxygen species (ROS) production and endothelial NO syntase (eNOS) inactivation via conventional protein kinase C, resulting in impaired endothelium-dependent vasodilation (Shuto et al., 2009). Furthermore, dietary phosphate loading can deteriorate flow-mediated vasodilation in healthy men, suggesting that dietary phosphate loading or elevation of serum phosphorus level may be a risk factor for cardiovascular disease in healthy persons as well as CKD patients (Takeda et al., 2006; Shuto et al., 2009). Di Marco et al. also reported that high phosphate loading increased ROS production via phosphate influx and induced apoptosis in endothelial cells (Di Marco et al., 2008). Association of serum phosphorus level and vascular dysfunction has been well investigated, because fasting serum phosphorus level could not increase in healthy persons, even if dietary phosphate was overloaded. However, postprandial phosphorus elevation was associated with %FMD in young healthy men (Shuto et al., 2009). Thus, dietary phosphate loading can cause endothelial dysfunction within a short time. Oxidative stress and decreased NO production in endothelial cells are possible mechanisms for the impaired endothelial function mediated by phosphate loading (Fig. 2).

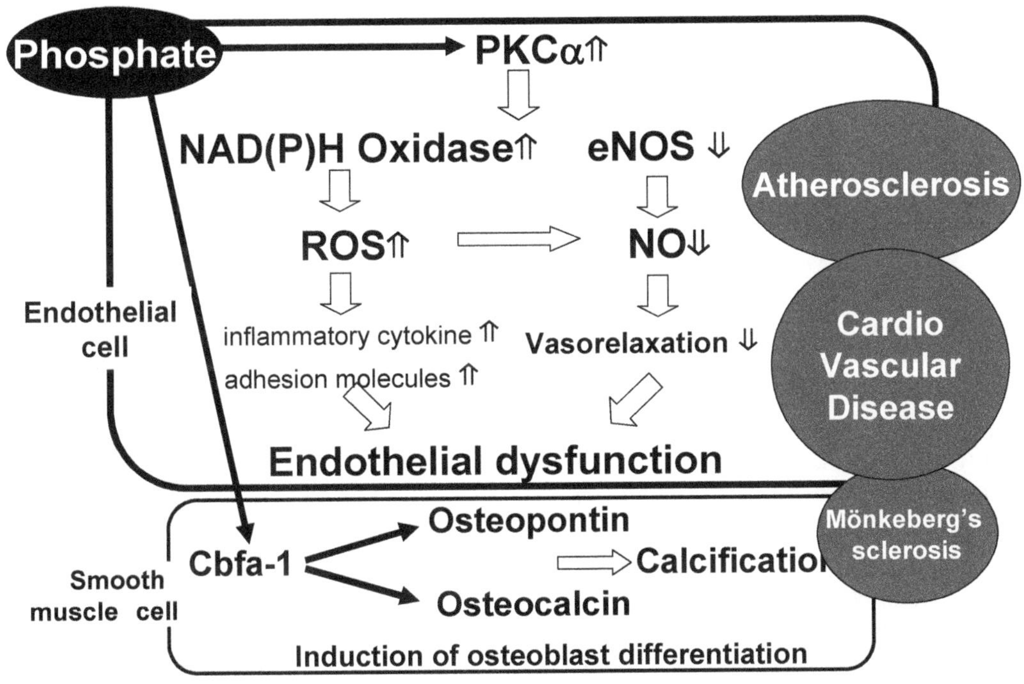

Fig. 2. Dual pathways for vascular dysfunction caused by hyperphosphatemia

3.4 Arterial stiffness

Arterial disease observed in end-stage kidney disease patients is characterized by extensive intimal as well as medial calcification. Histological changes in coronary arteries from dialysis patients, compared with age matched controls, reveal a similar magnitude of atherosclerotic plaque burden and intimal thickness but markedly increased medial calcification (arteriolosclerosis) (Schwarz et al., 2000). Medial calcification has been shown to affect vascular elasticity and leads to increased arterial wall stiffness of large capacity, elastic-type arteries like the aorta and the common carotid artery, increased pulse pressure and decreased perfusion of coronary arteries during diastole (Blacher et al., 1998; London, 2003; Speer & Giachelli, 2004). Recent studies also demonstrated that elevated FGF23 levels were associated with arterial stiffness, increased left ventricular mass index and increased prevalence of left ventricular hypertrophy in patients with CKD (Hsu & Wu, 2009; Mirza et al., 2009; Gutierrez et al., 2009).

4. Management of hyperphosphatemia in hemodialysis patients

4.1 Target of management

As elevated serum phosphorus and calcium levels are associated with vascular calcification and cardiovascular mortality in CKD, priority should be given to normalization of these parameters. It is generally accepted that adequate control of serum phosphorus remains a cornerstone in the clinical management of patients with CKD not only to attenuate the progression of secondary hyperparathyroidism but also possibly to reduce the risk for vascular calcification and cardiovascular mortality. A Ca x P more tan 72 mg^2/dl^2 is associated with a significant increase in the relative risk (RR) of mortality (RR = 1.34) compared with Ca x P less than 50 mg^2/dl^2 (Cozzolino et al., 2001). In a study in patients on hemodialysis, those who did not experience valvular calcification had maintained Ca x P at an average of 51 mg^2/dl^2 in the 6 months prior to the study, while those who did experience valvular calcification had an average Ca x P of 60 mg^2/dl^2 (Ribeiro et al., 1998). The target of treatment should be to maintain serum phosphorus level less than 5 mg/dl with serum calcium level less than 10 mg/dl to prevent cardio vascular consequences. This will allow the maintenance of Ca x P less than 50 mg^2/dl^2, a level which available evidence has so far shown not to promote calcification or increase mortality (Ribeiro et al., 1998).

High FGF23 levels are more strongly associated with kidney disease progression, left ventricular hypertrophy, vascular disease, and mortality than serum phosphorus levels, and were most predictive of adverse events in patients with normal serum phosphorus (Thadhani et al., 2008; Oliveira et al., 2010). Dietary phosphate binders can lower FGF23 in CKD (Oliveira et al., 2010). Management of hyperphosphatemia relies on dietary restriction, the use of phosphate binders and dialysis.

4.2 Dietary restriction of phosphate intake

The average diet in North America and Europe contains approximately 1,000 to 1,500 mg of phosphorus per day (Willett & Buzzard, 1998). Dietary approach to phosphate retention in advanced renal failure patients, dietary approach to phosphate reduction is an important step in the treatment of hyperphosphatemia. The level of expression of klotho mRNA was greatly reduced in the kidneys of all chronic renal failure patients. Dietary phosphate restriction induced klotho expression, which enhances the beneficial effect of phosphate restriction in patients with chronic renal failure and or on hemodialysis. However, dietary restriction cannot considerably reduce the level of phosphate retention. As dialysis patients tend to need higher levels of protein due to the losses via dialysis, tight restriction on phosphate is difficult without compromising a patient's nutritional status. Because most dietary phosphate is contained in protein-rich foods, there is some concern about excessive protein restriction. In fact, the minimum amount of protein of 1.2 g/kg body weight/day, recommended to prevent malnutrition makes planning a diet with less than 1 g of phosphorus impossible (Kopple, 2001; Eknoyan et al., 2003). Recommendations that call for 1.0 to 1.2 g/kg/day protein will usually obligate a phosphorus intake of 800 to 1,400

mg/day. Net phosphorus absorption averages 60% to 70% of intake (Delmez & Slatopolsky, 1992; Sheikh et al., 1989), however, this percentage can rise as high as 86% of ingested phosphate with calcitriol use and decrease to 30% to 40% of ingested phosphate with optimal binder usage.(Sheikh et al., 1989; Delmez & Slatopolsky, 1992).
Other foods that are high in phosphate are processed foods such as processed meats which have phosphate based additives to improve the consistency and appearance of the food. Since 1990, intake of phosphate from additives has doubled and has been 1,000 mg in USA (Calvo & Park, 1996). This is the amount that some renal patients are advised for the whole day from all food groups (James & Jackson, 2002). As people are becoming more reliant on processed and packaged meals due to convenience, phosphate from these sources needs to be considered when advising on diet. Fresh meat is considered suitable for someone following a phosphate restriction, however processed foods may in fact be providing much more phosphate than realised (Sullivan et al., 2007). Beverages such as sodas, juices and sport drinks also contain phosphate additives (Murphy-Gutekunst, 2007). It has been estimated that for a person on hemodialysis the average phosphate removal per day is 300 mg (Vaithilingham et al., 2004). This leaves the patient with a positive balance for phosphate.

4.3 Hemodialysis

The clearance of phosphate varies among the different modalities of dialysis. Ideally, adequate dialysis in any form would remove adequate amounts of all uremic toxins, including phosphate. Unfortunately, conventional thrice-weekly hemodialysis (4 h duration) removes approximately 900 mg of phosphorus each treatment (an average of only 300 mg/day) (Gotch et al., 2003). Increasing the dosage of dialysis, preferably to lengthy three times per week dialysis, hemodiafiltration, or, even better, daily/nightly dialysis may prevent phosphorus retention and even require no dietary phosphate restriction or the withdrawal of phosphate binders (Maduell et al., 2003; Benaroia et al., 2008). However, regular dialysis treatment is not able to remove all the phosphorus ingested with a diet containing protein of 1.0 - 1.2 g/kg/day (Mallick & Gokal, 1999).

4.4 Phosphate binders

Isakova et al analyzed a prospective cohort study of 10,044 incident hemodialysis patients at Fresenius Medical Care facilities in 2004 and 2005 comparing 1-year all-cause mortality among patients who were treated with phosphate binders (Isakova et al., 2009). In an intention-to-treat analysis, they compared patients who began treatment with any phosphate binder during the first 90 days after initiating hemodialysis, with those who remained untreated during that period. Treatment with phosphate binders was independently associated with decreased mortality compared with no treatment. In the unmatched cohort, the phosphate binder-treated group had a relative risk reduction of 42%, while in the intention-to-treat and as-treated analyses, the magnitude of the survival benefit ranged between 18% and 30% in multivariate models. The association between use of phosphorus binders and survival was observed within each quartile of baseline serum phosphorus except the lowest. Results from human data suggest that lowering of phosphorus levels by intake of phosphate binders will substantially reduce serum FGF-23 levels (Koiwa et al., 2005; Pande et al., 2006). In this prospective observational study, treatment with phosphate binders was associated with a reduced 1-year mortality among incident hemodialysis patients (Isakova et al., 2009).

Sevelamer hydrochloride and lanthanum carbonate are a phosphate binders containing neither calcium nor aluminium, and are useful in those being administered concurrent vitamin D to reduce the potential for hypercalcemia. Attenuation in the progression of coronary artery calcification, after 6 and 12 months, was shown in hemodialysis patients treated with sevelamer, with reduced serum calcium, compared with patients on calcium carbonate (Chertow et al., 2002). A more recent randomized study of 114 incident hemodialysis patients demonstrated a survival advantage for patients on sevelamer compared with calcium carbonate after 18-month follow up (Block et al., 2007). A further beneficial effect of sevelamer has been proved on markers of coronary artery and aortic calcification compared with calcium based phosphate binders (Chertow et al., 2002). The attenuation of vascular and, in particular, coronary calcifications compared with calcium-based phosphate binders in end-stage kidney disease patients under dialysis has been studied by electron beam computed tomography (Raggi, 2002; Raggi, 2004). High doses of sevelamer (3.2–8 g/day) are necessary to bring hyperphosphatemia back to target level, and the number of pills per day (about 8 x 800 mg tablets) may certainly be a conditioning factor for the patient's compliance (Chertow et al., 2002).

Patients with end-stage kidney disease treated with lanthanum carbonate up to 2.5–3.8 g/day for up to 2 years have been reported to obtain effective reduction of serum phosphorus level (Finn, 2006). Lanthanum-carbonate-treated patients have, also been shown to reach a significantly reduced calcium/phosphate product and parathyroid hormone level compared with the placebo (Joy & Finn, 2009). Lanthanum carbonate, therefore, is an effective, at least as effective as calcium carbonate, well-tolerated phosphate binder (Hutchison, 2004; Hutchison et al., 2006). However, despite the very encouraging results, further studies involving larger numbers of patients are needed to definitively establish the long-term safety of lanthanum regarding tissue deposition, as well as its efficacy on vascular calcifications or outcomes in treated patients, which also need to be confirmed in the long term.

4.5 Combination in treatment

A multiple-factor approach can be used to reduce serum phosphate including reduced phosphorus intake in the diet, using phosphate binders efficiently and avoidance of under- dialysis. The patient's diet should be high in nutrition but with the lowest possible phosphorus content. Since dietary control of phosphorus intake and dialysis removal are usually not sufficient, phosphate binders are usually needed as adjuvants to increase fecal excretion (Bover et al; 2005). For an optimal protein diet of 1-1.2 g/kg/day, the phosphorus intake was 778-1,444 mg/day and 5,500-10,000 mg/week. Dialysis has limited ability for phosphate control, although phosphate removal by hemodialysis is very much a time-dependent process. The amount of phosphorus removed by hemodialysis, extrapolated to an average week, is 250-300 mg/day. The introduction of non-calcium-based phosphate binders has enabled a reduction in the total phosphate load and provides a useful tool in the prevention of vascular calcification in CKD. The use of phosphate binders may decrease the phosphorus absorbed from the diet to 40% (Llach & Bover, 2000). In these circumstances, 320 mg of phosphorus and 21g of protein (0.3-0.35g of protein/kg/day) intake should be the critical value above which a positive balance of phosphate may occur (Fig. 3).

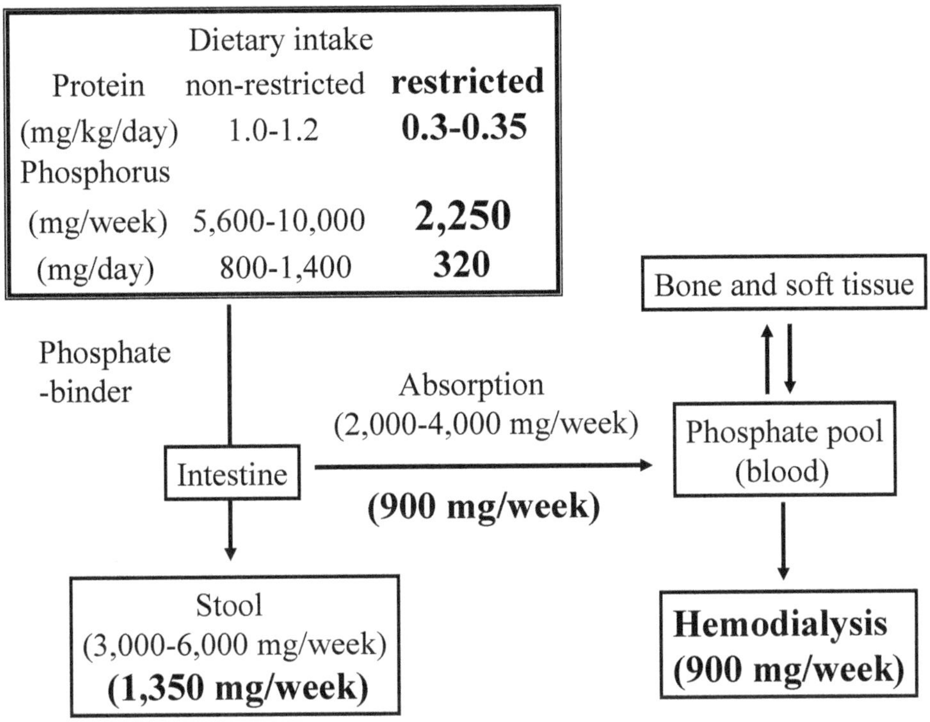

Fig. 3. Phosphate balance in hemodialysis patient
Those in restricted protein and phosphate intake are shown in bold.

Successful control of phosphate is one of the key aspects in the management of dialysis patients (Rodriguez-Benot et al., 2005; Young et al., 2004, Young et al., 2005), However, numerous studies have revealed the difficulty in achieving phosphorus targets less than 5.5 mg/dl (Arenas et al., 2006; Lorenzo et al., 2006: Wei et al., 2006), despite the wide variety of drugs available for its treatment (Joy & Finn, 2003; Sprague, 2007; Arenas et al., 2008). Both endothelial dysfunction and medial calcification are closely associated with development of cardiovascular disease. It is well known that long-term exposure to phosphate, generally observed in end-stage renal failure patients, can mediate vascular calcification (Jono et al., 2000; Giachelli, 2003). Dietary high phosphate loading can be involved in the postprandial elevation of serum phosphorus level, and this short-term exposure to phosphate was enough to decrease endothelium-dependent vasodilation.

5. Conclusion

The goals of therapy have been to reduce phosphorus intake with low protein diet and phosphate binders. Since low protein diet is thought to be induce malnutrition, it is thought that strict adherence to a low protein diet is not practical. A diet rich in proteins is usually also rich in phosphorus. However, proteins with very different phosphorus contents can provide equivalent nutritional value, as can be seen from the difference in phosphorus content between meat, cheese, and eggs. Egg white is an excellent example of food with a high level of protein but low phosphorus content. Moe et al. demonstrates the importance of the protein source of phosphate in overall mineral metabolism after only 7 days of controlled diets. Despite equivalent protein and phosphorus concentrations in the diets, subjects had lower serum phosphorus levels, a trend toward decreased urine 24-hour phosphorus excretion, and significantly decreased FGF23 levels in the vegetarian diet compared with the meat-based diet (Moe et al., 2011).

Lafage et al. (Lafage et al., 1992) used a very low protein diet (0.3 g/kg/d) supplemented with amino acids and ketoanalogues and with only 1 g of calcium carbonate and 1,000 IU of vitamin D_2 in 17 patients with advanced renal failure. They have shown not only a beneficial effect related to the control of hyperphosphatemia on the biologic and histologic parameters of hyperparathyroidism but also a correction of acidosis, which resulted in the disappearance of the osteomalacic component. Thus, dietary control often considered to be of minor importance, is actually one of the major keys to success in the management of hyperphosphataemia.

6. Acknowledgements

The work described in this publication was supported by Grants-in-Aid for Scientific Research from the Ministry of Education, Culture, Sports, Science and Technology in Japan (to ET, HY, and YT).

7. References

Achinger SG, Ayus JC. (2006) Left ventricular hypertrophy: is hyperphosphatemia among dialysis patients a risk factor? *J Am Soc Nephrol* 17(12 suppl 3): S255-S261.

Amann K, Törnig J, Kugel B, Gross ML, Tyralla K, El-Shakmak A, Szabo A, Ritz E. (2003) Hyperphosphatemia aggravates cardiac fibrosis and microvascular disease in experimental uremia. *Kidney Int* 63: 1296–1301.

Arenas MD, Alvarez-Ude F, Gil MT, Soriano A, Egea JJ, Millán I, Amoedo ML, Muray S, Carretón MA. (2006) Application of NKFK/DOQI clinical practice guidelines for bone metabolism and disease: changes of clinical practices and their effects on outcomes and quality standards in three haemodialysis units. *Nephrol Dial Transplant.* 21: 1663-1668.

Arenas MD, Malek T, Gil MT, Moledous A, Nunez C, Alvarez-Ude F. (2008) Use of aluminum-based phosphate-chelators in hemodialysis in the era of ultrapure water. *Nefrologia.* 28: 168-173.

Benaroia M, Pierratos A, Nesrallah GE. (2008) A primer for the prescription of short-daily and nocturnal hemodialysis. *Hemodial Int* 12: 23-29.

Biber J, Hernando N, Forster I, Murer H. (2009) Regulation of phosphate transport in proximal tubules. *Pflu¨gers Arch* 458: 39–52.

Blacher J, Demuth K, Guerin AP, Safar ME, Moatti N, London GM, (1998) Influence of biochemical alterations on arterial stiffness in patients with end-stage renal disease. *Arterioscler Thromb Vasc Biol* 18: 535-541.

Block GA, Hulbert-Shearon TE, Levin NW, Port FK. (1998) Association of serum phosphorus and calcium x phosphate product with mortality risk in chronic hemodialysis patients: A national study. *Am J Kidney Dis* 31: 607–617.

Block GA, Port FK. (2000) Re-evaluation of risks associated with hyperphosphatemia and hyperparathyroidism in dialysis patients: recommendations for a change in management. *Am J Kidney Dis* 35: 1226–1237.

Block GA, Klassen PS, Lazarus JM, Ofsthun N, Lowrie EG, Chertow GM. (2004) Mineral metabolism, mortality, and morbidity in maintenance hemodialysis. *J Am Soc Nephrol* 15: 2208–2218.

Block GA, Raggi P, Bellasi A, Kooienga L, Spiegel DM. (2007) Mortality effect of coronary calcification and phosphate binder choice in incident hemodialysis patients. *Kidney Int.* 71: 438–441.

Blumsohn A. (2004) What have we learnt about the regulation of phosphate metabolism? *Curr Opin Nephrol Hypertens.* 13: 397- 401.

Bover J, Ortiz-Herbener F, Ballarín J, Andrés E, Barceló P. (2005) New therapy strategies in secondary hyperparathyroidism on dialysis (I): new concepts, new treatments. *Nefrologia.* 25 Suppl 2: 100-108.

Braun J, Oldendorf M, Moshage W, Heidler R, Zeitler E, Luft FC. (1996) Electron beam computed tomography in the evaluation of cardiac calcification in chronic dialysis patients. *Am. J. Kidney Dis.* 27: 394–401.

Bringhurst FR, Demay BM, Krane SM, Kronenberg HM. (2004) Bone and mineral metabolism in health and disease. In: Kasper DL, Braunwald E, Fauci AS, Hauser SL, Longo DL, Jameson L, Isselbacher KJ, eds. *Harrison's Principles of Internal Medicine.* New York, NY: McGraw-Hill.

Calvo & Park 1996. Calvo MS, Park YK. (1996).Changing phosphorus content of the U.S. diet: potential for adverse effects on bone. *J Nutr.* 126(4 Suppl):1168S-1180S.

Chertow GM, Burke SK, Raggi P. (2002) Sevelamer attenuates the progression of coronary and aortic calcification in hemodialysis patients. *Kidney Int.* 62: 245–52.

Cozzolino M, Dusso AS, Slatopolsky D. (2001) Role of calciumphosphate product and bone-associated proteins on vascular calcification in renal failure. *J Am Soc Nephrol* 12: 2511–2516.

Delmez JA, Slatopolsky E. (1992) Hyperphosphatemia: its consequences and treatment in patients with chronic renal disease. *Am J Kidney Dis.* 19(4):303-317.

Di Marco GS, Hausberg M, Hillebrand U, Rustemeyer P, Wittkowski W, Lang D, Pavensta¨dt H. (2008) Increased inorganic phosphate induces human endothelial cell apoptosis in vitro. *Am J Physiol Renal Physiol* 294: F1381–1387.

Eknoyan G, Levin A, Levin NW. National Kidney Foundation. (2003) Bone metabolism and disease in chronic kidney disease. *Am J Kidney Dis* 42 [Suppl 3]: S1–S201

Ferrari SL, Bonjour JP, Rizzoli R. (2005) Fibroblast growth factor-23 relationship to dietary phosphate and renal phosphate handling in healthy young men. *J Clin Endocrinol Metab.* 90: 1519-1524.

Finn WF. SPD 405–307 Lanthanum Study Group. (2006) Lanthanum carbonate versus standard therapy for the treatment of hyperphosphatemia: safety and efficacy in chronic maintenance hemodialysis patients. *Clin Nephrol* 65(3): 191-202.

Floege J, Ketteler M. (2004) Vascular calcification in patients with endstage renal disease. *Nephrol Dial Transplant.* 19 [Suppl 5]: V59–V66.

Foley RN, Parfrey PS, Sarnak MJ. (1998) Clinical epidemiology of cardiovascular disease in chronic renal disease. *Am. J. Kidney Dis.* 32: S112–19.

Fukagawa M, Kurokawa K, Papadakis MA. (2004) Fluid and electrolyte disorders. In: Tierney LM, McPhee SJ, Papadakis MA, eds. *Current Medical Diagnosis and Treatment 2005*. New York, NY: McGraw-Hill/Appleton & Lange; 837–867.

Furgeson SB. (2008) Chonchol: Beta-blockade in chronic dialysis patients. *Semin Dial* 21: 43-48.

Ganesh SK, Stack AG, Levin NW, Hulbert-Shearon T, Port FK. (2001) Association of elevated serum PO(4), Ca x PO(4) product, and parathyroid hormone with cardiac mortality risk in chronic hemodialysis patients. *J Am Soc Nephrol* 12: 2131–2138.

Giachelli SM, Jono S, Mori K, Morii H, (2001) Vascular calcification and inorganic phosphate. *Am J Kidney Dis* 38: S34-37.

Giachelli CM. (2003) Vascular calcification: In vitro evidence for the role of inorganic phosphate. *J Am Soc Nephrol* 14: S300–S304.

Goldsmith D, Ritz E, Covic A. (2004) Vascular calcification: a stiff challenge for the nephrologist. *Kidney Int* 66: 1315–1333

Goodman WG, Goldin J, Kuizon BD, Yoon C, Gales B, Sider D, Wang Y, Chung J, Emerick A, Greaser L, Elashoff RM, Salusky IB. (2000) Coronary-artery calcification in young adults with end-stage renal disease who are undergoing dialysis. *N Engl J Med* 342: 1478–1483

Gotch FA, Panlilio F, Sergeyeva O, Rosales L, Folden T, Kaysen G, Levin NW. (2003) A kinetic model of inorganic phosphorus mass balance in hemodialysis therapy. *Blood Purif* 21: 51–57.

Gutierrez O, Isakova T, Rhee E, Shah A, Holmes J, Collerone G, Jüppner H, Wolf M. (2005) Fibroblast growth factor-23 mitigates hyperphosphatemia but accentuates calcitriol deficiency in chronic kidney disease. *J Am Soc Nephrol.* 16: 2205-2215.

Gutiérrez OM, Mannstadt M, Isakova T, Rauh-Hain JA, Tamez H, Shah A, Smith K, Lee H, Thadhani R, Jüppner H, Wolf M. (2008) Fibroblast growth factor 23 and mortality among patients undergoing hemodialysis. *N Engl J Med.* 359(6): 584-592.

Gutiérrez OM, Januzzi JL, Isakova T, Laliberte K, Smith K, Collerone G, Sarwar A, Hoffmann U, Coglianese E, Christenson R, Wang TJ, deFilippi C, Wolf M. (2009) Fibroblast growth factor-23 and left ventricular hypertrophy in chronic kidney disease. *Circulation.* 119: 2545-2552.

Henry RM, Kostense PJ, Bos G, Dekker JM, Nijpels G, Heine RJ, Bouter LM, Stehouwer CD: (2002) Mild renal insufficiency is associated with increased cardiovascular mortality: the Hoorn Study. *Kidney Int* 62: 1402–1407.

Hruska KA, Mathew S, Lund R, Qiu P, Pratt R. (2008) Hyperphosphatemia of chronic kidney disease. *Kidney Int* 74: 148-157.

Hsu HJ, Wu MS. (2009) Fibroblast growth factor 23: a possible cause of left ventricular hypertrophy in hemodialysis patients. *Am J Med Sci.* 337:116-122.

Hutchison AJ. (2004) Improving phosphate-binder therapy as a way forward. *Nephrol Dial Transplant* 19 [Suppl 1]: i19–i24.

Hutchison AJ, Maes B, Vanwalleghem J, Asmus G, Mohamed E, Schmieder R, Backs W, Jamar R, Vosskühler A. (2006) Long-term efficacy and tolerability of lanthanum carbonate: results from a 3-year study. *Nephron Clin Pract* 102: c61–c71.

Imanishi Y, Inaba M, Nakatsuka K, Nagasue K, Okuno S, Yoshihara A, Miura M, Miyauchi A, Kobayashi K, Miki T, Shoji T, Ishimura E, Nishizawa Y. (2004) FGF-23 in patients with end-stage renal disease on hemodialysis. *Kidney Int.* 65: 1943-1946.

Isakova T, Gutiérrez OM, Chang Y, Shah A, Tamez H, Smith K, Thadhani R, Wolf M. (2009) Phosphorus binders and survival on hemodialysis. *J Am Soc Nephrol.* 20: 388-396.
James G, Jackson H: European guidelines for the nutritional care of adult renal patients. (2002) *EDTNA/ERCA*, pp1-52.
Jono S, McKee MD, Murry CE, Shioi A, Nishizawa Y, Mori K, Morii H, Giachelli CM. (2000) Phosphate regulation of vascular smooth muscle cell calcification. *Circ. Res.* 87: E10–17.
Joy MS, Finn WF. (2003) Randomized, double-blind, placebocontrolled, dose-titration, Phase III study assessing the efficacy and tolerability of lanthanum carbonate: a new phosphate binder for the treatment of hyperphosphatemia. *Am J Kidney Dis* 42: 96–107.
Ketteler M, Bongartz P, Westenfeld R, Wildberger JE, Mahnken AH, Böhm R, Metzger T, Wanner C, Jahnen-Dechent W, Floege J. (2003) Association of low fetuin-A (AHSG) concentrations in serum with cardiovascular mortality in patients on dialysis: a cross-sectional study. *Lancet* 361: 827–833.
Koiwa F, Kazama JJ, Tokumoto A, Onoda N, Kato H, Okada T, Nii-Kono T, Fukagawa M, Shigematsu T; ROD21 Clinical Research Group. (2005) Sevelamer hydrochloride and calcium bicarbonate reduce serum fibroblast growth factor 23 levels in dialysis patients. *Ther Apher Dial* 9: 336–339.
Komori T, Yagi H, Nomura S, Yamaguchi A, Sasaki K, Deguchi K, Shimizu Y, Bronson RT, Gao YH, Inada M, Sato M, Okamoto R, Kitamura Y, Yoshiki S, Kishimoto T. (1997) Targeted disruption of Cbfa1 results in a complete lack of bone formation owing to maturational arrest of osteoblasts. *Cell.* 89(5):755-764.
Kopple JD. (2001) National Kidney Foundation K/DOQI clinical practice guidelines for nutrition in chronic renal failure. *Am J Kidney Dis* 37 [Suppl 2]: S66–S70.
Kuro-o M, Matsumura Y, Aizawa H, Kawaguchi H, Suga T, Utsugi T, Ohyama Y, Kurabayashi M, Kaname T, Kume E, Iwasaki H, Iida A, Shiraki-Iida T, Nishikawa S, Nagai R, Nabeshima YI. (1997) Mutation of the mouse klotho gene leads to a syndrome resembling ageing. *Nature* 390: 45–51.
Lafage MH, Combe C, Fournier A, Aparicio M. (1992) Ketodiet, physiological calcium intake and native vitamin D improve renal osteodystrophy. *Kidney Int.* 42(5): 1217-1225.
Larsson T, Nisbeth U, Ljunggren O, Jüppner H, Jonsson KB. (2003) Circulating concentration of FGF-23 increases as renal function declines in patients with chronic kidney disease, but does not change in response to variation in phosphate intake in healthy volunteers. *Kidney Int.* 64: 2272-2279.
Llach L, Bover J. (2000) Renal osteodystriphies; in Brenner BM (ed): *The Kidney.* Philadelphia, Saunders, pp2103-2186.
London GM. (2000) Alterations of arterial function in end-stage renal disease. *Nephron* 84: 111-118.
London GM. (2003) Cardiovascular Calcifications in Uremic Patients: Clinical Impact on Cardiovascular Function. *J Am Soc Nephrol* 14: S305–S309.
London GM, Guérin AP, Marchais SJ, Métivier F, Pannier B, Adda H. (2003) Arterial media calcification in end-stage renal disease: Impact on all-cause and cardiovascular mortality. *Nephrol. Dial. Transplant* 18: 1731–1740.

Longenecker JC, Coresh J, Powe NR Levey AS, Fink NE, Martin A, Klag MJ. (2002) Traditional cardiovascular disease risk factors in dialysis patients compared with the general population: The CHOICE Study. *J. Am. Soc. Nephrol.* 13: 1918–1927.

Lorenzo V, Martin-Malo A, Perez-Garcia R, Torregrosa JV, Vega N, de Francisco AL, Cases A. (2006) Prevalence, clinical correlates and therapy cost of mineral abnormalities among haemodialysis patients: a cross-sectional multicentre study. *Nephrol Dial Transplant.* 21: 459-465.

Maduell F, Navarro V, Torregrosa E, Rius A, Dicenta F, Cruz MC, Ferrero JA. (2003) Change from three times a week on-line hemodiafiltration to short daily on-line hemodiafiltration. *Kidney Int* 64: 305-313.

Mallick NP, Gokal R. (1999) Haemodialysis. *Lancet* 353: 737–742

Mirza MA, Larsson A, Lind L, Larsson TE. (2009) Circulating fibroblast growth factor-23 is associated with vascular dysfunction in the community. *Atherosclerosis.* 205: 385-390.

Miyamoto K, Ito M, Tatsumi S, Kuwahata M, Segawa H. (2007) New aspect of renal phosphate reabsorption: the type IIc sodium-dependent phosphate transporter. *Am J Nephrol* 27: 503–515.

Miyamoto K, Segawa H, Ito M, Kuwahata M. (2004) Physiological regulation of renal sodium-dependent phosphate cotransporters. *Jpn J Physiol* 54: 93–102.

Moe SM, Duan D, Doehle BP, O'Neill KD, Chen NX. (2003) Uremia induces the osteoblast differentiation factor Cbfa1 in human blood vessels. *Kidney Int.* 63: 1003–1011.

Moe SM, Zidehsarai MP, Chambers MA, Jackman LA, Radcliffe JS, Trevino LL, Donahue SE, Asplin JR. (2010) Vegetarian compared with meat dietary protein source and phosphorus homeostasis in chronic kidney disease. *Clin J Am Soc Nephrol.* 6(2): 257-264.

Murer H, Hernando N, Forster I, Biber J. (2000) Proximal tubular phosphate reabsorption: molecular mechanisms. *Physiol Rev* 80: 1373–1409.

Murphy-Gutekunst L. (2007) Hidden phosphorus: where do we go from here ? *J Ren Nutr* 4: e31-e36.

Nishida Y, Taketani Y, Yamanaka-Okumura H, Imamura F, Taniguchi A, Sato T, Shuto E, Nashiki K, Arai H, Yamamoto H, Takeda E. (2006) Acute effect of oral phosphate loading on serum fibroblast growth factor 23 levels in healthy men. *Kidney Int.* 70: 2141-2147.

Oliveira RB, Cancela AL, Graciolli FG, Dos Reis LM, Draibe SA, Cuppari L, Carvalho AB, Jorgetti V, Canziani ME, Moysés RM.. (2010) Early control of PTH and FGF23 in normophosphatemic CKD patients: a new target in CKD-MBD therapy? *Clin J Am Soc Nephrol.* 5(2): 286-291.

Owen WF, Lowrie EG: (1998) C-reactive protein as an outcome predictor for maintenance hemodialysis patients. *Kidney Int* 54: 607–617.

Pande S, Ritter CS, Rothstein M, Wiesen K, Vassiliadis J, Kumar R, Schiavi SC, Slatapolsky E, Brown AJ. (2006) FGF-23 and sFRP-4 in chronic kidney disease and post-renal transplantation. *Nephron Physiol* 104: 23–32.

Perwad F, Azam N, Zhang MY, Yamashita T, Tenenhouse HS, Portale AA. (2005) Dietary and serum phosphorus regulate fibroblast growth factor 23 expression and 1,25-dihydroxyvitamin D metabolism in mice. *Endocrinology.* 146: 5358-5364.

Raggi P. (2000) Detection and quantification of cardiovascular calcifications with electron beam tomography to estimate risk in hemodialysis patients. *Clin Nephrol* 54: 325–333.

Raggi P. (2002) Effects of excess calcium load on the cardiovascular system measured with electron beam tomography in end-stage renal disease. *Nephrol Dial Transplant* 17: 332–335.

Ribeiro S, Ramos A, Brandão A, Rebelo JR, Guerra A, Resina C, Vila-Lobos A, Carvalho F, Remédio F, Ribeiro F. (1998) Cardiac valve calcification in haemodialysis patients: role of calcium-phosphate metabolism. *Nephrol Dial Transplant* 13: 2037–2040.

Rodriguez-Benot A, Martin-Malo A, Alvarez-Lara MA, Rodriguez M, Aljama P. (2005) Mild hyperphosphatemia and mortality in hemodialysis patients. *Am J Kidney Dis.* 46: 68-77.

Ross R. (1999) Atherosclerosis-an inflammatory disease. *N Engl J Med* 340: 115–126.

Schwarz U, Buzello M, Ritz E, Stein G, Raabe G, Wiest G, Mall G, Amann K. (2000) Morphology of coronary atherosclerotic lesions in patients with end-stage renal failure. *Nephrol. Dial. Transplant.* 15: 218–223.

Segawa H, Kaneko I, Setsuko Y, Ito M, Kuwahata M, Inoue Y, Kato S, Miyamoto K. (2004) Intestinal Na-Pi cotransporter adaptation to dietary Pi content in vitamin D receptor null mice. *Am J Physiol Renal Physiol* 287: F39–F47.

Seiler S, Reichart B, Roth D, Seibert E, Fliser D, Heine GH. (2010) FGF-23 and future cardiovascular events in patients with chronic kidney disease before initiation of dialysis treatment. *Nephrol Dial Transplant.* 25(12): 3983-3989.

Sheikh MS, Maguire JA, Emmett M, Santa Ana CA, Nicar MJ, Schiller LR, Fordtran JS. (1989) Reduction of dietary phosphorus absorption by phosphorus binders. A theoretical, in vitro, and in vivo study. *J Clin Invest.* 83(1): 66-73.

Shimada T, Hasegawa H, Yamazaki Y, Muto T, Hino R, Takeuchi Y, Fujita T, Nakahara K, Fukumoto S, Yamashita T. (2004) FGF-23 is a potent regulator of vitamin D metabolism and phosphate homeostasis. *J Bone Miner Res.* 19: 429-435.

Shimada T, Yamazaki Y, Takahashi M, Hasegawa H, Urakawa I, Oshima T, Ono K, Kakitani M, Tomizuka K, Fujita T, Fukumoto S, Yamashita T. (2005) Vitamin D receptor-independent FGF23 actions in regulating phosphate and vitamin D metabolism. *Am J Physiol Renal Physiol.* 289: F1088-F1095.

Shuto E, Taketani Y, Tanaka R, Harada N, Isshiki M, Sato M, Nashiki K, Amo K, Yamamoto H, Higashi Y, Nakaya Y, Takeda E. (2009) Dietary phosphorus acutely impairs endothelial function. *J Am Soc Nephrol.* 20(7): 1504-1512.

Slatopolsky E, Brown A, Dusso A. (2002) Role of phosphorus in the pathogenesis of secondary hyperparathyroidism. *Am J Kidney Dis* 37: S54–S57.

Speer MY, Giachelli CM, (2004) Regulation of cardiovascular calcification. *Cardiovascular Pathology* 13: 63-70.

Sprague SM. (2007) A comparative review of the efficacy and safety of established phosphate binders: calcium, sevelamer, and lanthanum carbonate. *Curr Med Res Opin.* 23: 3167-3175.

Sullivan CM, Leon JB, Sehgal AR. (2007) Phosphorus-containing food additives and the accuracy of nutrient databases: implications for renal patients. *J Ren Nutr.* 17(5): 350-354.

Takeda E, Taketani Y, Morita K, Tatsumi S, Katai K, Nii T, Yamamoto H, Miyamoto K. (2000) Molecular mechanisms of mammalian inorganic phosphate homeostasis. *Adv Enzyme Regul* 40: 285-302.

Takeda E, Taketani Y, Nashiki K, Nomoto M, Shuto E, Sawada N, Yamamoto H, Isshiki M. (2006) A novel function of phosphate-mediated intracellular signal transduction pathways. *Adv Enzyme Regul* 46: 154–161.

Tenenhouse HS. (2006) Regulation of phosphorus homeostasis by the type IIa Na/phosphate cotransporter. *Annu Rev Nutr* 25: 197–214.

US Renal Data System Annual Data Report Bethesta (2005) *National Institutes of Health National Institute of Diabetes and Digestive and Kidney Diseases.*

Vaithilingam I, Polkinghorne KR, Atkins RC, Kerr PG. (2004) Time and exercise improve phosphate removal in hemodialysis patients. *Am J Kidney Dis.* 43(1): 85-89.

Wang AY, Wang M, Woo J, Lam CW, Li PK, Lui SF, Sanderson JE. (2003) Cardiac valve calcification as an important predictor for all-cause mortality and cardiovascular mortality in long-term peritoneal dialysis patients: A prospective study. *J. Am. Soc. Nephrol.* 14: 159–168.

Wei M, Taskapan H, Esbaei K, Jassal SV, Bargman JM, Oreopoulos DG. (2006) K/DOQI guideline requirements for calcium, phosphate, calcium phosphate product, and parathyroid hormone control in dialysis patients: can we achieve them? *Int Urol Nephrol.* 38: 739-743.

Willett WC, Buzzard M. (1998) *Nature of Variation in Diet in Nutritional Epidemiology,* 2nd Ed., edited by Willett WC, New York, Oxford University Press, pp33-49.

Xu H, Bai L, Collins JF, Ghishan FK. (2002) Age-dependent regulation of rat intestinal type IIb sodium-phosphate cotransporter by 1,25-(OH2) vitamin D3. *Am J Physiol Cell Physiol* 282: C487–C493.

Yoshida T, Fujimori T, Nabeshima Y. (2002) Mediation of unusually high concentrations of 1,25-dihydroxyvitamin D in homozygous klotho mutant mice by increased expression of renal 1 alpha-hydroxylase gene. Endocrinology 143: 683–689.

Young EW, Akiba T, Albert JM, McCarthy JT, Kerr PG, Mendelssohn DC, Jadoul M. (2004) Magnitude and impact of abnormal mineral metabolism in hemodialysis patients in the Dialysis Outcomes and Practice Patterns Study (DOPPS). *Am J Kidney Dis.* 44(Suppl 2): 34-38.

Young EW, Albert JM, Satayathum S, Goodkin DA, Pisoni RL, Akiba T, Akizawa T, Kurokawa K, Bommer J, Piera L, Port FK. (2005) Predictors and consequences of altered mineral metabolism: The Dialysis Outcomes and Practice Patterns Study. *Kidney Int.* 67: 1179–1187.

Yu X, White KE. (2005) Fibroblast growth factor 23 and its receptors. *Ther Apher Dial* 9: 308–312.

Yu X, White KE. (2005) FGF23 and disorders of phosphate homeostasis. Cytokine Growth Factor Rev 16: 221–232.

Zoccali C. (2000) Cardiovascular risk in uraemic patients – Is it fully explained by classical risk factors? *Nephrol. Dial. Transplant.* 15: 454–457.

7

The Importance of Exercise Programs in Hemodialysis Patients

Susanne Heiwe[1], Andrej Ekholm[2] and Ingela Fehrman-Ekholm[3,4]
[1]*Dept of Physiotherapy, Karolinska Institutet, Dept of Medicine & Dept of Clinical Sciences,*
[2]*Karolinska Institutet*
[3]*Dept of Renal Medicine, Karolinska University Hospital,*
[4]*Stockholm and Transplantation Centre, Sahlgrenska Academy, Göteborg,*
Sweden

1. Introduction

The lifestyle today is new. We sit with our computers, televisions etc. Usually, we do not carry heavy things. We gain weight and loose muscle strength. Through history the life has included moments with physical efforts. The body has not changed. It still needs physical training and efforts. The person who is untrained gets quickly tired. Therefore it is important to make the efforts regularly. The capacity of the heart to transport oxygen increases and the energy increases with physical training. The muscle condition is important. The mitochondria in the muscles cells may increase with 30-40 % after one month of exercise. With more mitochondria more fat is consumed and less carbohydrate is needed. Consequently, less lactic acid is formed and the blood does not change the pH towards acidosis as easily.

Thus, modern people need exercise. You need not to go to a gym or run every day. It is more about having an active life. Take the cycle or walk to the job or to the shop, take the stairs instead of escalator or elevator. The exercise is a part of the natural common life and the body is a tool which needs to be used. It could be enough with 30 minutes of activity to reach physical efforts the heart rate has to increase, maybe to 120 beats/minute. This could be a dilemma for many patients since they have decreased maximal capacity and interacting medication. The training program has to be individualized but the goal is to improve the capacity. If success the daily normal activities feel easier and the patients get more improved trust and comfort. Physical activities mean also better control and less fear of having fall accidents. With a feeling of control there are fewer obstacles.

Thus exercise and effort are important to all of us which are true for many people with different diseases. For patients with cardiac diseases, hypertension, diabetes mellitus there are often exercise programs but for patients with different stages of chronic kidney disease, CKD, there is no obvious exercise treatment program. However, more and more evidence exists that exercises are important for these patients. The dialysis treatment hours have increased more and more to increase KT/V, the dialysis dose, but this also means less time for activities like exercise, work, family life and spear time. How could we help these patients?

Hence, this chapter is chosen with the intention to provide the reader with information concerning exercise capacity and level of physical activity in adults with chronic kidney disease. It also has the aim to make health-care providers within renal medicine aware of exercise training as an evidence-based intervention to improve health and well-being in adults with CKD. Despite the fact that exercise training is easy, cost effective and preventive, exercise training has not been implemented into clinical practice. We hope that this chapter will stimulate to action and provide some knowledge about these patients and their problems in order to understand why exercise training should be included in the standard care for adults with CKD. The chapter also contains general information about exercise and expected effects in healthy individuals.

2. What is a training program for grown-up people?

It is important to consider the training models, methodology, and expected changes that happen at regular physical activity in general. We consider different measures to describe the activities.

- *Frequency* - That means how often we do the training. A daily dosage of effort like taking walks, taking stair-cases is basic.
- *Intensity* - This is how the levels of efforts are. A common used definition is RM that is repetition maximum. One RM is the weight or load you are able to lift once but not twice. It has been shown that 60-70% of 1 RM could be enough for the starter to give an increase of muscle strength. For the well-trained it is necessary with almost 70-84% for the increase of muscle mass and strength (Kramer et al 1997).
- *Duration* - It is the length of the exercise period at a time. A 30 minute period of physical exercise is nowadays a common, recommended duration. A simple and common instrument is the pedometer, which could quantify the number of steps and calculate the calories, the walking distance one could obtain during a period.

Concerning intensity this could be varied by adding different muscle groups. The level of effort and the muscle groups involved are important for the results. If you add walking with sticks, the shoulder and arm muscles become involved and increase the results. In these moments also the important coordination becomes involved.
The general effects of training are many. Below are some aspects and findings.

Muscles

Skeletal muscle is not a simple homogenous group of fibers. Type I fibers are characterized by slow speed of contraction, low activity of myosin ATPase and are well suited for prolonged aerobic exercise. Type II fibers have the ability to generate energy for quick and forceful contractions. At training there is an increase in both muscle fibre size and muscle number, the largest effect being increase of muscle size. The number of mitochondria and the small vessels in the muscles increase. Interestingly, even very old people could increase the strength. In an interesting study it was shown that 90-year old persons living at a nursing home could double the muscle strength, increase the quadriceps muscular volume with 10 % as well as increase the daily function after 8 weeks of bodybuilding (Fiatarone et al 1990).

Cardiosvascular system

The cardiac output will increase. The normal pulse will be reduced. The small arteries will dilate which contribute to decreasing blood pressure. The blood circulation to the heart and muscles will increase and both the blood volume and the haemoglobin level will increase.

Many patients with CKD have hypertension. In dialysis the hypertension is most linked to salt and water over load. After kidney transplantation the immunosuppressive drugs CNI (calcineurin inhibitors such as tacrolimus and ciclosporin) and corticosteroids contribute to hypertension. In transplants patients with CAN (chronic allograft nephropathy) ischemia in the kidneys aggravate the situation and give severe hypertension with often therapy resistant blood pressure.

The basis of treatment in hypertension is life style changes, exercise, stop smoking habits and decrease of the sodium chloride in the diet. These are basic advice applicable also to the CKD patients. Many patients have treatment with diuretics to decrease salt and water. Beta-blockers protect the heart from stress and lower the pulse rate, sometimes hamper maximal training efforts. Calcium blockers are frequently used, cause relaxation of the muscles and vasodilatation.

ACE-inhibitors block the angiotensin system and are often well tolerated. It could however be important to be aware of the fact that severe dehydration could be dangerous due to risk of high serum potassium and loss of blood pressure which is a severe condition. This information is important to give to the patient in case of any situation with loss of water like gastrointestinal acute diseases.

Regular physical activity lowers the blood pressure but the blood pressure increases during exercise, mostly the systolic blood pressure. With a stress ECG the individual patient could get information about the level of blood pressure and ECG changes during efforts. There are recommended levels not to exceed.

Nerve system

Regular physical activity affects the nerves. The coordination, the balance and the ability to react becomes better. Most of the persons who do regular exercise have better sleep, less depressions and more self-esteem.

Hormone system

The exercise increases the insulin sensitivity in the skeletal muscle and decreases the insulin in the blood. This means less adiposities and a more healthy profile of the lipids with increased HDL-cholesterol and decreased triglycerides. For body builders the growth hormone may increase. Also testosterone levels have been found to increase and androgen receptors which increase the effect of testosterone (Kraemer et al 2005). Added testosterone has a much stronger effect, both increasing the muscle mass and adding new cells. However, this substance is classified as doping preparation. Cortisol is a catabolic substance and could be increased at stress caused by some exercises and exercisers. However, cortisol is a life-necessary substance. Catecholamine (noradrenalin and adrenalin) are also produced in the moments of stress, fight and flight response. There is probably an anabolic effect on the skeletal muscles which has been shown in certain animal studies. That is why these preparations are on the doping list. Insulin-like growth factor (IGF-1) could also be produced locally in the muscle but the systemic effect is unclear.

3. Physical fitness and physical functioning and self-evaluation in patients with CKD

The physical fitness and physical functioning (= the ability and capacity to perform activities of daily living) is severely reduced in adults with CKD (Kettner-Melsheimer et al 1987;

Kouidi et al 1998; Heiwe et al 2003; Johansen et al 2003; Heiwe et al 2005). It is declining from 70% of the expected norm in a pre-uremic phase to 50% of the expected norm when starting dialysis therapy (Painter et al 1986; Kettner-Melsheimer et al 1987; Brodin et al 2001). However, also ageing decreases muscle mass. The median age at dialysis start in Sweden is 66 years. The muscle mass in 70-year old person is 25% lower compared with 25-year old persons (Klitgaard et al 1990).

Patients with a renal transplant have a lower physical fitness of approximately 70-80% of the age-matched controls (Painter et al 1986). Here, the corticosteroids, still a basic immunosuppressive treatment, contribute to muscular atrophy. Thus, the physical fitness in adults with CKD is reduced and affects the capacity of the patients to perform activities in everyday life and occupational tasks.

Physical functioning in patients with CKD is affected by several factors like consequences of CKD in it-self, the original disease process that brought about the patient's kidney disease and the treatment of CKD which may have further detrimental effects (Marlowe et al 2001). The main factors causing reduced physical fitness are anaemia (Clyne et al 1987; McMahon et al 1999) and muscular weakness (Bohannon et al 1994; Johansen et al 2003). This results in fatigue and increasing inactivity, which in turn reduces physical fitness even further and increases impairments in physical functioning (Bohannon et al 1994; Nielens et al 2001; Johansen et al 2003).

Today, anaemia is successfully corrected by erythropoietin treatment and results in an improved, but not normalised, physical fitness (McMahon et al 1999). When analysing muscle biopsies it has been shown that adults with CKD have muscular histopathological abnormalities already in the pre-uremic phase (Heiwe et al 2005). The causes of muscular weakness in patients with CKD have, however, not been fully elucidated. Muscle atrophy, a neuropathic process and myopathy are potential causes of the muscular weakness. It is suggested that myopathy is due to abnormal energy metabolism (Thompson et al 1993), secondary hyperparathyreoidism (Ritz et al 1980), malnutrition (Guarnieri et al 1983), prolonged physical inactivity (Jones et al 1990) and to uraemia itself (Sakkas et al 2003).

It is important that the consultant renal physiotherapist, renal nurse, renal dietician and renal physician have an understanding of limitations in physical fitness and physical functioning that adults with CKD are expected to face and how various unique issues may alter the treatment approach. All training methods have to start with cautions and feed-back to the patients.

It has been shown that adults with CKD experience limitations in their daily life due to insufficient physical fitness. In a previous study (Heiwe et al 2003) it was shown that adult with CKD experience fatigue both mental and physical fatigue. This results in a reduced physical fitness and reduced physical functioning in terms of impact on performance and endurance. The experienced fatigue appeared frequently and varied in strength.

The informants described having a more or less always-present mental fatigue, which was experienced as something that they really had to fight to overcome. Feeling listless and paralysed by fatigue was a common trait of this group of descriptions. The feeling of physical fatigue appeared as soon as they started performing a physical activity and could vary in extent from day to day. They experienced muscular weakness and rapid onset of tiredness. Pagels et al (2006) have shown that when asked to rate the level of physical activity 40% of the adults being in a pre-uremic phase had a low activity and 11% were mostly sitting or lying down. Thus, the daily basic walks became an effort.

Many adults with CKD experience difficulties in walking if the ground is not level, as in the case of stairs or steps, uphill slopes, etc. In such conditions, they experience physical resistance very quickly. Many elderly with CKD also have difficulties in performing everyday chores, such as managing their personal hygiene, making their bed, hanging up laundry, vacuum-cleaning, lifting things, rising from a squatting position, cleaning, etc. They also experience difficulty in performing a physical activity over a prolonged period of time, for instance, hanging up laundry, without having to pause several times, which they have not had to do prior to the disease. Most of the patients also have difficulties in performing physical activities at the same pace as they did prior to the CKD.

Adults with CKD may also experience temporal stress since they cannot do as much as they would have liked to. They need more time to perform various activities, partly due to "internal demands", like the need for physical rest and partly due to their experiences of external demands as a result of all the medical appointments and other appointments. All these factors may have a negative impact on the patients' level of activity and participation as well as their social life (Heiwe et al 2003). It seems urgent to do something for these patients.

Rehabilitation has a positive effect on physical fatigue and improves both 'endurance' and physical 'performance', which, in turn, could reduce the need for more time to be able to perform everyday chores or other physical activities. It would then be possible for the patients to find more time for their own activities, increasing their physical activity level. It is important to make clear to patients that just by putting time and effort into physical exercise or activity they can improve several aspects of their experience of fatigue, reduced physical fitness and temporal stress. It is, though, important that appointments for physical exercise training are co-ordinated, as far as possible, with the patients' other medical appointments. This would give the patients more time to perform their own physical activities.

It is also important that physiotherapists consider patients' views when reflecting upon and interpreting how they can support and strengthen patients in their effort to be able to perform physical activities as well as social activities that are of importance to them.

Adults with CKD are subjected to multiple physiological and psychological stressors. Welch et al (1999) have for instance showed that the most common treatment-related stressors in patients with haemodialysis are fluid limitations, the length of dialysis and vacation limitations. When adults with CKD rank the stressors that they are subjected to, it is limitation of physical activity which is the number one stressor (Lok et al 1996). Therefore, it is important to include questions concerning physical activity when meeting these patients.

Coping has been proposed as an important mediating factor with regard to adaptation to illness. Coping refers to 'an individual's efforts to master demands that are appraised (or perceived) as exceeding or taxing his or her resources. It is a process that may consist of behaviours and intra-psychic responses designed to overcome, reduce or tolerate these demands (Lazarus et al 1984). There are many ways in which coping responses can be grouped, but the two general categories of coping strategies are problem-solving efforts and strategies aimed at the regulation of emotions (Lazarus et al 1984). Problem-focused coping refers to efforts to improve the troubled person-environment relationship by changing things, for instance by seeking information about what to do. Emotional-focused (or palliative) coping refers to thoughts or actions whose goal is to relieve the emotional impact of stress (for example, bodily or psychological disturbances). Although both sets of strategies are brought to bear on most stressful events, problem-solving efforts are especially useful for managing controllable stressors, and emotional-regulation efforts are well suited to managing the impact of uncontrollable stressors.

It has been shown that in order to cope with the limited physical fitness three coping activities are used: 1) avoiding physical activities, 2) adjusting pace and 3) scheduling. The strategies were problem-focused, and patients used active-, avoidant- and social-support coping strategies. When coping with limited physical fitness, adults with CKD tend to use coping strategies that have a positive short-term outcome. These strategies are, however, also associated with negative long-term outcomes. The individual is placed in an evil circle where the physical functioning decreases as the experience of mental and physical fatigue increases (Heiwe et al 2004). It is therefore important that renal physicians and renal nurses identify these patients and refer them to a renal physiotherapist at an early stage, so that they can get information and help with physical exercise training. This could contribute to the patients' own resources which can then be used to improve the level of participation and also to improve some parts of the patient's social life.

All people employ different combinations of problem-focused and emotion-focused methods to cope with stress. The conditions determining our coping methods in specific situations are complex and at present largely unknown, but they are likely to depend on the conditions being faced, the options available to us and our personality. An issue often emerging in discussions about coping is whether some coping processes are more effective than others. For instance, whether avoidant responses to stressful events are more adaptive or whether more confrontational coping methods are superior. However, coping processes have both positive and negative consequences for an individual. A behaviour that might be effective from, say, the physiological perspective might have devastating consequences for the psychological or sociological domains. Moreover, what is an optimal response in one situation at a particular point in time may be damaging in some other situation or at a different point in time. Most people appear to use a variety of coping strategies to deal with a stressor. Successful coping may depend more on a match of different coping strategies to the features of the stressful event than on the relative efficacy of one coping strategy over another. Therefore, when meeting a patient with CKD and evaluating his or her coping and adaptation, the health-care provider must take into account diverse levels of analysis (physiological, psychological, sociological), short versus long-term consequences and the specific nature of the situation in question.

4. Evidence based effects of exercise training in patients with CKD

There is scientific evidence showing that if adults with CKD do not exercise only having a certain level of physical activity in their daily living:

- The muscle mass and physical fitness will continue to decrease (Painter et al 1986; Kettner-Melsheimer et al 1987; Bohannon et al 1994; Brodin et al 2001; Heiwe et al 2001; Sakkas et al 2003; Heiwe et al 2005; McIntyre et al 2006; Zamojska et al 2006)
- The patient's possibility to maintain, for him or her, a satisfyingly active and social life will be reduced = reduced health-related quality of life (Brodin et al 2001; Fukuhara et al 2003; Heiwe et al 2003; Heiwe et al 2004)

- An already high cardiovascular risk factor and co-morbidity burden (Yao et al 2004; Venkataraman et al 2005) will increase even more due to the severely reduced level of physical activity

Published articles concerning effects of physical exercise on patients with CKD started to appear in the 1980s. Since then, interest in effects of physical exercise has increased in renal medicine, and today there are numerous published articles showing positive effects of exercise training. Data from previously and recently published studies have shown that exercise training in adults with CKD can affect the following factors:

- Muscular hypotrophy, -strength, -endurance & physical functioning (Kouidi et al 1998; Mercer et al 2002; Painter et al 2002; DePaul et al 2002; Sakkas et al 2003; Heiwe et al 2005; McIntyre et al 2006; Heiwe & Jacobson 2011)
- The structure and number of capillaries and mitochondria (Kouidi et al 1998; Sakkas et al 2003, Cheema et al 2010)
- Glucose metabolism (Goldberg et al 1983)
- Aerobic capacity (Painter et al 1986; Painter et al 2002; DePaul et al 2002)
- Blood pressure (Goldberg et al 1983; Pechter et al 2003)
- Cardiac performance (i.e. augmentation of cardiac vagal activity, decrease of vulnerability to arrhythmias) and improvement of coronary risk profiles (Venkataraman et al 2005)
- Depression, performance of pleasant activities in daily living and health-related quality of life (Suh et al 2002; Molsted et al 2004; van Vilsteren et al 2005)
- Circulating cytokines (Cheema BS et al 2010)
- Nutritional parameters and energy expenditure using SWA, SenseWear™ Armband (Cupusti A el al 2011)

A review article, based on 29 trials on this issue, shows that exercise training in dialysis patients improves arterial compliance, cardiac autonomic control and left ventricular systolic function. Moreover, exercise diminishes oxidative stress, blood pressure and inflammation. As shown in Table 1, significant effects of exercise and training were found.

It is interesting to notice that haemoglobin levels, s-albumin, PCR (protein catabolic rate) and KT/V increase. This tells us that less erythropoietin is needed, which means that training is cost-effective. The patients have better protein intake. They probably eat more to get energy. The recommended protein intake at training in general is 1.6-1.7 g/kg. The recommendations for uremic patients in dialysis are a protein intake above 1.3 g/kg body weight.

Also, the decrease in CRP is an interesting finding. CRP is connected to residual renal function (Pecoits-Filho et al 2003). The low inflammatory process in the dialysis patients becomes thus better after 6 months of repeated cycle training and this might be an adequate prescription! Actually, today the physiotherapists give prescriptions on physical activities like the doctors do on medication. The difficulties could be the compliance or adherence of the patient to the physical program suggested but the same problem exists with the prescribed drugs.

Here is a prescription or suggestions to patients with CKD. To obtain improvements it is, however, important that the exercise program has an adequate intensity, frequency and duration. Examples and type of exercises are given (Table 2).

prescription	duration	variable	% change	significance
Cycle ergometer, walking, jogging	8-9 months	HDL cholesterol Hemoglobin Plasma insulin fasting Plasma glucose	+23% +29% -40% -6.3%	< 0.05 < 0.05 <0.01 <0.01
Cycle ergometer 3 times/week	12 weeks	Max workload	Increase	< 0.05
Aerobic strength training 90 min 3 times per week	6 months	VO2 peak Peak blood lactate Isometric strength Type muscle fibre area I Type muscle fibre area II	Increase Decrease Increase Increase	< 0.05 < 0.05 < 0.05 < 0.05
Cycle ergometer 30 min 3 times per week	6 months	Albumin CRP PCR KT/V	Increase Decrease Increase Increase	< 0.024 < 0.046 < 0.001 < 0.026
Treadmill walking or cycle ergometer	3 months	Arterial stiffness Pulse pressure Systolic blood pressure	Decrease Decrease Decrease	0.01 <0.05 <0.05

Table 1. 29 studies and effects of physical activity in dialysis patients on metabolic and nutritional parameters. (Cheema BS, Sing MA 2005).

Activity	Example	Intensity	Duration	Frequency
Muscular Sustained training	Sequential exercise Individual program with weight cuffs as resistance	50 % 1RM	Maximal number of correctly performed repetitions. Corresponding to self-rated total exertion 13-15 according to Borg's RPE-scale	3 times/w
Functional training (including walking-, balance- and coordination-training)	Walking, eg on treadmill or balance carpet. Standing on balance plate Knee bow Stairs Standing up from knee bow		Maximal walking and number of correctly performed repetitions. Corresponding to self-rated total exertion 13-15 according to Borg's RPE-scale	3 times/w
Isometric strength	Sequence training Individual training with weight cuffs or other things as resistance	80% 1RM	1 set á 8-10 reps	3 times/w

Borg´s RPE scale = Borg rating of perceived exertion. It was constructed in the 60-ties by Gunnar Borg, professor in perception and psychophysics in Stockholm. The scale indicates different degrees of effort from 6 to 20. The rated RPE shows a linear relation to workload and heart pulse frequency. It is used within rehabilitation and training (Borg 1970).

VO2 peak: This is the oxygen uptake which reflects the maximal performance of the individual. This has to be measured before start of programme and this helps to adjust the programme for each individual.

Reps = repetitions, **RM** repetition maximum see page 2

Table 2. Prescription on physical activities in patients with CKD and explanations

5. Details and aim of physical training

- Get the patient informed about the importance of physical training in CKD both in dialysis and after kidney transplantation.
- To make the patient independent in the daily life and to keep/increase the quality of life.
- Diminish the risk of cardiovascular disease, osteoporosis and loss of muscle mass. Increase/maintain muscular strength and endurance, balance as well as the sub maximal oxygen uptake.
- Minimize the risk of fall accident.
- Minimize depression.

Dynamic muscular endurance	• Maximal number of muscle contractions with a strain corresponding to 50 % of 1RM and at fixed frequency. • Standing heel-rise test. • Sit-to-stand-to-sit
Static muscular endurance	• Maximal number of seconds the patient is able to maintain an isometric muscle contraction, for example knee extension, with loading corresponding to 50% of 1RM. • Unilateral isotonic shoulder flexion, bilateral isometric shoulder abduction
Functional capacity	• 6-minutes walking test with patient's experienced leg fatigue, breathlessness and possible cardiac pain is rated by the patient according to Borg's CR-10 scale and the total effort according to Borg's RPE-scale before and after the test performed • Walking 30 meters in self-selected normal rate and maximal rate • Timed "Up & Go" • Stand on one leg Functional reach • Stairs
Muscular strength	• One repetition maximum (1RM) • GRIPPIT(grip strength), Jamar hand dynamometer: correlating to muscular mass • Isometric leg strength.
Self-rated physical level of activity	• Disability Rating Index (DRI). Activity rating according to Grimby Frändin
Physical capacity	• Standardized, symptom limited ergometer cycling with patient's experienced leg fatigue, breathlessness and possible cardiac pain is rated by the patient according to Borgs CR-10 scale and the total effort according to Borg's RPE-scale.
Quality of life	• SF-36

Notes: **General about CKD 4-5**

- For patients with secondary kidney diseases it is important to consider the original disease at assessment of physical capacity, general advice and follow-up. For patients with diabetes mellitus for instance it is important to consider the present foot status and the insulin regimen.

- Patients with polycystic kidney disease should avoid contact sports like karate since hard hits against the kidneys may cause bleeding and pain. There is also a higher risk of hernia of the abdominal wall in this disease. Patients with kidney transplants should also avoid contact sports like ice-hockey and land-hockey due to risk of tackling moments.
- Patients with CKD 4 and 5 suffer more easily from tendinitis. Treatment with chinolones means increased risk of tendinitis. Because of this it is important with heating and cool-down to be prolonged. Also the training of mobility and agility should be prolonged and the training intensity and duration increase smoothly.

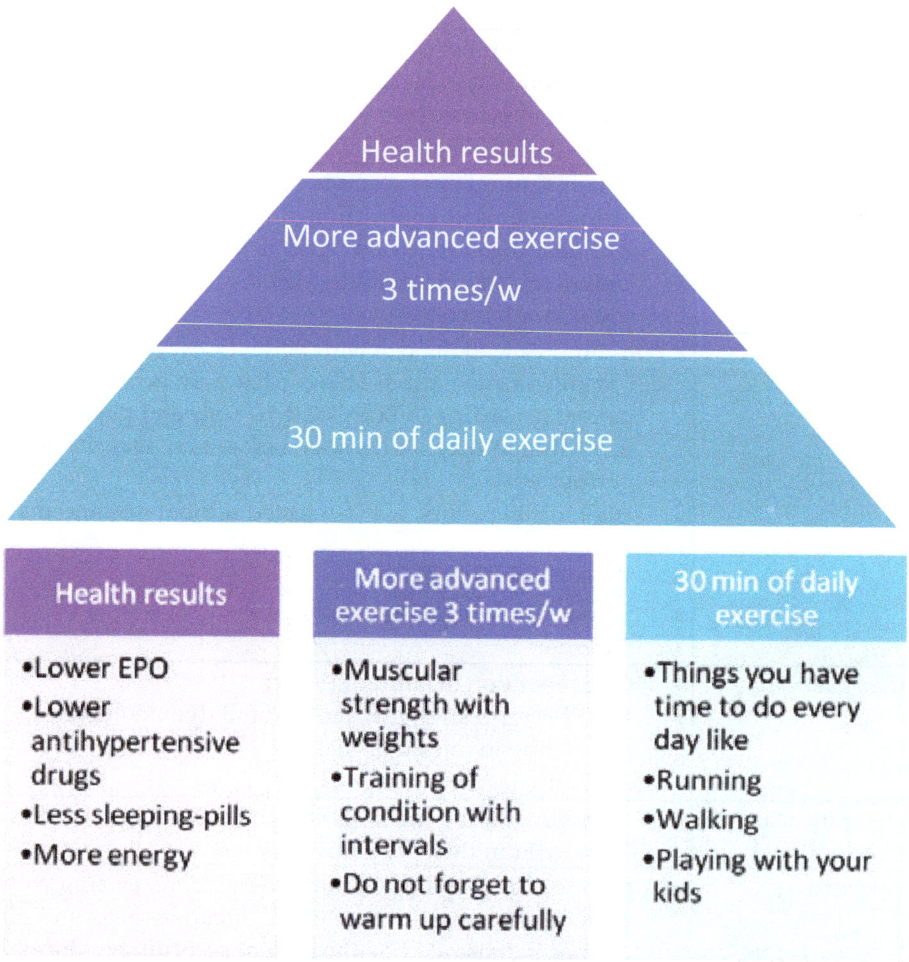
Health results
More advanced exercise
3 times/w
30 min of daily exercise
Health results
•Lower EPO
•Lower antihypertensive drugs
•Less sleeping-pills
•More energy
More advanced exercise 3 times/w
•Muscular strength with weights
•Training of condition with intervals
•Do not forget to warm up carefully
30 min of daily exercise
•Things you have time to do every day like
•Running
•Walking
•Playing with your kids

Fig. 1. The amount of training and training effects in CKD patients in a schematic form

Concerning haemodialysis patients:

- When is the physical training to be performed? It is the medical condition of the patient and the desire of the patient which decide the optimal timing for the training. The most optimal training effect is obtained with the physical activity on dialysis free days. If this is a problem for the patient, for instance far distance to travel, confinement to the hospital etc, the training may be performed before the dialysis treatment or during the first two hours in dialysis. It is not recommended to do the exercise after dialysis treatment since the patients are dehydrated and there is great risk of hypotensive episodes. Since the patients often have lack of time, it is important to coordinate the different treatments within the team.

- The amount of fluid, sodium, potassium and blood pressure is constantly variable in a dialysis patient. As a physical therapist it is important to consider these factors in planning the training schedule and in every training opportunity. Consider the restriction of water in individual patients! However, in jogging and running all need water. The simplest method is to instruct the patient to weigh himself/herself before and after the running episodes.
- The signs of exercise-induced hyponatremia should be recognized by everyone handling dialysis patients. These are symptoms of cerebral over hydration: nausea, malaise when sodium is below 125-130 mmol/L. If plasma sodium falls below 115 to 120 mmol/L there are adding symptoms with headache, lethargy, seizures, and coma. This is a risk identified in marathon runners (Ayes et al 2000).
- Avoid circular pressure in the arm with arteriovenous (AV)-fistula/graft. The blood pressure should not be measured in that arm because of risk to strangle and destroy the important blood flow to the access.
- Before surgery of AV-fistula/graft it is important to perform endurance training of the muscles in the forearm and the hand. This may increase the size of the vena cephalica which is valuable. During a short period after the surgery the patient should not use watches, bracelets or carry heavy bags which may hamper the blood flow in the important AV access. Training the arm with squeezing a soft ball could be important to increase the blood flow in the vein. This makes the AV-fistula more strong and useful. Shoulder and elbow move ability should be alerted and the arm/hand could be used for easier house and family work. Depending on the surgeon's prescription and the status of the patient it may be valuable to start strength training after 3-4 weeks to maintain muscular fitness.
- Patients with central dialysis catheters (CDK) on the neck or frontal thorax may start training of muscle and motility. If the sutures cause pain or prevent movements in the neck/shoulder, the physician is consulted for possible adjustment. Considering the risk of infection the patient with CDK is not allowed to exercise in a pool.

6. Nutrition and exercise

Nutrition is a most important issue in CKD patients. Before start of dialysis many patients have protein restricted diet. This has to be changed as soon as dialysis treatment is initiated. The protein intake has instead to be increased. Both the dialysis process and the physical activities need proteins and amino acids. We usually calculate the PCR = protein catabolic rate every month in the dialysis patients based on urea determinations before and after dialysis session and urea before the next dialysis. The patients could get feedback on their protein intake and add protein supplements if needed.

Carbohydrates are important to refill the glycogen stores in the liver and the muscles. The more glycogen, the more energy is available for the exercise. It is considered that 5-7 g/kg/day on training days are needed. If we eat too much more fat is stored instead.

Fats are needed, in the first hand, the essential fatty acids. But any fat to get the important energy balance is important.
Fruit and vegetables are recommended to sportsmen and sportswomen. However, due to risk of hyperpotassemia and high water content in fruits, caution is needed for patients in dialysis. The patients should have lists from dieticians to find the most proper fruits.
Vitamins are needed. Especially C-vitamins since they are removed at hemodialysis or hemofiltration (Fehrman-Ekholm et al 2008). D-vitamins are needed for the skeleton and in treatment of secondary hyperparathyroidism. Iron is necessary in anemia treatment and today most patients have intravenous iron supply at dialysis sessions.
General recommendation is to eat often and to eat after the exercise to fill up the glycogen stores again.
In co work with other team members the physical therapist works to motivate the patient to continue exercises for the rest of life. Regular check-ups by physiotherapist with knowledge of renal medicine and transplant medicine are of greatest importance to maintain maximal physical performance whatever CKD treatment the patient has. We also know that there are several national guidelines that include exercise training and physical activity as part of the treatment for problems that are common in patients with CKD, i.e. high blood pressure, hyperlipidemia and cardiovascular diseases. Within renal care and -medicine we spend a lot of time trying to find ways to optimise the outcome of the care that is given to our patients. But there is already an easy, low-tech intervention that has multiple advantages for these patients' health and well-being, but which hasn't been implemented as a part of the standard care for patients with CKD: Exercise training and physical activity in daily living! Another question is if aerobic exercise and strength training starting early in renal disease could play an important role in prevention or progression of CKD (Moinuddin et al 2008).

7. Conclusion

- The physical fitness is severely reduced among adults with haemodialysis treatment
- Physical exercise programs should be initiated with gentle start and preferably non-dialysis days or before dialysis treatment
- Exercise training including various programs improves aerobic capacity, muscular strength and endurance, physical functioning, physical- and psychological well-being if the program is regular and monitored
- Exercise training has positive effects on the cardiovascular risk profile, oxidative stress and inflammation
- Exercise training improves protein intake (PCR), dialysis effects (KT/V), haemoglobin and the endothelial function which are important treatment parameters in hemodialysis patients.

We need to encourage our patients with CKD to get more physically active and to start exercising. We need to refer them to physiotherapists with special knowledge in renal medicine that can give them adequate, individually adapted exercise recommendations.

8. References

Ayus JC, Varon J, Arieff AI. Hyponatremia, cerebral edema, and noncardiogenic pulmonary edema in marathon runners. Ann Intern Med 2000; 132:711

Bohannon RW, Hull D, Palmeri D. Muscle strength impairments and gait performance deficits in kidney transplantation candidates. Am J Kidney Dis. 1994 Sep;24(3):480-5.

Borg G. Perceived exertion as an indicator of somatic stress. Scandinavian J Rehabilitation Medicine 1970;2:92.

Brodin E, Ljungman S, Hedberg M, Sunnerhagen KS. Physical activity, muscle performance and quality of life in patients treated with chronic peritoneal dialysis. Scandinavian journal of urology and nephrology. 2001 Feb;35(1):71-8.

Cheema BS, Abas H, Smith B, O'Sullivan AJ, Chan M, Patwardhan A, Kelly J, Gillin A, Pang G, Lloyd B, Berger K, Baune BT, Fiatarone Singh MA. Investigation of skeletal muscle quantity and quality in end-stage renal disease. Nephrology (Carlton). 2010 Jun;15(4):454-63.

Cheema BS and Singh MA. Exercise of training in patients receiving maintenance hemodialysis: a systematic review of clinical trials. Am J Nephrol 2005; 25: 352-364.

Cheema BS, Abas H, Smith B, O'Sullivan AJ, Chan M, Patwardhan A, Kelly J, Gillin A, Pang G, Lloyd B, Berger K, Baune BT, Fiatarone Singh MA. Effects of resistance training during hemodialysis on circulating cytokines: a randomised controlled trial. Eur J Appl Physiol 2010 Dec (Epub ahead of print).

Clyne N, Jogestrand T, Lins LE, Pehrsson SK, Ekelund LG. Factors limiting physical working capacity in predialytic uraemic patients. Acta medica Scandinavica. 1987;222(2):183-90.

Cupisti A, Capitanini A, Betti G, D´Allesasandro C and Barsotti G. Assessment of habitual physical activity and energy expenditure in dialysis patients and relationships to nutritional parameters. Clin Nephrology 2011; 75:218-25.

DePaul V, Moreland J, Eager T, Clase CM. The effectiveness of aerobic and muscle strength training in patients receiving hemodialysis and EPO: a randomized controlled trial. Am J Kidney Dis. 2002 Dec; 40(6):1219-29.

Fehrman-Ekholm I, Lotsander A, Logan K, Dunge D, Odar-Cederlöf I and Kallner A. Concentrations of vitamin C, vitamin B12 and folic acid in patients treated with hemodialysis and on-line hemodiafiltration or hemofiltration. Scand J Urology and Nephrology 42: 74-80, 2008.

Fiatarone M, Marks E, Ryan N, Meredith C, Lipsitz L et al. High intensity strength training in nonagenarians. Effects on skeletal muscle. JAMA 1990; 263; 3029-34.

Fukuhara S, Lopes AA, Bragg-Gresham JL, Kurokawa K, Mapes DL, Akizawa T, et al. Health-related quality of life among dialysis patients on three continents: the Dialysis Outcomes and Practice Patterns Study. Kidney Int. 2003 Nov;64(5):1903-10.

Goldberg AP, Geltman EM, Hagberg JM, Gavin JR, 3rd, Delmez JA, Carney RM, et al. Therapeutic benefits of exercise training for hemodialysis patients. Kidney International. 1983 Dec; 16: 303-9.

Guarnieri G, Toigo G, Situlin R, Faccini L, Coli U, Landini S, et al. Muscle biopsy studies in chronically uremic patients: evidence for malnutrition. Kidney international. 1983 Dec;16: 187-93.

Heiwe S & Jacobson H S. Effects of regular exercise training in adults with chronic kidney disease - a Cochrane Collaboration meta-analysis. In publication 2011.

Heiwe S, Abrandt-Dahlgren M. Living with chronic renal failure: coping with physical activities of daily living. Advances in Physiotherapy. 2004;6:147-57.

Heiwe S, Clyne N, Dahlgren MA. Living with chronic renal failure: patients' experiences of their physical and functional capacity. Physiother Res Int. 2003;8(4):167-77.

Heiwe S, Clyne N, Tollback A, Borg K. Effects of regular resistance training on muscle histopathology and morphometry in elderly patients with chronic kidney disease. American journal of physical medicine & rehabilitation / Association of Academic Physiatrists. 2005 Nov; 84(11):865-74.

Johansen KL, Shubert T, Doyle J, Soher B, Sakkas GK, Kent-Braun JA. Muscle atrophy in patients receiving hemodialysis: effects on muscle strength, muscle quality, and physical function. Kidney Int. 2003 Jan;63(1):291-7.

Jones D, Round J. Skeletal muscle in health and disease. Manchester: University Press 1990.

Kettner-Melsheimer A, Weiss M, Huber W. Physical work capacity in chronic renal disease. The International journal of artificial organs. 1987 Jan;10(1):23-30.

Klitgaard H, Mantoni M, Schiaffino S, Ausoni S, Gorza et al. Function, morphology and protein expression of ageing skeletal muscle: a cross-sectional study of elderly men with different training backgrounds. Acta Physiol Scand 1990; 140:41-54.

Kouidi E, Albani M, Natsis K, Megalopoulos A, Gigis P, Guiba-Tziampiri O, et al. The effects of exercise training on muscle atrophy in haemodialysis patients. Nephrol Dial Transplant. 1998 Mar;13(3):685-99.

Kraemer WJ, Ratamess NA. Hormonal responses and adaptations to restistance exercise and training. Sports Med 2005;35; 339-61.

Kramer J, Stone M, O´bryant H et al. Effects of single vs multiple sets of weight training: impact of volume, intensity, and variation. J Strength Cond Res 1997;11: 143-147.

Lazarus R, Folkman S. Stress, Appraisal, and Coping. New York: Springer 1984.

Lok P. Stressors, coping mechanisms and quality of life among dialysis patients in Australia. Journal of advanced nursing. 1996 May;23(5):873-81.

Marlowe E. Rehabilitation concerns in the treatment of patients with chronic renal failure. American journal of physical medicine & rehabilitation / Association of Academic Physiatrists. 2001 Oct;80(10):762-4.

McIntyre CW, Selby NM, Sigrist M, Pearce LE, Mercer TH, Naish PF. Patients receiving maintenance dialysis have more severe functionally significant skeletal muscle wasting than patients with dialysis-independent chronic kidney disease. Nephrol Dial Transplant. 2006 Aug;21(8):2210-6.

McMahon LP, McKenna MJ, Sangkabutra T, Mason K, Sostaric S, Skinner SL, et al. Physical performance and associated electrolyte changes after haemoglobin normalization: a comparative study in haemodialysis patients. Nephrol Dial Transplant. 1999 May;14(5):1182-7.

Moinuddin I, Leehey DJ. A comparison of aerobic exercise and resistance training in patients with and without chronic kidney disease. Adv Chronic Kidney Dis 2008; 15: 83-89

Molsted S, Eidemak I, Sorensen HT, Kristensen JH. Five months of physical exercise in hemodialysis patients: effects on aerobic capacity, physical function and self-rated health. Nephron Clin Pract. 2004; 96(3): 76-81.

Nielens H, Lejeune TM, Lalaoui A, Squifflet JP, Pirson Y, Goffin E. Increase of physical activity level after successful renal transplantation: a 5 year follow-up study. Nephrol Dial Transplant. 2001 Jan;16(1):134-40.

Nilsen T, Hermann M, Eriksen CS, Dagfinrud et al. Grip force and pinch grip in adult population: Reference values and factors associated with grip force. Scand J Occup Ther 2011 Feb 28 (Epub ahead of print).

Pagels A, Heiwe S, Hylander B. Nutritional status and handgrip strength in pre-dialysis patients. Journal of Renal Care. 2006;XXXII:151-55.

Painter P, Messer-Rehak D, Hanson P, Zimmerman SW, Glass NR. Exercise capacity in hemodialysis, CAPD, and renal transplant patients. Nephron. 1986;42(1):47-51.

Painter PL, Hector L, Ray K, Lynes L, Dibble S, Paul SM, et al. A randomized trial of exercise training after renal transplantation. Transplantation. 2002 Jul 15;74(1):42-8.

Pechter U, Ots M, Mesikepp S, Zilmer K, Kullissaar T, Vihalemm T, et al. Beneficial effects of water-based exercise in patients with chronic kidney disease. International journal of rehabilitation research Internationale Zeitschrift fur Rehabilitationsforschung. 2003 Jun;26(2):153-6.

Pecoits-Filho R, Heimburger O, Barany P, Suliman M, Fehrman-Ekholm I, Lindholm B and Stenvinkel P. Associations between circulating inflammatory markers and residual renal function in CRF patients. American Journal of Kidney Diseases. 2003 Vol 41, 6: 1212-1218.

Ritz E, Boland R, Kreusser W. Effects of vitamin D and parathyroid hormone on muscle: potential role in uremic myopathy. The American journal of clinical nutrition. 1980 Jul 33(7):1522-9.

Sakkas GK, Ball D, Mercer TH, Sargeant AJ, Tolfrey K, Naish PF. Atrophy of non-locomotor muscle in patients with end-stage renal failure. Nephrol Dial Transplant. 2003 Oct;18(10):2074-81.

Sakkas GK, Sargeant AJ, Mercer TH, Ball D, Koufaki P, Karatzaferi C, et al. Changes in muscle morphology in dialysis patients after 6 months of aerobic exercise training. Nephrol Dial Transplant. 2003 Sep;18(9):1854-61.

Sonn U, Frändin K, Grimby G. Instrumental activities of dailys living related to impairments and functional limitations in 70-year-olds and changes between 70 and 76 years of age. Scand J Rehabil Med 1995;27: 119-28.

Thompson CH, Kemp GJ, Taylor DJ, Ledingham JG, Radda GK, Rajagopalan B. Effect of chronic uraemia on skeletal muscle metabolism in man. Nephrol Dial Transplant. 1993;8(3):218-22.

van Vilsteren MC, de Greef MH, Huisman RM. The effects of a low-to-moderate intensity pre-conditioning exercise programme linked with exercise counselling for sedentary haemodialysis patients in The Netherlands: results of a randomized clinical trial. Nephrol Dial Transplant. 2005 Jan;20(1):141-6.

Venkataraman R, Sanderson B, Bittner V. Outcomes in patients with chronic kidney disease undergoing cardiac rehabilitation. American heart journal. 2005 Dec;150(6):1140-6.

Welch JL, Austin JK. Factors associated with treatment-related stressors in hemodialysis patients. ANNA journal / American Nephrology Nurses' Association. 1999 Jun;26(3):318-25; discussion 26.

Yao Q, Pecoits-Filho R, Lindholm B, Stenvinkel P. Traditional and non-traditional risk factors as contributors to atherosclerotic cardiovascular disease in end-stage renal disease. Scandinavian Journal of urology and nephrology. 2004;38(5):405-16.

Zamojska S, Szklarek M, Niewodniczy M, Nowicki M. Correlates of habitual physical activity in chronic haemodialysis patients. Nephrol Dial Transplant. 2006 May;21(5):1323-7.

8

Lipid and Lipoprotein Abnormalities in Chronic Renal Insufficiency

Oliver Rácz[1], Rudolf Gaško[2] and Eleonóra Klímová[3]
[1]*Šafárik University, Medical School, Košice*
[2]*Railway Hospital, Košice*
[3]*University of Prešov,*
Faculty of Health Care, Prešov
Slovak Republic

1. Introduction

1.1 Kidney disease and cardiovascular mortality

Cardiovascular disease is a leading case of mortality not only in the whole population but also in groups with different, noncardiovascular chronic conditions. Kidney disease is one of these and many patients with kidney disease paradoxically do not die from end stage kidney failure but from cardiovascular causes. Already mild or moderate renal impairment represents a considerable excess risk of cardiovascular mortality. The probability of premature death is even more striking in some subgroups of kidney patients - e.g. the cardiovascular mortality rate of young end stage renal disease (ESRD) patients is 500 times higher as compared with an age-matched control group. The situation is moreover complicated by the fact that traditional risk factors (the "Framingham factors") are of lesser predictive value in kidney disease than in general population (Foley et al, 1998, Magnus and Beaglehole, 2001, Go et al, 2004).

To explain this dismal picture it is not sufficient to disclose that chronic kidney disease (CKD) and chronic renal insufficiency (CRI) is associated with accelerated atherosclerosis and abnormal lipid/lipoprotein metabolism (Felström et al., 2003, Lacquaniti, 2010). One should keep in mind that "CKD", "CRI" and "ESRD" are collective terms and the actual diseases and conditions behind them are manifold (Table 1). Some of them (e.g. diabetes mellitus and hypertension) have a profound effect on lipid metabolism and atherosclerosis independently from kidney function already before the manifestation of renal impairment. From the data in Table 1 is evident that diabetes and hypertension is behind ESRD in one quarter (Great Britain) or even two thirds (USA) of cases.

The natural history of each underlying disease is dependent on a wide range of factors and although the K/DOQI classification based on glomerular filtration rate is a very useful one from practical point of view it does not reveal anything about the pathogenesis of the particular condition.

Etiology of ESRD	Great Britain	Australia	USA	Japan
Chronic glomerulonephritis	30%	30%	9%	47%
Diabetic nephropathy	16%	22%	43%	31%
Hypertension	12%	14%	26%	10%
Chronic interstitial nephritis	8%	10%	2%	2%
Polycystic degeneration	6%	6%	2%	2%
Other/unkown	28%	18%	13%	8%

Table 1. Etiology of end stage renal disease in different regions of word. (According to Viklický, 2006)

1.2 Accelerated atherosclerosis in CKD

Despite all above mentioned uncertanities concerning the causal association between renal disease and accelerated atherosclerosis there is a considerable amount of knowledge in the field of pathophysiology and pathobiochemistry of this topic (Felström et al, 2003, Vaziri, 2006, Kwan et al, 2007, Saland &t Ginsberg, 2007, Tsimihodimos et al. 2008 and 2011, Basnakian at al, 2010; Karumanchi & Thadhani, 2010). An overview of different factors influencing the rate of atherosclerosis in CKD, CRI and ESRD is summarized in Table 2. These factors however do not act independently but in the frame of a complicated and not yet fully understood network (Fig 1.). They are present already in the early phases of kidney diseases and in many cases other pathological conditions associated with accelerated atherosclerosis (obesity, diabetes, hypertension, etc.) are present, too.

Dyslipidemia (increased triglycerides and LDL-cholesterol, decreased HDL-cholesterol)
Atherogenic lipid fractions (oxidized and carbamylated LDL, small dense LDL, triglyceride rich particles)
Abnormal values and forms of apolipoproteins (apoB, apoAI, $Lp_{(a)}$)
Uremic toxins
Alterations of calcium and phosphorus metabolism
Oxidative stress (increased formation of reactive oxygen species and advanced glycation endproducts, decreased acitivty of antioxidants)
Immunodeficiency
Inflammation
Malnutrition, hypalbuminemia and proteinuria
Anaemia
Physical inactivity
Ethnicity and genetic polymorphism
Drug treatment
Hemodialysis modalities
Peritoneal dialysis

Table 2. Factors influencing atherosclerosis development in CKD, CRI and ESRD

1.3 The aim of this chapter

In this chapter the authors try to answer some question conserning accelerated atherosclerosis and its assessment in CRI patients. In the subsequent parts they:

1. Describe and analyze the lipid and lipoprotein abnormalities in CRI, ESRD and HD.
2. Show the results of a metaanalysis dealing with methodological problems measuring LDL-cholesterol in CRI, ESRD and HD patients and results from a study on analytical quality of LDL-cholesterol assessment in real word laboratories.
3. Give simple advice how to assess cardiovascular risk in CRI, ESRD and HD patients in everyday clinical practice.

Therapeutic attempts and possibilities to normalize the lipid abnormalities and decrease the high risk of cardiovascular events in CRI, ESRD and HD patients are not the topics of this chapter.

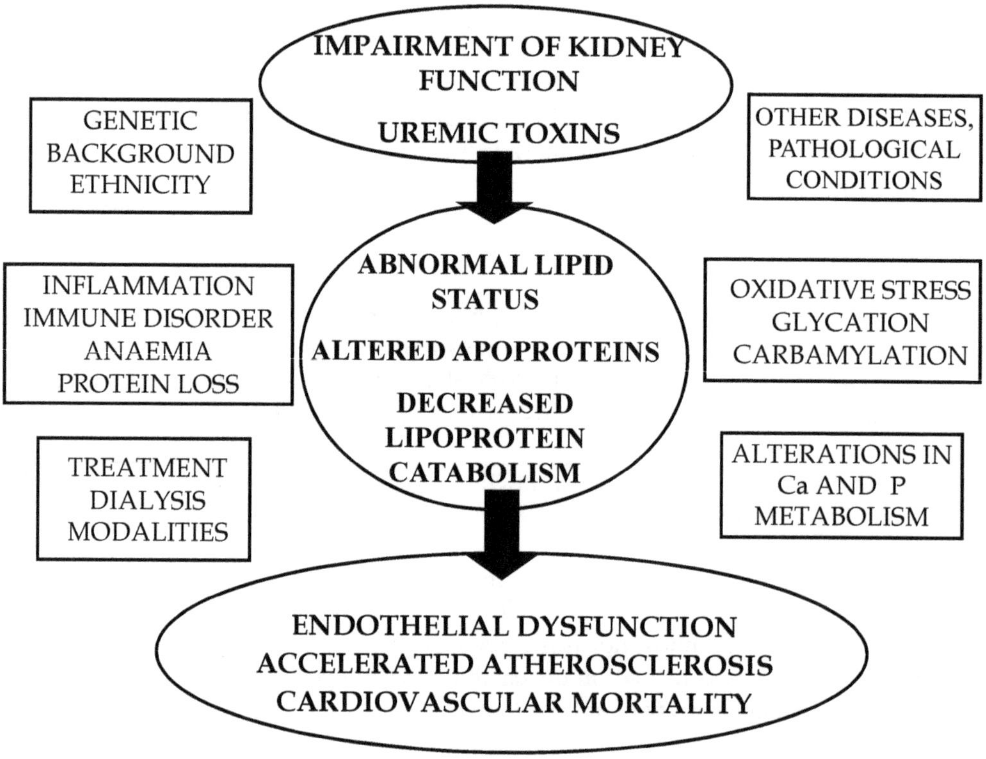

Fig. 1. Factors responsible for abnormal lipid metabolism and accelerated atherosclerosis in kidney disease form a complicated and intertwined network

2. Lipid and lipoprotein abnormalities in kidney disease

2.1 Changes of routinely measured lipid parameters in CRI and HD

The changes of two basic lipid parameters – the concentration of triglycerides (TG) and total cholesterol (TC) in different forms of renal disease are in Table 3. Increased triglyceride concentration is a general feature of kidney disease whereas increased cholesterol is not. Assesment the risk of atherosclerosis related morbidity from these two parameters is of course not possible because they do not reflect the real metabolic situation sufficiently. Lipids are insoluble in blood plasma and therefore they can circulate only in the form of lipoproteins. On the other side increased TG alone is an important warning sign of the presence of highly atherogenic triglyceride rich lipoprotein particles (TRL). The concentration of total cholesterol on the other side does not provide a valuable information because its carriers can be less and more atherogenic or even antiatherogenic. In table 4 data on changes of HDL-cholesterol, non-HDL-cholesterol and the highly atherogenhic $Lp_{(a)}$ in CRI are shown. LDL-cholesterol is not involved in this table for reasons of its analytical uncertainity which is further analyzed in part 3 of this chapter. From data in Table 3 and 4 the shift towards accelerated atherosclerosis is evident - high amount of triglycerides in the lipoproteins and a low level of antiatherogenic HDL particles regardless on the form and stage of kidney disease (Vazari, 2006, Saland et Ginsberg, 2007, Tsimihodimos et al., 2008, Attman et al., 2010).

Condition	Triglycerides	Total cholesterol
Minimal proteinuria	Increased	No change or decrease
Heavy proteinuria	Increased	Highly increased in nephrotic syndrome
Chronic renal insufficiency	Increased	No change
Hemodialysis	Increased	Controversial data - mostly no change
Peritoneal dialysis	Increased	Increased

Table 3. Triglycerides and total cholesterol in different conditions associated with kidney disease

Condition	Non-HDL cholesterol	HDL-cholesterol	$Lp_{(a)}$
Chronic renal insufficiency	Increased	Decreased	Increased
Hemodialysis	Increased	Decreased	Increased
Peritoneal dialysis	Increased	Decreased	Increased

Table 4. Non-HDL cholesterol, HDL cholesterol and $lipoprotein_{(a)}$ in chronic renal insufficiency, hemodialysis and peritoneal dialysis

2.2 Lipoprotein metabolism in health and kidney disease

Lipoproteins are complex particles consisting from lipids transferred from and to the tissues and a phospholipid envelope containing different proteins. They are not passive containers of TG and cholesterol but dynamic particles with variable composition. Both lipoprotein turnover and composition is altered in kidney diseases and therefore basic knowledge about it is essential for the proper assessment of cardiovascular risk in this special case. Lipoprotens are divided int three families: Chylomicrons and their remnants, the VLDL-IDL-LDL family and the HDL family. Their composition and apoprotein content is in Tables 5 and 6.

Chylomicrons produced in enterocytes are carriers of lipids from guts to liver. There are much bigger than the other lipoproteins and during ultracentrifugation they do not sediment at all. Chylomicrons contain one molecule of apoprotein is B48 and some apoprotein molecules A I, A II and A IV. During their life span they acquire apo E and apo C from HDL particles. In contact with muscle and fat tissue capillary endothelial cells they release fatty acids through triglyceride lipolysis catalyzed by endothelium-bound lipoprotein lipase. Remnants of chylomicrons are removed by the liver.

Lipoprotein	Size, nm	Density, g/l	Lipid content, %		
			TG	CH	PL
Chylomicrons **Chylomicron remnants**	80 – 500 > 50	< 0,940	80 – 95	2-7	3-9
VLDL **IDL** **LDL**	30 – 80 25 – 35 18 – 25	0,950 – 1,005 1,000 – 1,019 1,019 – 1,063	55 – 80 20 – 50 5 – 15	5 – 15 20 – 40 40 – 50	10 – 20 15 –25 20 – 25
HDL_2 **HDL_3**	9 – 12 5 - 9	1,063 – 1,125 1,125 – 1,210	5 – 10	15 – 25	20 – 30

Table 5. Basic characteristics of lipoproteins (According to Žák, 2002, modified; PL = phospholipids)

Apoprotein, function	Gene	Finding
A I - activator of LCAT	11q23-qter	HDL, CHY
A II – activator of liver lipase, Inhibitor of LCAT	11q21-q23	HDL, CHY
A IV - activator of LCAT	11q23-qter	HDL, CHY
B 100 - key protein for assembly and receptor binding	2p23-24	LDL, IDL, VLDL
B 48 - short form of B 100	The same as B100	CHY
C I -Cofactor of LCAT	19q12-q13.2	CHY, VLDL
C II – activator of lipoprotein lipase	19q12-q13.2	CHY, VLDL, HDL
C III – inhibitor of VLDL transfer into liver	11q23-qter	CHY, VLDL, IDL
D – regulator of cholesterol ester transfer	3q14.2-qter	HDL
E – Transfer of CHY remnants into liver	19q12-q13.2	CHY, VLDL, IDL

Table 6. Apoprotein function and their occurence in lipoproteins

After a meal rich in fat the peak value of chylomicrons occurs approximately in 3 hours and they disappear in 8 – 9 hours. Visible plasma turbidity is a clear sign of chylomicron presence (mostly caused when blood sampling is not realized in fasting state). Chylomicrons are not involved singificantly in atherogenesis but in the case of their decreased catabolism (which is a case in kidney disease) the accumulated remnants can be atherogenic (Chan et al, 2009).

Endogenous lipid carrier particles are formed in the liver as VLDL. They contain a bigger variant of apoB (apoB100) but the function of this protein is the same as in chylomicrons. Apoproteins B are of key importance during the assembly of lipoprotein particles and also serve as a docking structure when the lipoprotein binds to the LDL-receptor. The interaction of VLDL with HDL and with the tissues is similar to that of chylomicrons and during their circulation they became smaller – known as IDL and LDL. LDL particles during their relatively long life span ($t_{1/2}$ = 2 – 4 hours and in CRI probably even more) can undergo oxidation, glycation and carbamylation. These random postsynthetic events alter the quality of liporoteins with a profound effect on their cellular metabolism – e.g. the uptake of damaged LDL particles through the scavenger receptor and not through the LDL-receptor. Another important topic important for the rate of atherosclerosis (not only) in CRI patients is the presence of small dense LDL particles and (Table 7) and increased levels of abnormal particles as $Lp_{(a)}$ - Tables 4 and 8. All these features render the interpretation of basic laboratory parameters of lipid/lipoprotein metabolism in regard to the assessment of atherosclerosis difficult (Table 9).

Despite the complicated and sometimes contradictory data on LDL metabolism in CRI, ESDR and HD it is possible to summarize the underlying picture in a relatively simple way. According to Ikerwaka et al (2005) and Chan et al (2009) all lipid and lipoprotein alterations associated with LDL particles have a common soil - their decreased catabolism. Increased synthesis can play an additonal role in the case of massive proteinuria.

Class	Density, g/ml	Size, nm	% of LDL
I	1.026	27.5 - 26.0	3
II	1.028	26.0 - 25.5	16
III	1.034	25.5 - 24.2	50
IV	1.048	24.2 - 21.8	22
V	> 1.048	< 21.8	9

Table 7. Normal density distribution of LDL particles

Lipoprotein $Lp_{(a)}$ has a similar structure and composition as LDL particles	
Density:	1,050 - 1,100
Size:	25 - 35 nm
Proteins:	ApoB 100 and an abnormal protein, $Apo_{(a)}$ attached to the B 100 $Apo_{(a)}$ has a variable molecular weight between 300 - 800 kDa, its structure is similar to the plasminogen (involved in fibrinolysis).
Subtypes:	6 different forms - F, B and S1 - S4
Concentration:	0 - 1200 mg/l with abnormal distribution of values. As atherogenic are considered concentrations above 200 - 300 mg/l
Lp(a) in CRI:	Increased but the cause of increase is not clear. The basic level of $Apo_{(a)}$ is probably associated with gene polymorphisms and the kidney disease is a provocative factor for further increase (Danesh et al, 2000)

Table 8. Structure of $Lp_{(a)}$

The basic function of HDL is the reverse transport of surplus cholesterol from the tissues to liver. HDL particles are synthetized as discoid particles poor in lipids. Nascent HDL (or HDL_3) particles contain a lot of different apoproteins (70 % of total protein is Apo A-I and 20 % Apo A-II) crucial in TG and cholesterol metabolism which they exchange with chylomicrons and VLDL. Cholesterol bound to the surface of HDL is esterified by the enzyme LCAT and the esters are internalized. The cholesterol-ester loaded HDL_2 particles unload their content through a specific receptor into the liver. The low number and decreased function of LDL particles (manifest as "low HDL-C") is probably a consequence of the enzyme LCAT and the apoprotein A-I. Recently Rosenson et al (2011) highlighted the topic of HDL heterogeneity and its possible role in the pathophysiology of accelerated atherosclerosis in kidney disease. According to this concept not the low level of "good cholesterol" but rather the altered constellation of HDL structure and function is of importance in atherogenesis.

Tiacylglycerols and cholesterol are insoluble in water. They circulate in the blood exclusively as lipoproteins. Lipoproteins are complex particles; their cholesterol content (measured or calculated as HDL-C and LDL-C) does not reflect their real composition and structure. Lipoproteins are dynamic, changing their lipid and protein composition during their life span in the circulation. Lipoproteins are heterogeneous and their different density is not a simple biological variation but it has profound effect on their metabolism. Small dense lipoproteins are more atherogenic than those with low density. In some people and in some pathological conditions there are also abnormal lipoproteins in the blood. One of them is $lipoprotein_{(a)}$ which is highly aterogenic and its concentration is increased in renal disease. Some of the assay methods for lipids and lipoproteins are not bulletproof from analytical point of view - see part 3 of this chapter

Table 9. Pitfalls in interpretation of basic lipid parameters from clinical point of view

3. Methods for measurement and lipids, lipoproteins with special attention to LDL-cholesterol measurement

3.1 Basic lipid assays and the short history of lipid and lipoprotein measurement

The first cumbersome but at that time reliable colorimetric methods for cholesterol and triglyceride assays were developed in the first half of the last century. From today's point of view obsolete methods were crucial for understanding the association between lipid metabolism and cardiovascular disease. Later there were replaced with enzymatic assays and adjusted for the use in automatic analyzers. Isolation of lipoproteins by ultracentrifugation giving basis for the today lipoprotein terminology was introduced in the 40's of the last century. Analytical and preparative ultracentrifugation is also today the gold standard method for quantification, separation and research on lipoproteins. About the same time paper electrophoresis (later replaced by agarose and polyacrylamide gel) gave the rise not only to an alternative nomenclature (alpha, pre-beta and beta lipoproteins) but also to the epoch-making phenotypic classification of dyslipoproteinemias by Fredrickson & Lees in 1965 and a better understanding of the pathobiochemistry of atherosclerosis. This methodology is currently reserved only for specialized applications. (For an excellent review on this topic see Mcnamara et al., 2006).

Triglyceride and total cholesterol assays are the starting points of lipid status assessment also today but their information value is different. Strictly speaking both are "artefacts" but whereas total triglycerides provide an important information about the presence of TRLs, total cholesterol itself has a limited diagnostic value.

3.2 Estimation of LDL-cholesterol

Lipoproteins are prone to differential precipitation in arteficial conditions (e.g. heparin-manganese or dextran-magnesium solutions) and this allowed to develop methods to separate them without ultracentrifugation or electrophoresis. Based on this procedure in 70's first the direct measurement of HDL-C was developed and introduced into clinical chemistry. On the other side direct measurement of LDL-C was not possible until the end of the century. In the 25 year long interim period there was only one possibility to estimate the

concentration of LDL-C in everyday practice. It was the calculation according to Friedewald formula (Friedewald et al, 1972). The formula was based on the analysis of a large LDL database created in research laboratories using ultracentrifugation. It was however clear that a calculation from three (TC, TG, HDL-C) measured values with their own analytical uncertainity is only a recourse from necessity.
The uncertainity of the currently employed 3rd generation methods is much lower than that of the Friedewald formula or the older methods but from strictly analytical point of view they are also not sufficient to obtain accurate results (Bairaktari et al., 2005). Another unsolved problem is that the assay methods from different providers are not yet harmonized at all (Fuentes-Arderiu et al, 2009, Miller et al, 2010).

3.3 Apoprotein measurements

The discovery of immunochemical methodology in 70's made apoprotein assays possible. In the same time their function and their role in lipid metabolism was identified. According to recent view some of them belong to parameters providing important information when assessing cardiovascular disease risk (Ritz & Wanner, 2004, Batista et al, 2005) There are three apoproteins which should be measured in each patiens with elevated risk of cardiovascular disease: Apoprotein B100, apoprotein A-I and lipoprotein$_{(a)}$.
Only one molecule of ApoB100 is present in each LDL-type particle (Fig 2). ApoB100 is a big molecule (m.w. 550 kDa) crucial already in the synthesis of VLDL and playing an essential role in the removal of LDL from the circulation. Measurement of ApoB100 in routine clinical practice is possible and in contrast to dynamic and heterogenous entities as "HDL-cholesterol" and "LDL-cholesterol" is an unambiguously defined analyte. The concentration of ApoB100 therefore provides the best information about the presence of LDL-type particles circulating in the blood (Olofsson et al, 2007). Elevated concentration apoB100 and normal or slightly elevated LDL-C or nonHDL-C is an indirect but valuable marker of small dense LDL particles
Apoprotein A-I is a small molecule (28 kDa) and HDL particles contain several of them. They are activators of LCAT, that means the concentration of Apo A-I is a marker of HDL particle function and the metabolic activity of the particles and not their size or number.

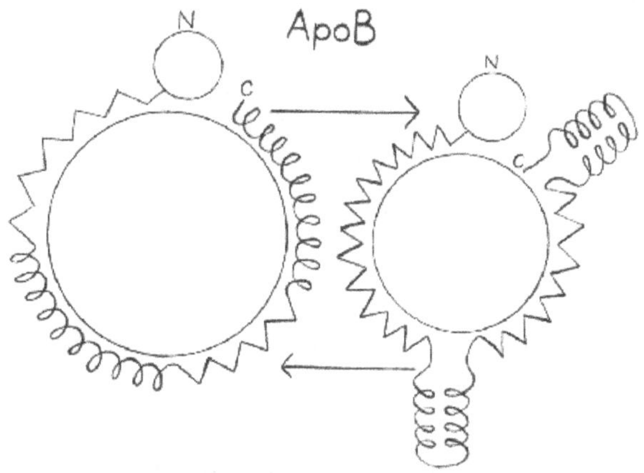

Fig. 2. Apoprotein B100 is a big ringlike flexible molecule holding the whole particle together in its different stages of metabolism and making its binding to LDL-receptor

4. Analytical accuracy of LDL-C in kidney disease and hemodialysis

4.1 Metaanalysis of results achieved with Friedewald equation compared to reference ultracentrifugation method

Our metaanalysis contains data from all available published papers dealing (entirely or as a part of broader study) with analytical accuracy of LDL-C assessment according to the Friedewald equation as compared with the reference UC method in CRI patients. The methodology of the metanalysis is described in our previous paper (Gaško et Sánchez-Meca, 2009). It includes studies from 1990 until the end of year 2010. Four studies were found but two of them were further divided according to the details of the study. The basic data of the studies are summarized in Table 10 and the results of metaanalysis in Fig 3.

Study, Year	Probands	Location	% Weight	Inclusion criteria
Nauck & al 1, 1996	887	Germany	0.0%	healthy (not included)
Nauck & al 2, 1996	136	Germany	23.2%	HD, TG < 4.56 mmol/l
Nauck & al 3, 1996	171	Germany	29.2%	CAPD, TG < 4.56 mmol/l
Pedro-Botet & al, 1996	101	Spain	17.2%	HD, age 20 - 80 years
Bairaktari & al 1, 2001	54	Greece	9.2%	HDs, TG < 2.26 mmol/l
Bairaktari & al 2, 2001	38	Greece	6.5%	HD, TG 2,26 – 4.52 mmol/l
Bairaktari & al, 2004	86	Greece	14.7%	HDs TG < 4.5 mmol/l
	586		100.0%	

Table 10. Studies included in metaanalysis, divided into subgroups according to inclusion criteria.

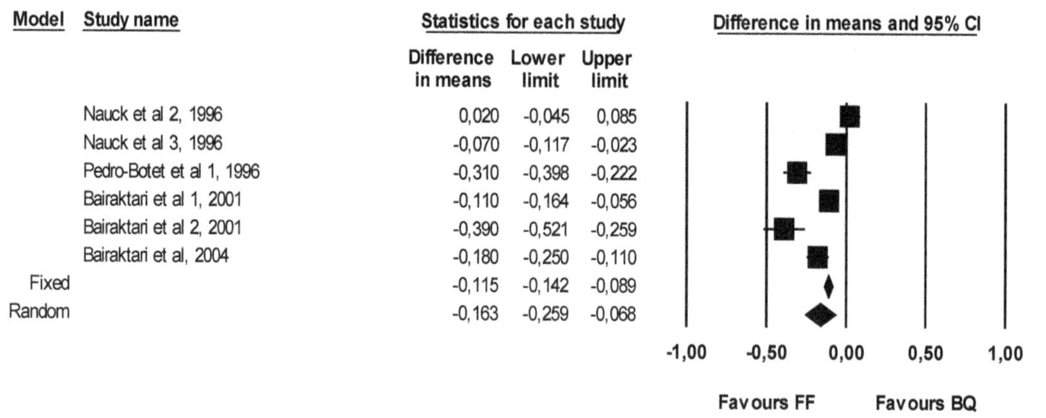

Fig. 3. Difference in means LDL-C with 95% CI in 4 studies included with 6 subgroups of patients with severe nephropathy on different forms of dialysis, with fixed and random effects model summary difference. Forest plot. Units: mmol/l. Patients included 586.

For patients in different dialysis regimes the summary differences of means of LDL-C is 0.234 mmol/l, what presents a bias of -4.9%. The information value of this result is much higher when compared with results on healthy probands od with results of patients with other diseases. We identified 23 publications including 17 213 patients analyzing accuracy of LDL-C assessment on healthy probands or in patients with hyperlipidemia from 1990 until 2009. The summary differences of means in this setting is 0.108 mmol/l and the bias is +2.3%. Furhter 3 papers followed analytical accuracy LDL-C in 350 patients with I and II diabetes mellitus or with hepatopathy. Total difference in means in this group was 0.234 mmol/l, (bias +6.8%; Fig 4).

From these findings it is possible to conclude that calculated concentrations of LDL-C according to the Friedewald equation can differ from the true values by almost 12 % systemic error. For clinical practice this analytical error can have a unwelcome situation because in approximately 7% of patients proper and necessary treatment according to guidelines is not prescribed and in another 5 % superfluous treatment is prescribed. This second group however is not in a danger of non-treated dyslipidemia because but there is problem of pharmacoeconomy.

Model	Study name	Statistics for each study		
		Difference in means	Lower limit	Upper limit
	Matas et al 2, 1994	0,370	0,214	0,526
	Matas et al 3, 1994	0,310	0,215	0,405
	Hirany et al 1, 1997	0,180	0,099	0,261
	Hirany et al 2, 1997	0,280	0,234	0,326
	Wägner et al, 2000	0,240	0,197	0,283
	Wägner et al, 2003	0,090	0,038	0,142
Fixed		0,220	0,196	0,245
Random		0,234	0,160	0,309

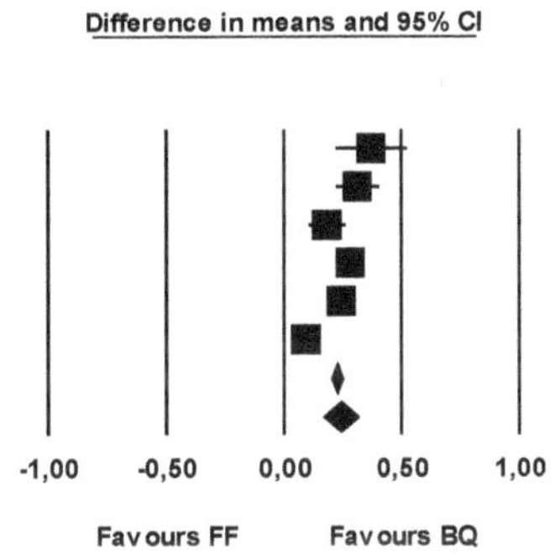

Fig. 4. Difference in means LDL-C with 95% CI in 3 studies included with 6 subgroups of patients with diabetes mellitus or hepatopathy, with fixed and random effects model summary difference. Forest plot. Units: mmol/l. Patients included 350. Figure from Gaško & Sánchez-Meca, 2009, with permision.

4.2 Unreliability of LDL-C assessment in everyday laboratory practice

There is only one method providing a true picture about the composition of the particles ultracentrifugation with subsequent chemical analysis of their composition. This method is the golden standard and the anchor of all methods used in routine clinical practice.

For a couple of years there was only one indirect way to estimate the cholesterol content of LDL particles. Despite modern methods estimating total cholesterol, HDL-cholesterol and triglycerides with a high level of precision and accuracy they have a certain degree of uncertainity and the overall uncertainity is too high to give a reliable picture on LDL-cholesterol even in probands without any confounding factors. In CRI patients the situation is even worse.

Recently clinical chemistry laboratories can use one commercial kits based on 7 different method for direct LDL-C assays. Some laboratories however calculate LDL-C according to the Friedewald formula or use both procedures (e.g. direct assay only in the case of elevated total cholesterol or in patients with otherwise elevated cardiovascular risk). According to

Agrawal et al (2010) in USA in 2009 approximately 2200 laboratories used direct assays but 3300 calculated LDL-C according to Friedewald. In Czech and Slovak republics the ratio was different (159 laboratories on direct assays and only 83 on formula (Gaško et al, 2011).
There is no official recommendation on international level about the methodology of LDL-C estimation. The choice depends solely on the decision of the laboratory and/or the health care provider. Another confounding factor is that the same laboratory can change the actual type of the direct method or use alternatively a direct method or the calculation mostly without any warning towards the clinician.
We realized a multicentric prospective study to compare the results achieved by different direct method compared with the results of Friedewald calculation (Gaško et al, 2011) in 13 laboratories. All of them were controlled also in the frame of an external quality assesment system. All of them diclosed results of the control sera in the appropriate range. Results of the direct assay and the calculation were compared on a set of randomly selected 200 patient samples with a broad range of diseases including CRI. In Fig 5. the average difference between the results of direct (considred in this study as reference) method and the calculated results are shown. The differences are in the range from -8 % ap to + 30 %. Of course the evident limitation of this study is the lack of comparison with the reference ultacentrifugation method. Despite this limitation the results of this simple study combined with the results of metanalysis (4.1.) show an unacceptable degree of uncertainity of LDL-C estimation in individual patients not to mention those who are at special risk.

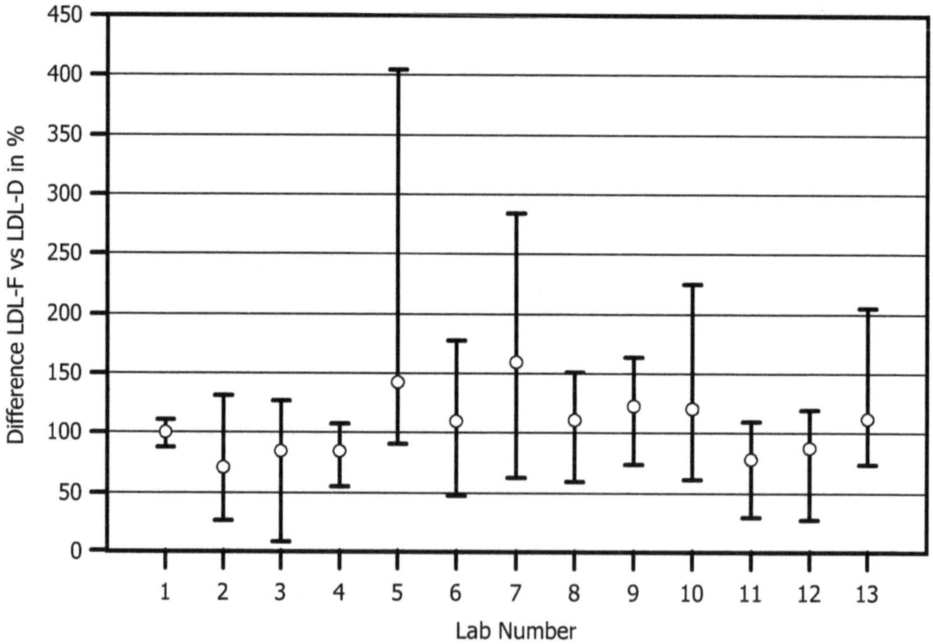

Fig. 5. Average differences (n = 200) in calculated LDL-C compared with results of the direct assay in 13 different laboratories. Value measured by the direct method in each laboratory is considered 100%. Data are shown as median and 2.5 to 97.5 percentiles.

A very interesting question is the situation after kidney transplatation. These patients at the first sight are „cured" but as a matter of fact they are far from being „healthy" beacause of the long-life immunosuppression therapy and of the slightly decreased kidney function in most of them. Balal et al (2010) compared results from 103 renal transplant recipients and the sum of differences between the calculation according to Friedewaldovho and the direct method was - 6,5 % ± 6,6 % (mean ± SD). According to Tsimihodimos et al (2008) after transplantation one very important atherogenic factor disappears - the increased level of Lp(a).

5. Conclusions

5.1 Where we stand today?

From our metaanalysis and the study on the unreliability of LDL-C estimation we conclude that the Friedewald formula seems to be no longer a viable test for appropriate targeted therapy in chronic renal failure and hemodialysis. Direct assays of LDL-C are not absolutely without error but they provide considerably more reliable results as a calculation from three measurements.

Clinicians should be aware that despite our gradually better understanding of the pathobiochemistry, pathobiochemistry and genetic background of atherosclerosis and kidney disease laboratories are not able to provide full explanation about the situation in individual patients. According to McNamara et al (2006) "we are still only scratching the surface, and mich more research and discovery remains to fully understand these critically important particles". As is depicted in Fig. 6 the scientist are looking on the different visible parts of the problem. The situation in clinical chemistry is even more problematic because the currently available methods are showing only the footprints of the real situation, not its essence.

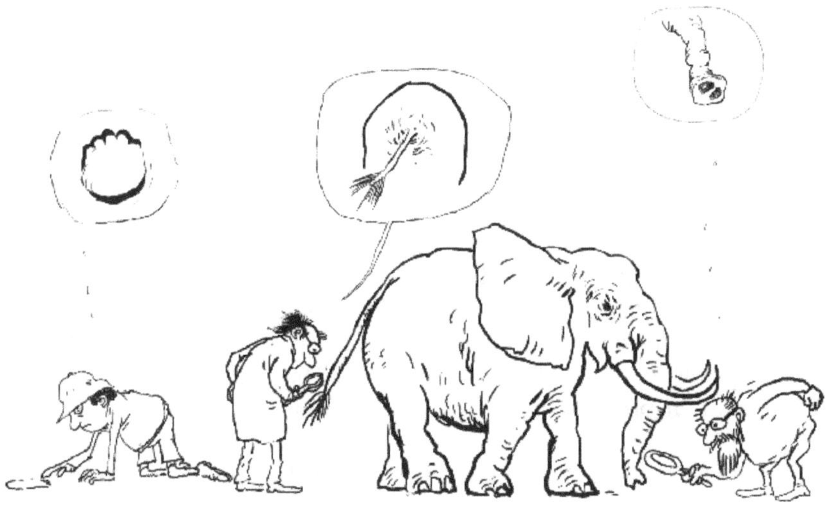

Fig. 6. Scientist looking at miscellaneous aspects of the problem and a clinical chemist trying to gain some information from the footseps.

5.2 Conclusion

In patients with CRI and/or ESRD, HD the pace of atherosclerosis development should be estimated as follows:

Proper clinical and biochemical evaluation of the underlying kidney disease and continuous monitoring of its progression. Special attenttion should be devoted to proteinuria and hypalbuminemia because they directly influence the metabolism of LDL-type particles and their concentration in the blood.
Evaluation of the risk factors not directly associated with the kidney disease (smoking, obesity, diabetes, hypertension, etc.)
Evaluation of lipid parameters - total cholesterol, LDL-cholesterol measured directly, HDL-cholesterol, triglycerides, apoprotein B100, apoporotein AI and Lp(a). The evaluation should not be a mechanistical process but should be based on pathophysiology of atherosclerosis in renal disease and should consider the strengths and weaknesses of the employed methods.
Measurement of other parameters not fully validated yet from analytical point of view and from their clinical usefulness (small dense LDLs, parameters of the oxidative stress and antioxidant systems) is possible for research purposes.

6. List of abbreviations

C	Cholesterol (as LDL-C, HDL-C, nonHDL-C)
CHY	Chylomicron
CKD	Chronic kidney disease
CRI	Chronic renal insufficiency
ESRD	End stage renal disease
HD	Hemodialysis
HDL	High-density lipoprotein
IDL	Intermediate-density lipoprotein
LCAT	Lecithin-cholesterol acyltransferase
LDL	Low-density lipoprotein
TC	Total cholesterol
TG	Triglyceride
TRL	Triglyceride rich particle
VLDL	Very low-density lipoprotein

7. References

Agrawal, M., Spencer, H.J., Fass, F.H. (2010) Method of LDL cholesterol measurement influences classification of LDL cholesterol treatment goals: Clinical research study. *Journal of Investigative Medicine*, Vol.58, No.8, pp. 945-949, ISSN 1081-5589

Attman, P.O., Samuelson, O. & Alaupovic P. (2011) The effect of decreasing renal function on lipoprotein profiles. *Nephrol Dialysis Transplant* doi:10.1093/ndt/gfq762, ISSN 1460 - 2385

Bairaktari, E., Tzallas, C., Kalientzidou, M. & al. (2004) Evaluation of alternative calculation methods for determining low-density lipoprotein cholesterol in hemodialysis patiens. *Clinical Biochemistry*, Vol.37, No.10, pp. 937-940, ISSN 0009-9120

Bairaktari, E., Elisaf, M., Tzallas, Ch. & al. (2001) Evaluation of five methods for determining low-density lipoprotein cholesterol (LDL-C) in hemodialysis patients. *Clinical Biochemistry*, Vol.34, No.8, pp. 593-602, ISSN 0009-9120

Balal, M., Paydas, S., Inal, T. & al. (2010) Validation of the Friedewald formula for the determination of low-density lipoprotein cholesterol in renal transplant recipients. Renal Failure, Vol.32, No. 4, pp. 455-458, ISSN 1525-6049

Basnakian, A.G., Shah, S.V. & Ok, E. (2010) Carbamylated LDL. Advances in Clinical Chemistry, Vol.51, pp. 25-52, ISSN 0065-2423

Batista MC, Welty FK, Diffenderfer MR et al (2004) Apolipoprotein A-I, B-100, and B-48 metabolism in subjects with chronic kidney disease, obesity and the metabolic syndrome. *Metabolism Clin Exp* Vol 53, No, 10, pp. 1255-1261, ISSN 1532 - 8600

Chan, D.T., Dogra, G.K., Irish A.B. et al (2009) Chronic kidney disease delays VLDL-apoB-100 particle catabolism: potential role of apolipoprotein C-III. *J Lipid Res* Vol. 50, pp. 2524-2531, ISSN 1539 - 7262

Danesh, J., Collins, R. & Peto, R. (2000) Lipoprotein(a) and coronary heart disease: Meta-analysis of prospective studies. *Circulation* Vol. 102, pp. 1082-1085, ISSN 0009 - 7322

Felström, B.C., Holdaas, H. & Jardine, A.G. (2003) Why do we need a statin trial hemodialysis patiens? *Kidney International,* Vol. 63, No. S84, pp. S204–S206, ISSN 0085-2538

Foley, R.N., Parfrey, R.S., Sarmak M.J. (1998) Clinical epidemiology of cardiovascular disease in chronic renal disease. *Am J Kidney Dis* Vol. 32, pp. S112-S119, ISSN 0272-6386

Fredrickson, D.S. & Lees, R.S. (1965) A system for phenotyping hyperlipoproteinemias. *Circulation* Vol. 31, pp. 321-327, ISSN 0009-7322

Friedewald, W.T., Levy, R.I., Fredrickson, D.S. (1972) Estimation of the concentration of low-density lipoprotein cholesterol in plasma, without use of the preparative ultracentrifuge. *Clin Chem* Vol. 18, pp. 499–502, ISSN 0009-9147

Fuentes-Arderiu, X., Braga-Fernández, S., Freire-Campo, L. & al. (2009) Comparison of measurement uncertainties in direct plasma low-density lipoprotein cholesterol method of measurement and indirect estimation according to Friedewald equation. *Accreditation and Quality Assurance,* Vol.14, No.2, pp. 179-183, ISSN 1432 0517

Gaško, R. & Sánchez-Meca, J. (2009) LDL cholesterol: A critical assessment of analytical accuracy of Friedewald's formula. Meta-analysis. *Kardiológia/Cardiology,* Vol.18, No.5, pp. 244–255, ISSN 1210-0048

Gaško, R., Rácz, O., Jedličková, B. & al. (2011) Methods for measurement of LDL-cholesterol: a critical assessment of direct measurement versus calculation in the treatment goals by European guidelines (2007), a multicenter study. *Cardiology Letters,* ISSN 1210-0048, accepted

Go, A.S., Chertow, G.M., Fan, D. & al (2004) Chronic kidney disease and the risks of death, cardiovascular events, and hospitalization. N Engl J Med Vol. 351, pp. 1296-1305, ISSN 1533-4406

Ikewaki, K., Schaefer, J.R., Frischmann, M.E. et al (2005) Delayed in vivo catabolism of intermediate-density lipoprotein and low-density lipoprotein in hemodialysis patients as potential cause of premature atherosclerosis. *Arteriosclerosis, Thrombosis & Vasc Biol* Vol 25, pp. 2615-2622, ISSN 1079 - 5642

Karumanchi, S.A. & Thadhani, R. (2010) Kidney complications: Why don´t statins always work? Nature Medicine, Vol.16, pp. 38-40, ISSN 1546-170X

Kwan, B.C.H., Kronenberg, F., Beddhu, S. & Cheing, A.K. (2007) Lipoprotein Metabolism and Lipid Management in Chronic Kidney Disease. *Journal of the American Society of Nephrology,* Vol.18, No.4, pp. 1246-1261, ISSN 1533-3450

Lacquaniti, A., Bolignano, D., Donato, V. & al. (2010) Alterations of lipid metabolism in chronic nephropathies: Mechanisms, diagnosis and treatment. *Kidney&Blood Pressure Research,* Vol.33, pp. 100-110. ISSN 1420-4096

Magnus, P. & Beaglehole, R. (2001) The real contribution of the major risk factors to the coronary factors to the coronary epidemics: time to end the "only 50%" myth. *Arch Intern Med* Vol. 161, pp. 2657-2669, ISSN 1538-3679

McNamara, J.R., Warnick, G.R & Cooper, G.R. (2006) A brief hisstory of lipid and lipoprotein measurements and their contribution to clinical chemistry. *Clin Chim Acta* 369, No 2, pp. 158-167, ISSN 0009-8981

Miller, W.G., Myers, G.L., Sakurabayashi, I. & al. (2010) Seven direct methods for measuring HDL and LDL cholesterol compared with ultracentrifugation. Reference measurement procedures. *Clin Chem* Vol. 56, pp. 1007-1014, ISSN 0065-2423

Nauck, M., Kramer-Guth, A., Bartens, W. & al. (1996) Is the determination of LDL cholesterol according to Friedewald accurate in CAPD and HD patients? *Clinical Nephrology,* Vol.46, No.3, pp. 319-325, ISSN 0301-0430

Olofsson, S.E., Wiklund, O. & Borén, J (2007) Apolipoproteins A-I and B: biosynthesis, role in the development of atherosclerosis and targets for intervention against cardiovascular disease. *Vasc Health Risk Manag* Vol. 3, pp. 491 – 503, ISSN 1178-2048

Pedro-Botet, J., Sentí, M., Rubiés-Prat, J. & al. (1996) When to treat dyslipidaemia of patients with chronic renal failure on haemodialysis ? A need to define specific guidelines. *Nephrology Dialysis Transplantation,* Vol.11, No.2, pp. 308-313, ISSN 1460-2385

Rosenson, R.S., Brewer, H.B., Chapman, M.J. et al (2011) HDL measures, particle heterogeneity, proposed nomenclature, and relation to atherosclerotic cardiovascular events. *Clin Chem* Vol. 57, No 1, pp. 392-410, ISSN ISSN 1530 - 8561

Ritz, E. & Wanner, C. (2008) Lipid abnormalities and cardiovascular risk in renal disease. *J Am Soc Nephrol* Vol 18, pp. 1065-1070, ISSN 1533 - 3450

Saland, J.M. & Ginsberg H.N. (2007) Lipoprotein metabolism in chronic renal insufficiency. *Pediatr Nephrol* Vol 22, pp. 1095-1112, ISSN 1432-198X

SHARP Collaborative Group. (2010) Study of Heart and Renal Protection (SHARP): Randomized trial to assess the effects of lowering low-density lipoprotein cholesterol among 9,438 patients with chronic kidney disease. *American Hearth Journal,* Vol.160, No.5, pp. 785-794, ISSN 1097-6744

Viklický O. (2006) Chronické selhání ledvin a uremický syndrom. *In: Tesař, V. Schück, O. (Eds) Klinická nefrologie. Grada Publishing Praha* pp. 477-511 ISBN 80-247-0503-6

Tsimihodimos, V., Dounousi, E., Siamopoulos, K.C. (2008) Dyslipidemia in chronic kidney disease: An approach to pathogenesis and treatment. *Am J Nephrol* Vol. 28, pp. 958-973, ISSN 1421-9670

Tsimihodimos, V., Mitrogianni Z., Elisaf M. (2011) Dyslipidemia associated with chronic kidney disease. *Open Cardiovasc Med J* Vol. 5, pp. 41-49, ISSN 1874-1924

Vaziri, N.D. (2006) Dyslipidemia of chronic renal failure: the nature, mechanisms, and potential consequences. *Am J Physiol Renal Physiol* Vol. 290, pp. F262-F272, ISSN 1522-1466

9

Malnutrition, Inflammation and Reverse Epidemiology in Hemodialysis Patients

Rodney G. Bowden, Neil A. Schwarz and Brian D. Shelmadine
Baylor University , Waco, TX
USA

1. Introduction

Reverse epidemiology, or risk factor paradox, has been used to describe the observed effect that traditional risk factors for cardiovascular disease may not necessarily signify the same risk for hemodialysis patients (HP) as for healthy populations. In fact, recent published findings have suggested counter-intuitive outcomes (Chavalitdhamrong, Danovitch, & Bunnapradist, 2007; Tsirpanlis et al., 2009) regarding the role cholesterol may play in disease progression in HP with chronic inflammation and malnutrition comorbidities (Dungan, Guster, DeWalt, & Buse, 2007). However, contemporary experimental studies regarding reverse epidemiology are lacking. The few published findings on this topic suggest chronic inflammation, as measured by C-reactive protein (CRP), and malnutrition, as measured by albumin, is associated with normal cholesterol levels yet higher levels of mortality (Chavalitdhamrong, et al., 2007; Chmielewski, Carrero, Nordfors, Lindholm, & Stenvinkel, 2008).

In contrast, traditional risk factors such dyslipidemia, hyperhomocysteinemia, obesity, or hypertension may provide protective effects in HP, at least in the short term (Kalantar-Zadeh, Block, Humphreys, & Kopple, 2003). Important predictors of clinical outcomes in HP are protein-energy wasting (malnutrition) (PEM) and inflammation (Fleischmann, Bower, & Salahudeen, 2001; Kalantar-Zadeh & Kopple, 2001; Kopple, 1997; Kopple, Zhu, Lew, & Lowrie, 1999; Lowrie & Lew, 1990; Nishizawa, Shoji, Ishimura, Inaba, & Morii, 2001). Because inflammation and PEM are interconnected and similarly affect markers of nutritional status both are considered part of a malnutrition inflammation complex (MIC) (Kalantar-Zadeh, et al., 2003; Kalantar-Zadeh & Kopple, 2001; Kalantar-Zadeh, Kopple, Block, & Humphreys, 2001). Thus, this chapter will address inflammation, malnutrition, cholesterol, and the overall concept of reverse epidemiology in HP relative to MIC as well as the implications of this information on short- and long-term treatment.

2. Inflammation in hemodialysis patients

2.1 Acute vs. chronic inflammation

Initially, the inflammatory response is a defense mechanism to cellular injury or pathogenic invasion. The acute response includes vasodilatation, hyperemia and vascular permeability and can be detected within a relatively short amount of time (minutes to days) via an increase in neutrophils and the presence of fluid protein exudates (Sprague & Khalil, 2009).

Additional responders involved in the inflammatory response are cytokines (Sprague & Khalil, 2009) and acute phase proteins, which reach peak circulating levels within two days in the acute setting (Ceciliani, Giordano, & Spagnolo, 2002). Typically, the inflammatory process ceases when the mechanism responsible for cellular injury is removed, subsequent cellular intermediaries are inhibited, and healing takes place (Sprague & Khalil, 2009). However, in some instances that inflammatory process is not resolved. Thus, the response remains active and proceeds into a chronic process, which can result in necrosis and/or loss of functional tissue.

2.2 Markers of inflammation in hemodialysis patients

In HP the inflammatory response and markers of inflammation, namely CRP and the inflammatory cytokine interleukin-6 (IL-6), are predictive of mortality (Barreto et al., 2009; Pecoits-Filho, Barany, Lindholm, Heimburger, & Stenvinkel, 2002; Stenvinkel, Barany, Heimburger, Pecoits-Filho, & Lindholm, 2002; Yeun, Levine, Mantadilok, & Kaysen, 2000; Zimmermann, Herrlinger, Pruy, Metzger, & Wanner, 1999). In addition to CRP and IL-6, albumin and the inflammatory cytokine tumor necrosis factor-alpha (TNF-α) are markers of inflammation commonly found in the literature. Each marker can provide evidence regarding the inflammatory state of HP, but there is debate as to which marker should be used and even debate as to the role in the inflammatory process of certain markers, namely CRP. For example, IL-6 and TNF-α are known pro-inflammatory cytokines and are also associated with declining kidney function. Various cells including, macrophages and mast cells, produce TNF-α and IL-6 (Sprague & Khalil, 2009). Among the numerous effects of TNF-α are the stimulation of a febrile response, up-regulation of other cytokines, such as IL-6, and stimulation of acute phase reactants (Sprague & Khalil, 2009). IL-6, in turn, has pleiotropic effects that include antibody secretion, the acute phase response and has also been shown to be pro-atherogenic, to name a few. However, TNF-α and IL-6 are not typically used in clinical medicine and are more often found in research; therefore other means of assessing inflammation are used as these tests can become costly. Conversely, albumin and CRP are measurements of inflammation readily available to physicians. Interestingly, albumin levels are also commonly used to assess nutritional status as both nutrition and inflammation can affect albumin (more on this topic will be presented later in the chapter).

CRP, however, is frequently used to confirm the presence of inflammation, as it is an acute phase protein produced by the liver and greatly regulated by IL-6. Additionally CRP is associated with reduction in nitric oxide production, induces monocyte recruitment and plays a strong role in foam cell formation. However, the causal role of CRP in cardiovascular events is still being debated (Genest, 2010; Lippi, Favaloro, Montagnana, & Franchini, 2010; Sattar & Lowe, 2006) and the use of CRP must be justified as it incurs added cost (Kaysen, 2009). Regardless, it is a marker of inflammation that in the native form consists of five noncovalently bonded subunits and is termed pentameric CRP or pCRP. This is typically the CRP measured in plasma or serum, and is also known as high sensitivity CRP (hsCRP). High sensitivity CRP can dissociate into monomeric CRP (mCRP) after binding with activated platelets (Eisenhardt et al., 2009). New evidence suggests that mCRP, through the interaction of hsCRP with activated platelets, may play a more dominant role in the inflammatory process than hsCRP as mCRP was found to colocalize with macrophages and platelets (Eisenhardt, Habersberger, Murphy, et al., 2009). High sensitivity CRP has also been found in atherosclerotic lesions (Sun et al., 2005), but the antibodies used to detect CRP in this study detected both pCRP and mCRP (Eisenhardt, Habersberger, & Peter, 2009). It has been reported that once pCRP dissociates into mCRP, mCRP stimulates monocytes to a greater extent than pCRP, leads to increased monocyte adhesion, and exerts proinflammatory properties (Eisenhardt, Habersberger, Murphy, et al., 2009). Additionally, mCRP may be more effective at regulating LDL metabolism than pCRP (Ji, Wu, Potempa, Qiu, & Zhao, 2006).

2.3 Causes of inflammation in hemodialysis patients

Aside from the primary reason for the patient being placed on hemodialysis, often a disease associated with inflammation, dialysis and the integral pieces of hemodialysis can be sources of inflammation. Kaysen (2009) indicates that the type of vascular access used in dialysis, the insertion of the catheters, biofilm on catheters, bacterial components present in dialysate, and water supply can all be sources of inflammation (Kaysen, 2009). Markers of inflammation associated with vascular access alone include albumin (Chand, Teo, Fatica, & Brier, 2008; Wystrychowski et al., 2009), CRP (Costa et al., 2008; Movilli et al., 2006; Sachdeva, Kovalchuk, Bitzer, & Mokrzycki, 2009), and IL-6 (Costa, et al., 2008; Sachdeva, et al., 2009). As Kaysen (2009) points out, the type of vascular access in HP is associated with mortality (Xue, Dahl, Ebben, & Collins, 2003). Acutely, initial insertion of vascular access, especially catheter or arteriovenous graft (AVG), resulted in transient elevations of CRP and IL-6 whereas arteriovenous fistulas (AVF) did not demonstrate a transient rise in inflammatory markers (Sachdeva, et al., 2009). In regards to chronic inflammation, changing vascular access type from a catheter to AVG was shown to cause an increase in albumin, where as a change from AVG to catheter caused a decrease in albumin (Wystrychowski, et al., 2009). Similarly, catheter and AVG use have been demonstrated to result in elevated levels of CRP and IL-6 and lower levels of albumin than AVF (Costa, et al., 2008; Movilli, et al., 2006). Thus, the type of vascular access has an impact on inflammation levels. An additional impact on inflammation levels is adipose tissue as adipocytes produce IL-6 (Fasshauer, Klein, Lossner, & Paschke, 2003), which is also a strong predictor of mortality in HP (Barreto, et al., 2009; Pecoits-Filho, et al., 2002; Stenvinkel, et al., 2002).

3. Malnutrition in hemodialysis patients

3.1 Albumin as a marker of nutritional status

Albumin is the most abundant plasma protein with a half-life of about twenty-one days. It is a negative acute-phase protein that functions to maintain oncotic pressure and act as a transport protein (Carlson, 2004). Normal serum albumin concentration is between 3.5 and 5.2 g/dL, and this reference range is often utilized as a marker of nutritional status in healthy older populations (Carlson, 2004; Covinsky, Covinsky, Palmer, & Sehgal, 2002). The cutoff point for low serum albumin concentration (hypoalbuminemia) has been proposed to be even higher at about 3.9 g/dL in HP (Trivedi, Xiang, & Klein, 2009). However, it must be noted that conclusions derived from measures of serum albumin concentration are not always in agreement with the conclusions derived from clinical assessments regarding nutritional status (Covinsky, et al., 2002). Forty HP with CRP levels below 0.80 mg/dL were evaluated for malnutrition by measuring serum albumin and through the use of the Subjective Global Assessment (SGA) described by Detsky, McLaughlin, and Baker et al. (1987). The SGA was used to determine whether a patient was classified as well-nourished or malnourished. Using 3.5 g/dL as the cutoff point for hypoalbuminemia resulted in a sensitivity of just 14.3% compared to the results of the SGA. Raising the hypoalbuminemia cutoff point to 4.1 g/dL increased the sensitivity of the measurement to 64%. Furthermore, the mean albumin concentrations for the well-nourished and malnourished groups were 4.3 g/dL and 4.0 g/dL, respectively, with considerable overlap between the two groups. These data suggest that serum albumin alone may not be a sensitive marker of malnutrition in the absence of inflammation in HP (Santos et al., 2003). Regardless, serum albumin is a very important marker of mortality risk in HP (Iseki, Kawazoe, & Fukiyama, 1993). Despite the lack of total agreement with clinical assessments of nutritional status, hypoalbuminemia has been demonstrated to be an independent risk factor for all-cause mortality in older persons especially when combined with measures of physical disability (Corti, Guralnik, Salive, & Sorkin, 1994). Additionally, hypoalbuminemia is associated with mortality in various disease populations including cardiovascular, cancer, and HP (Iseki, et al., 1993; Phillips, Shaper, & Whincup, 1989). A 1 g/dL reduction in serum albumin has been associated with a 47% greater risk of mortality in HP, with the serum albumin concentration in these particular HP being linked to inflammation more so than the presence of malnutrition (de Mutsert et al., 2009).

3.2 Regulation of serum albumin: malnutrition and inflammation

Serum albumin concentration is controlled by the rate of its synthesis, fractional catabolic rate (FCR), and distribution between intra and extravascular compartments. These three variables controlling albumin concentration are heavily influenced by both nutritional status and inflammation (Kaysen, 2003). In healthy individuals and HP without inflammation that are malnourished, albumin levels usually stay within a normal range until the degree of starvation is preterminal (Kaysen, 2009). Renal disease is associated with anorexia and PEM due to the build-up of uremic toxins. Additionally, hemodialysis for the removal of these toxins is also associated with anorexia and PEM because of the resulting nausea and post-dialysis fatigue (Bergstrom, 1996). PEM leads to a decreased rate of albumin synthesis. In normal individuals, the FCR of albumin and resting energy expenditure are also down-regulated in order to compensate for its decreased synthesis during periods of PEM. For HP that are in an inflammatory state, normal down-regulation of FCR is blunted leading to an imbalance between albumin synthesis and catabolism that result in hypoalbuminemia (Kaysen, 2009). Even in the absence of malnutrition, positive acute phase proteins that result from the production of pro-inflammatory cytokines are associated with decreased albumin synthesis. Additionally, inflammation leads to a greater than normal albumin FCR for a given serum albumin level (Kaysen, 2003). On top of the challenges presented by malnutrition and inflammation in HP, amino acid loss from hemodialysis itself may contribute further to nitrogen restriction and hypoalbuminemia (Kaysen, 2009).

3.3 Nutritional supplementation and hemodialysis patients

Recently, studies have investigated the effects of protein and amino acid supplements on serum albumin levels in HP (Bolasco, Caria, Cupisti, Secci, & Saverio Dioguardi, 2011; Moretti, Johnson, & Keeling-Hathaway, 2009; Taylor et al., 2011). When selecting an appropriate nutritional supplement for HP, phosphorus levels must be taken into consideration as it has been demonstrated that high-protein intake with concurrent low-phosphorus ingestion and normal serum phosphorus levels is associated with the lowest mortality rate among HP (Kalantar-Zadeh et al., 2010). Supplementation with 15 grams of liquid hydrolyzed collagen protein three times per week after each hemodialysis treatment in one crossover group increased serum albumin by month 3 of supplementation. However, this change was small (+0.03 g/dL) and was not sustained throughout the remaining 3 months of treatment (Moretti, et al., 2009). Conversely, two pilot studies have shown promising effects of nutritional supplementation on serum albumin. In one study, maintenance HP consumed eight ounces of egg whites (egg whites are low in phosphorus) once per day for six weeks (Taylor, et al., 2011). Mean serum albumin concentrations increased by 0.19 g/dL along with a fall in mean serum phosphorus of 0.94 mg/dL. In the other pilot study, four grams of oral amino acid supplementation three times daily increased mean serum albumin concentration by 0.50 g/dL after 3 months of treatment (Covinsky, et al., 2002). Also, inflammation was attenuated in the study group as demonstrated by a decrease in CRP levels. Based on these pilot studies, protein and amino acid supplementation may benefit HP, but more research including larger sample sizes with controlled trials is needed before a definite conclusion or treatment protocol can be formulated.

4. Cardiovascular disease and hemodialysis patients

The number of HP patients in the United States is approximately 350,000 with an expectation of reaching 1.5 million by 2016. Most HP have a significant decline in quality of life with two-thirds dying within 5 years of dialysis initiation; a survival rate worse than most cancers (Kilpatrick et al., 2007). Cardiovascular disease (CVD) is a leading cause of death in HP with rates higher than the general population and risk primarily associated with elevated lipids, inflammation, malnutrition, hypertension, hyperhomocysteinemia, obesity, and insulin resistance (Third Report of the National Cholesterol Education Program Expert Panel on Detection, Evaluation, and Treatment of High Blood Cholesterol in Adults (Adult Treatment Panel III) Final Report, 2002). Most HP patients' elevated lipid profiles are associated with a higher incidence of CVD morbidity and mortality (Vaziri, 2009) and all-cause mortality (Tsirpanlis, et al., 2009). Additionally, non-fatal CVD is 10-30 times higher in HP suggesting this population is more prone to heart disease (Nanayakkara & Gaillard, 2010). Though traditional treatment of CVD in HP has demonstrated promise, many large randomized trials in HP have not demonstrated a survival benefit from traditional treatment strategies (Nanayakkara & Gaillard, 2010). The challenge becomes understanding why traditional risk factors are less predictive and whether the progression of disease is so advanced in HP that risk factor management should be different in this patient population. It should be noted however, that traditional and non-traditional risk factors for CVD in HP do have some crossover, complicating our understanding of how risk factor management may assist in disease causation and association. Though this chapter focuses on HP, chronic kidney disease patients who are predialysis share some of the same counter-intuitive findings. Therefore it should be noted that progression of CVD begins well before HP begin dialysis and could be detected as early as stage I CKD. Finally, it has been suggested that plaque accumulation may occur differently in HP. In the general population arterial plaque is more associated with lipid accumulation, but with HP it is more likely to be associated with calcified plaques and increased arterial stenosis (Diepeveen, Wetzels, Bilo, van Tits, & Stalenhoef, 2008). Various research groups, including the National Cholesterol Education Program (NCEP) (Third Report of the National Cholesterol Education Program Expert Panel on Detection,

Evaluation, and Treatment of High Blood Cholesterol in Adults (Adult Treatment Panel III) Final Report, 2002) have established that lipids play a significant role in the progression of CVD and with reductions in cholesterol levels there is a similar and graded reduction in risk (Kalantar-Zadeh, et al., 2003). Dyslipidemia characterized in HP is primarily associated with hypertriglyceridemia, low HDL concentrations, elevated levels of LDL, elevated LDL particle numbers, a higher propensity of smaller and denser LDL particles which contain high levels of residual triglycerides, and elevated levels of lipoprotein (a) (Vaziri, 2009).

Cholesterol metabolism in HP can be significantly altered by dialysis protocol, lipid controlling medication, malnutrition, and inflammation (Montazerifar, Hashemi, Karajibani, & Dikshit, 2010). HDL can be significantly reduced in HP due to a reduced plasma concentration of ApoA-I and ApoA-II (Bowden, Hebert, Wilson, Gentile, & Lanning, 2007; Vaziri, 2009), reduced transporter proteins such as ABCA-1 (Vaziri, 2009), and the down-regulation of enzymatic process associated with HDL maturation (Malgorzewicz et al., 2010). Down-regulation also occurs with HDL paraoxonase which is associated with impaired protection against oxidative stress. Hypertriglyceridemia also occurs in HP, is normally associated with impaired VLDL and is the most prominent dyslipidemic abmormality reported in 70% of HP (Eisenhardt, Habersberger, & Peter, 2009). Additionally, hypertriglyceridemia is associated with increases in IDL, chylomicrons, and chylomicron remnants postprandial (Chmielewski, et al., 2008). Primarily a reduction in lipoprotein lipase, an enzyme associated with binding to VLDL and the release of the corresponding triglycerides, is associated with changes that cause a concomitant increase in plasma triglycerides that seems to correspond with a decrease in VLDL receptors. Finally, LDL in HP is normally more atherogenic as particles are usually smaller, denser and are more likely to be oxidized and engulfed by macrophages leading to more unstable arterial plaques (Kaysen, 2009). Oxidation can further cause LDL to no longer be recognizable to LDL receptors on the cell causing less deposition of LDL in intracellular pools. Less deposition can lead to the same amount of circulating LDL cholesterol being associated with smaller and denser LDL particles which can carry more risk for CVD. Excess LDL cholesterol is then removed from circulation primarily by being engulfed by macrophages which lead to more atherogenic foam cells leading to risk acceleration. Lipoprotein (a) is a LDL-like lipid with higher levels associated with increased risk of CVD and is associated with overproduction of apolipoproteins, specifically apoB. Apolipoprotein B is bound with LDL and is associated with increased numbers of LDL particles.

4.1 Reverse epidemiology

Though cholesterol metabolism in HP is associated with dyslipidemia and many CVD related deaths are associated with elevated levels of lipoproteins, recent evidence suggests that many HP have normal or reduced plasma cholesterol levels that are associated with a higher rate of mortality (Bowden & Wilson, 2010). CVD related mortality accounts for 40-45% of all-cause mortality in HP suggesting factors other than lipids may be associated with CVD in this patient population (Dungan, et al., 2007; Tsirpanlis, et al., 2009). Counter-intuitive outcomes regarding the role cholesterol may play in disease progression in HP may be affected by chronic inflammation and malnutrition with much of the published literature concerned with MIC (Bowden & Wilson, 2010; Chavalitdhamrong, et al., 2007). The term, though controversial, that has been used in the literature associated with this counter-intuitive finding is reverse epidemiology (Dungan, et al., 2007). Experimental studies are deficient, but the few published on this topic have suggested that HP with chronically elevated levels of inflammation, as measured by C-reactive protein (CRP) or interleukin-6 (IL-6), and malnutrition, as measured by albumin, are associated with normal cholesterol values but higher levels of mortality (Chavalitdhamrong, et al., 2007; Chmielewski, et al., 2008).

5. Malnutrition-inflammation complex

Cano et al. (2009) has reported that between 20-60% of HP may have MIC and that patients also have lower body weights, lower BMI, lower albumin levels, lower blood pressure and elevated CRP (Diepeveen, et al., 2008). Albumin has been specifically mentioned as a marker of nutritional status and identified as one of the criteria used to measure PEM which is associated with MIC. The association between hypoalbuminemia (< 3.9 mg/dL) and mortality has been well-established and albumin has been identified as a strong predictor of cardiovascular disease (Kaysen, 2009). Supporting this theory is the fact that most studies reporting on reverse epidemiology report no counter-intuitive findings with HDL. The cholesterol esters in HDL are primarily received from albumin (Vaziri, 2009) and therefore hypoalbuminemia would be associated with low HDL. This is also one possible explanation for why other lipoproteins would be low, yet still associated with a significantly higher mortality rate in HP. Challenging our understanding of how this might impact mortality and cholesterol is that albumin is also used as a measure of inflammation and may not necessarily be related a nutritional etiology (Trivedi, et al., 2009). Finally, CRP along with IL-6 are inflammatory markers that have been associated with higher rates of mortality as well (Bowden & Wilson, 2010).

5.1 Reverse epidemiology and cholesterol

In a subset of HP a decrease in baseline cholesterol levels, excluding HDL, has been associated with decreases in CVD mortality and all-cause mortality when patients have chronic levels of inflammation and poor nutritional status (Krane et al., 2009). Recent study authors have suggested the need to consider both malnutrition and inflammation simultaneously as albumin has been shown to be affected by inflammation levels. Inflammatory cytokines and acute phase reactants have been reported to decrease appetite, reduced albumin, increase catabolism (Liu et al., 2004) and quite possibly cause lower levels of cholesterol suggesting that low albumin levels may simply be a reflection of inflammation rather than malnutrition. Specifically most lipoproteins seem to be affected by MIC with the exception of HDL. In most studies where HDL was either low or unaffected most patients experience hypoalbuminemia and low protein intake in the diet (Kilpatrick, et al., 2007). Krane et al. (2009) in a study of 1,229 Type II diabetics who were HP reported that high levels of CRP strongly predicted all-cause mortality, sudden death and myocardial infarction when cholesterol levels were both low and high. Yet, when CRP levels were high and cholesterol levels were low, relative risks for CVD related deaths were even greater. It was further reported that CRP level and not LDL level was the variable more likely to predict risk for mortality and cardiovascular events. Another study confirmed the existence of reverse epidemiology in the presence of high inflammation suggesting the inflammation better predicted both morbidity and mortality (Tsirpanlis, et al., 2009). The study authors also reported that nutritional cachexia along with low cholesterol were good nutritional indices for malnutrition and may be the reason low cholesterol levels are associated with higher levels of mortality in HP. A more recent study reported on the cross-sectional association with MIC and the effects on cholesterol in HP (Bowden & Wilson, 2010). When comparing cholesterol levels, those classified as having hypoalbuminemia had a reverse epidemiological effect with LDL particle number. In the same study when HP were classified as having high inflammation, based on CRP, LDL, VLDL, and LDL particle number reported counter-intuitive findings. But, in patients classified as having both hypoalbuminemia and high inflammation, all lipid variables, with the exception of HDL, reported a reverse epidemiological effect. This suggests that though inflammation may play a more prominent role with reverse epidemiology, both inflammation and malnutrition can have a pronounced effect on lipids causing low cholesterol levels to be associated with more mortality. Additionally, other study authors have reported inverse associations with cholesterol and all-cause mortality, but also a U-shaped relationship with cholesterol in the presence of malnutrition and inflammation (Liu, et al., 2004). When malnutrition and inflammation were controlled for in the analysis, a strong, graded and positive association existed between high cholesterol levels and mortality further supporting the thought that reverse epidemiological associations with cholesterol in HP is associated with MIC. An additional review paper has suggested that previous studies that have controlled statistically for factors associated with MIC in HP, risk associated with cholesterol was the same as the general population and further speculates that cholesterol may be an additional marker of malnutrition (Chmielewski, et al., 2008). It should be noted that not all studies agree with these findings.

Another theory behind why low cholesterol in HP patients can be associated with high mortality has been called survival selection. It is well-established that most chronic kidney disease patients will not survive to kidney failure and End-Stage Renal Disease. Presently, it is suggested that only 10% (Trivedi, et al., 2009) of patients will live long enough to initiate dialysis. Therefore, since so few survive it is thought that only those who have a strong genetic predisposition for survival may be more likely to live but may also have a poorer risk profile. Additionally, simply stated, HP may not live long enough to die of the consequences of traditional CVD risk factors. Though this theory is not very new, it has yet to be confirmed with well controlled studies that take into consideration the age of the patients. Kalantar-Zadeh et al. (2003) also suggests that reverse epidemiology may be normal and that over-nutrition is primarily a 20th and 21st century phenomenon and that our understanding of traditional Framingham risk factors may in fact be new and the exception. Though over-nutrition is a problem in many countries it has been associated with longer living populations in Western nations. As one would expect this idea is highly controversial among scientist and nephrologists.

Additional study authors (Nanayakkara & Gaillard, 2010) have reported reverse epidemiology in HP concerning lipids could possibly be due oxidative stress. Reactive oxygen species (ROS) production that is not balanced by antioxidant control is associated with oxidative stress. Furthermore, oxidative injury has been reported to alter lipids in both the general population and HP and is involved in CVD acceleration (Diepeveen, et al., 2008). Though HP are normally supplemented with B vitamins and folic acid, many still have deficiencies in antioxidants with many patients shifting to a more pro-oxidative stress profile. High oxidized LDL is a well established comorbidity in both HP and CKD patients and is associated with small, dense LDL particles. Moreover, modification of LDL through oxidation is thought to be the first step in the development of CVD and specifically atherosclerosis. Oxidative stress occurs routinely in HP, especially in patients with a long-term dialysis vintage, making LDL smaller and denser and is associated with more endothelial dysfunction, inflammation, stenosis and intima media thickness. Therefore, the oxidative stress hypothesis may help to further explain reverse epidemiology. Oxidative stress in combination with MIC could cause lower levels of LDL and LDL particle numbers, but more atherogenic particles that can accelerate mortality and morbidity. Yet, those associations do exist, a causal relationship between oxidative stress, CVD, and reverse epidemiology has yet to be established suggesting the need for further study.

Chmielewski (2008) reports on an endotoxinlipoprotein hypothesis that suggests higher levels of cholesterol may be beneficial in HP. The theory suggests that higher levels of lipoproteins more readily bind bacterial lipopolysaccharide or endotoxins and modulate inflammatory immune responses. The authors continues to state that cholesterol levels and their ability to predict CVD fall on a continuum with lower and higher levels associated with mortality (Kalantar-Zadeh, 2007). Liu, et al. (2004) may help support this theory as they have reported a U-shaped curve regarding cholesterol levels and moratlity in HP. This theory is highly speculative and needs further study.

Finally, as mentioned previously, HP patients have been reported to have smaller, dense LDL particles that are more oxidized which may play a stronger role than LDL. Small LDL particle size has been identified as an emerging risk factor for CVD (*Third Report of the National Cholesterol Education Program Expert Panel on Detection, Evaluation, and Treatment of High Blood Cholesterol in Adults (Adult Treatment Panel III) Final Report,* 2002). A previous study (Bowden, Griggs, Wilson, & Gentile, 2009) has demonstrated that LDL particle number and LDL size can classify more HP at risk when compared to LDL and triglycerides. Since more HP have small, dense LDL particles there may be mortality associated with smaller LDL particles even when LDL particle number is lower. Therefore, though HP may have less LDL cholesterol and less of the smaller LDL particles, because smaller LDL particles are more atherogenic, more patients have increased morality with decrease levels of cholesterol.

6. Treatment

Reverse epidemiology has been associated with cholesterol but also body mass index (BMI), systolic and diastolic blood pressure, homocysteine, and creatinine levels (Balakrishnan & Rao, 2007) in HP suggesting the need for novel treatments. Since the counter-intuitive findings are prevalent in HP additional approaches are necessary to help identify novel treatments and to discover if new therapies are warranted. Though counter-intuitive findings are present in HP as well as advanced age, congestive heart failure, malignancies, and AIDS little data exists to support changes in non-traditional risk factors as a means to control CVD. To help increase albumin levels it has been proposed to increase protein content in the diet. But levels of protein augmentation with HP patients on chronic hemodialysis has not been sufficiently elucidated simply because dietary protein can be a significant source of uremic toxins and increase phosphate levels which can have deleterious effects on the health of HP patients (Stolic, 2010). It should be noted that hypercaloric consumption may take several years and even decades for serious health effects to occur, yet hypocaloric consumption, measured by albumin levels in HP patients, normally causes a more rapid deterioration in health. Combined with high inflammation levels, a decreased appetite and hypocaloric levels may cause a significant decrease in cholesterol but accelerated risk for mortality (Kalantar-Zadeh, et al., 2001). This short-term effect of malnutrition enhanced by inflammation may overcome the long-term impact of traditional risk factors for CVD and may cause the HP patients to not live long enough to develop elevated levels of cholesterol causing them die sooner than is expected. Also, evidence suggests that lipid levels become more elevated and more strongly associated with CVD the longer the HP receives dialysis and suggests that even though counter-intuitive cholesterol findings are evident in early dialysis traditional therapies such as statins, fibrates and niacin are necessary even with cholesterol levels are low (Chavalitdhamrong, et al., 2007). Therefore, treatment for HP patients with MIC needs to focus short-term on inflammation and malnutrition through dietary counseling and medication. Once MIC is controlled, a more long-term therapy may need to look at controlling lipids associated with CVD risk.

7. Conclusions

Reverse epidemiology in cholesterol levels associated with HP introduces a number of questions concerning our understanding of CVD and findings from the Framingham study. The questions becomes whether nephrologists should recommend the same cut-points for HP as is normally used in general populations. Should nephrologists attempt to control malnutrition and inflammation first and focus on lipids once HP have MIC under control? Though statins can help control lipids they may also help control inflammation which in turn may help to regulate appetite and increase albumin levels suggestions that statin therapy may still need to be used in most HP. Finally, more clinical trials are needed to discover if reverse epidemiology is "normal" in HP or simply a new understanding of traditional risk factors.

Author	Year	Sample	Population	Study Design	Study Findings
Bowden, et al	In Press	438	HP	Prospective ~ 3 years	Reverse epidemiological effects for total cholesterol, LDL, LDL particle number, LDL, triglycerides, and VLDL
Bowden, et al	2010	105	HP	Cross-sectional	Reverse epidemiology in number in hypoalbuminemia group; LDL, VLDL, and LDL particle number in inflamed group; total cholesterol, VLDL, large VLDL, triglycerides, Lp(a), LDL, and LDL particle number in hypoalbuminemia and inflamed group
Bowden, et al	2009	117	HP	Cross-sectional	Reverse epidemiology effect existed for LDL, large LDL, LDL particle size, and HDL
Krane, et al	2009	1255	HP with Type II Diabetes	Prospective ~ 4 years	Patients with low cholesterol and high inflammation had an

					adjusted relative risk equivalent to patients with high cholesterol and low inflammation in CVD death and all-cause mortality
Tsirpanlis, et al	2009	136	HP	Prospective ~ 2 years	Low cholesterol levels together with selected inflammatory markers predict CVD and all-cause mortality and morbidity
Kilpatrick, et al	2007	15,859	HP	Prospective ~ 3 years	Inverse associations between hyperlipidemia and survival, however, black HP with high LDL show almost two-fold increase in cardiovascular death risk
Liu, et al	2004	823	HP	Prospective ~ 3 years	Inverse association of cholesterol levels with all-cause mortality and a U-shaped relationship with CVD mortality in the presence of inflammation/malnutrition
Iseki, et al	2002	1167	HP	Prospective ~ 10 years	Hypercholesterolemia was an independent predictor on survival but was only evident in a sub-group of patients whose serum albumin was more than 4.5 g/dl

Table 1. Studies reporting a reverse epidemiology affect regarding cholesterol and HP (2002-Present).

8. References

Balakrishnan, V. S., & Rao, M. (2007). Genetics and reverse epidemiology among patients on chronic hemodialysis. *Seminars in Dialysis, 20*(6), 570-576.

Barreto, D. V., Barreto, F. C., Liabeuf, S., Temmar, M., Lemke, H. D., Tribouilloy, C., et al. (2009). Plasma interleukin-6 is independently associated with mortality in both hemodialysis and pre-dialysis patients with chronic kidney disease. *Kidney International, 77*(6), 550-556.

Bergstrom, J. (1996). Anorexia in dialysis patients. *Seminars in Nephrology, 16*(3), 222-229.

Bolasco, P., Caria, S., Cupisti, A., Secci, R., & Saverio Dioguardi, F. (2011). A novel amino acids oral supplementation in hemodialysis patients: a pilot study. *Renal Failure, 33*(1), 1-5.

Bowden, R. G., Griggs, J., Wilson, R. L., & Gentile, M. (2009). Cholesterol values are poor markers of disease risk in a chronic disease population. *Clinical Lipidology, 4*(5), 545-551.

Bowden, R. G., Hebert, S., Wilson, R., Gentile, M., & Lanning, B. A. (2007). Comparison of lipid measures and risk stratification among end-stage renal disease patients. *J Nephrol, 20*(2), 212-218.

Bowden, R. G., & Wilson, R. L. (2010). Malnutrition, inflammation, and lipids in a cohort of dialysis patients. *Postgraduate Medicine, 122*(3), 196-202.

Cano, N. J., Miolane-Debouit, M., Leger, J., & Heng, A. E. (2009). Assessment of body protein: energy status in chronic kidney disease. *Seminars in nephrology, 29*(1), 59-66.

Carlson, T. H. (2004). Laboratory Data in Nutrition Assessment. In L. K. Mahan & S. Escott-Stump (Eds.), *Krause's Food, Nutrition, & Diet Therapy* (11th ed., pp. 436-454). Philadelphia, PA: Saunders.

Ceciliani, F., Giordano, A., & Spagnolo, V. (2002). The systemic reaction during inflammation: the acute-phase proteins. *Protein and Peptide Letters, 9*(3), 211-223.

Chand, D. H., Teo, B. W., Fatica, R. A., & Brier, M. (2008). Influence of vascular access type on outcome measures in patients on maintenance hemodialysis. *Nephron Clinical Practice 108*(2), c91-98.

Chavalitdhamrong, D., Danovitch, G. M., & Bunnapradist, S. (2007). Is there a reversal of reverse epidemiology in renal transplant recipients? *Seminars in Dialysis, 20*(6), 544-548.

Chmielewski, M., Carrero, J. J., Nordfors, L., Lindholm, B., & Stenvinkel, P. (2008). Lipid disorders in chronic kidney disease: reverse epidemiology and therapeutic approach. *Journal of Nephrology, 21*(5), 635-644.

Corti, M. C., Guralnik, J. M., Salive, M. E., & Sorkin, J. D. (1994). Serum albumin level and physical disability as predictors of mortality in older persons. *The Journal of the American Medical Association, 272*(13), 1036-1042.

Costa, E., Rocha, S., Rocha-Pereira, P., Castro, E., Reis, F., Teixeira, F., et al. (2008). Cross-talk between inflammation,coagulation/fibrinolysis and vascular access in hemodialysis patients. *The Journal of Vascular Access, 9*(4), 248-253.

Covinsky, K. E., Covinsky, M. H., Palmer, R. M., & Sehgal, A. R. (2002). Serum albumin concentration and clinical assessments of nutritional status in hospitalized older people: different sides of different coins? *Journal of the American Geriatrics Society, 50*(4), 631-637.

de Mutsert, R., Grootendorst, D. C., Indemans, F., Boeschoten, E. W., Krediet, R. T., & Dekker, F. W. (2009). Association between serum albumin and mortality in dialysis patients is partly explained by inflammation, and not by malnutrition. *Journal of Renal Nutrition 19*(2), 127-135.

Detsky, A. S., McLaughlin, J. R., Baker, J. P., Johnston, N., Whittaker, S., Mendelson, R. A., et al. (1987). What is subjective global assessment of nutritional status? *Journal of Parenteral and Enteral nutrition, 11*(1), 8-13.

Diepeveen, S. H., Wetzels, J. F., Bilo, H. J., van Tits, L. J., & Stalenhoef, A. F. (2008). Cholesterol in end-stage renal disease: the good, the bad or the ugly? [Review]. *The Netherlands journal of medicine, 66*(2), 53-61.

Dungan, K. M., Guster, T., DeWalt, D. A., & Buse, J. B. (2007). A comparison of lipid and lipoprotein measurements in the fasting and nonfasting states in patients with type 2 diabetes. *Current Medical Research and Opinion, 23*(11), 2689-2695.

Eisenhardt, S. U., Habersberger, J., Murphy, A., Chen, Y. C., Woollard, K. J., Bassler, N., et al. (2009). Dissociation of pentameric to monomeric C-reactive protein on activated platelets localizes inflammation to atherosclerotic plaques. *Circulation Research, 105*(2), 128-137.

Eisenhardt, S. U., Habersberger, J., & Peter, K. (2009). Monomeric C-reactive protein generation on activated platelets: the missing link between inflammation and atherothrombotic risk. *Trends in Cardiovascular Medicine 19*(7), 232-237.

Fasshauer, M., Klein, J., Lossner, U., & Paschke, R. (2003). Interleukin (IL)-6 mRNA expression is stimulated by insulin, isoproterenol, tumour necrosis factor alpha, growth hormone, and IL-6 in 3T3-L1 adipocytes. *Hormone and Metabolic Research, 35*(3), 147-152.

Fleischmann, E. H., Bower, J. D., & Salahudeen, A. K. (2001). Risk factor paradox in hemodialysis: better nutrition as a partial explanation. *Asaio Journal, 47*(1), 74-81.

Genest, J. (2010). C-reactive protein: risk factor, biomarker and/or therapeutic target? *The Canadian Journal of Cardiology, 26 Suppl A*, 41A-44A.

Iseki, K., Kawazoe, N., & Fukiyama, K. (1993). Serum albumin is a strong predictor of death in chronic dialysis patients. *Kidney International, 44*, 115-119.

Ji, S. R., Wu, Y., Potempa, L. A., Qiu, Q., & Zhao, J. (2006). Interactions of C-reactive protein with low-density lipoproteins: implications for an active role of modified C-reactive protein in atherosclerosis. *The International Journal of Biochemistry & Cell Biology, 38*(4), 648-661.

Kalantar-Zadeh, K. (2007). What is so bad about reverse epidemiology anyway? *Seminars in Dialysis, 20*(6), 593-601.

Kalantar-Zadeh, K., Block, G., Humphreys, M. H., & Kopple, J. D. (2003). Reverse epidemiology of cardiovascular risk factors in maintenance dialysis patients. *Kidney International, 63*(3), 793-808.

Kalantar-Zadeh, K., Gutekunst, L., Mehrotra, R., Kovesdy, C. P., Bross, R., Shinaberger, C. S., et al. (2010). Understanding sources of dietary phosphorus in the treatment of patients with chronic kidney disease. *Clinical journal of the American Society of Nephrology : CJASN, 5*(3), 519-530.

Kalantar-Zadeh, K., & Kopple, J. D. (2001). Relative contributions of nutrition and inflammation to clinical outcome in dialysis patients. *American Journal of Kidney Diseases, 38*(6), 1343-1350.

Kalantar-Zadeh, K., Kopple, J. D., Block, G., & Humphreys, M. H. (2001). A malnutrition-inflammation score is correlated with morbidity and mortality in maintenance hemodialysis patients. *American Journal of Kidney Diseases, 38*(6), 1251-1263.

Kaysen, G. A. (2003). Serum albumin concentration in dialysis patients: why does it remain resistant to therapy? *Kidney international. Supplement*(87), S92-98.

Kaysen, G. A. (2009). Biochemistry and biomarkers of inflamed patients: why look, what to assess. *Clinical Journal of the American Society of Nephrology : CJASN, 4 Suppl 1*, S56-63.

Kilpatrick, R. D., McAllister, C. J., Kovesdy, C. P., Derose, S. F., Kopple, J. D., & Kalantar-Zadeh, K. (2007). Association between serum lipids and survival in hemodialysis

patients and impact of race. *Journal of the American Society of Nephrology 18*(1), 293-303.
Kopple, J. D. (1997). Nutritional status as a predictor of morbidity and mortality in maintenance dialysis patients. *Asaio Journal, 43*(3), 246-250.
Kopple, J. D., Zhu, X., Lew, N. L., & Lowrie, E. G. (1999). Body weight-for-height relationships predict mortality in maintenance hemodialysis patients. *Kidney Int, 56*(3), 1136-1148.
Krane, V., Winkler, K., Drechsler, C., Lilienthal, J., Marz, W., & Wanner, C. (2009). Association of LDL cholesterol and inflammation with cardiovascular events and mortality in hemodialysis patients with type 2 diabetes mellitus. *American Journal of Kidney Diseases, 54*(5), 902-911.
Lippi, G., Favaloro, E. J., Montagnana, M., & Franchini, M. (2010). C-reactive protein and venous thromboembolism: causal or casual association? *Clinical Chemistry and Laboratory Medicine 48*(12), 1693-1701.
Liu, Y., Coresh, J., Eustace, J. A., Longenecker, J. C., Jaar, B., Fink, N. E., et al. (2004). Association between cholesterol level and mortality in dialysis patients: role of inflammation and malnutrition. *The Journal of the American Medical Association, 291*(4), 451-459.
Lowrie, E. G., & Lew, N. L. (1990). Death risk in hemodialysis patients: the predictive value of commonly measured variables and an evaluation of death rate differences between facilities. *American Journal of Kidney Diseases, 15*(5), 458-482.
Malgorzewicz, S., Aleksandrowicz-Wrona, E., Owczarzak, A., Debska-Slizien, A., Rutkowski, B., & Lysiak-Szydlowska, W. (2010). Adipokines and nutritional status for patients on maintenance hemodialysis. *Journal of Renal Nutrition, 20*(5), 303-308.
Montazerifar, F., Hashemi, M., Karajibani, M., & Dikshit, M. (2010). Hemodialysis alters lipid profiles, total antioxidant capacity, and vitamins A, E, and C concentrations in humans. *Journal of Medicinal Food, 13*(6), 1490-1493.
Moretti, H. D., Johnson, A. M., & Keeling-Hathaway, T. J. (2009). Effects of protein supplementation in chronic hemodialysis and peritoneal dialysis patients. *Journal of Renal Nutrition, 19*(4), 298-303.
Movilli, E., Brunori, G., Camerini, C., Vizzardi, V., Gaggia, P., Cassamali, S., et al. (2006). The kind of vascular access influences the baseline inflammatory status and epoetin response in chronic hemodialysis patients. *Blood Purification, 24*(4), 387-393.
Nanayakkara, P. W., & Gaillard, C. A. (2010). Vascular disease and chronic renal failure: new insights. [Review]. *The Netherlands Journal of Medicine, 68*(1), 5-14.
Nishizawa, Y., Shoji, T., Ishimura, E., Inaba, M., & Morii, H. (2001). Paradox of risk factors for cardiovascular mortality in uremia: is a higher cholesterol level better for atherosclerosis in uremia? *American Journal of Kidney Diseases, 38*(4 Suppl 1), S4-7.
Pecoits-Filho, R., Barany, P., Lindholm, B., Heimburger, O., & Stenvinkel, P. (2002). Interleukin-6 is an independent predictor of mortality in patients starting dialysis treatment. *Nephrology Dialysis Transplantation, 17*(9), 1684-1688.
Phillips, A., Shaper, A. G., & Whincup, P. H. (1989). Association between serum albumin and mortality from cardiovascular disease, cancer, and other causes. *The Lancet, 334*(8677), 1434-1436.

Sachdeva, M., Kovalchuk, O., Bitzer, M., & Mokrzycki, M. H. (2009). Vascular access type and changes in inflammatory markers in incident dialysis patients: a pilot study. *The Journal of Vascular Access, 10*(3), 174-179.

Santos, N. S., Draibe, S. A., Kamimura, M. A., Canziani, M. E., Cendoroglo, M., Junior, A. G., et al. (2003). Is serum albumin a marker of nutritional status in hemodialysis patients without evidence of inflammation? *Artificial Organs, 27*(8), 681-686.

Sattar, N., & Lowe, G. D. (2006). High sensitivity C-reactive protein and cardiovascular disease: an association built on unstable foundations? *Annals of Clinical Biochemistry, 43*(Pt 4), 252-256.

Sprague, A. H., & Khalil, R. A. (2009). Inflammatory cytokines in vascular dysfunction and vascular disease. *Biochemical Pharmacology, 78*(6), 539-552.

Stenvinkel, P., Barany, P., Heimburger, O., Pecoits-Filho, R., & Lindholm, B. (2002). Mortality, malnutrition, and atherosclerosis in ESRD: what is the role of interleukin-6? *Kidney International Supplement*(80), 103-108.

Stolic, R. (2010). Obesity in renal failure--health or disease? *Medical Hypotheses, 75*(6), 497-500.

Sun, H., Koike, T., Ichikawa, T., Hatakeyama, K., Shiomi, M., Zhang, B., et al. (2005). C-reactive protein in atherosclerotic lesions: its origin and pathophysiological significance. *American Journal of Pathology, 167*(4), 1139-1148.

Taylor, L. M., Kalantar-Zadeh, K., Markewich, T., Colman, S., Benner, D., Sim, J. J., et al. (2011). Dietary egg whites for phosphorus control in maintenance haemodialysis patients: a pilot study. *Journal of Renal Care, 37*(1), 16-24.

Third Report of the National Cholesterol Education Program Expert Panel on Detection, Evaluation, and Treatment of High Blood Cholesterol in Adults (Adult Treatment Panel III) Final Report. (2002).

Trivedi, H., Xiang, Q., & Klein, J. P. (2009). Risk factors for non-fatal myocardial infarction and cardiac death in incident dialysis patients. *Nephrology, Dialysis, Transplantation : Official Publication of the European Dialysis and Transplant Association - European Renal Association, 24*(1), 258-266.

Tsirpanlis, G., Boufidou, F., Zoga, M., Triantafyllis, G., Fatourou, A., Stamatelou, K., et al. (2009). Low cholesterol along with inflammation predicts morbidity and mortality in hemodialysis patients. *Hemodialysis International, 13*(2), 197-204.

Vaziri, N. D. (2009). Causes of dysregulation of lipid metabolism in chronic renal failure. *Seminars in Dialysis, 22*(6), 644-651.

Wystrychowski, G., Kitzler, T. M., Thijssen, S., Usvyat, L., Kotanko, P., & Levin, N. W. (2009). Impact of switch of vascular access type on key clinical and laboratory parameters in chronic haemodialysis patients. *Nephrology Dialysis Transplantation, 24*(7), 2194-2200.

Xue, J. L., Dahl, D., Ebben, J. P., & Collins, A. J. (2003). The association of initial hemodialysis access type with mortality outcomes in elderly Medicare ESRD patients. *American Journal of Kidney Diseases, 42*(5), 1013-1019.

Yeun, J. Y., Levine, R. A., Mantadilok, V., & Kaysen, G. A. (2000). C-Reactive protein predicts all-cause and cardiovascular mortality in hemodialysis patients. *American Journal of Kidney Diseases, 35*(3), 469-476.

Zimmermann, J., Herrlinger, S., Pruy, A., Metzger, T., & Wanner, C. (1999). Inflammation enhances cardiovascular risk and mortality in hemodialysis patients. *Kidney International, 55*(2), 648-658.

10

Hemodialysis Vascular Access Dysfunction

Timmy Lee
Assistant Professor of Medicine
Department of Internal Medicine and Division of Nephrology and Hypertension, University of Cincinnati and Veterans Affairs Medical Center, Cincinnati, OH; United States of America

1. Introduction

A successful functioning vascular access is the "lifeline" for a hemodialysis patient. Hemodialysis vascular access dysfunction is a major cause of morbidity and mortality in hemodialysis patients[1-3]. Improving vascular access outcomes remains an ongoing challenge for nephrologists, vascular access surgeons, and interventionists. In arteriovenous fistulas (AVF) and grafts (AVG), the most common cause of this vascular access dysfunction is venous stenosis as a result of neointimal hyperplasia within the peri-anastomotic region (AVF) or at the graft-vein anastomosis (AVG) [4,5]. There have been few effective treatments to-date for venous neointimal hyperplasia in part because of the poor understanding of the pathogenesis of venous neointimal hyperplasia. Central venous catheters (CVC) are prone to frequent thrombosis and infection and the treatment of catheter-related bacteremia (CRB) remains on ongoing debate [6-8]. Therefore, this review will: (1) describe the pathology and pathophysiology of hemodialysis access stenosis in AVFs and AVGs, (2) discuss the pathogenesis of CRB and catheter thrombosis (3) discuss current and future novel therapies for treating venous neointimal hyperplasia, (4) discuss current strategies to treat CRB and catheter thrombosis, and (5) suggest future research areas in the field of hemodialysis vascular access dysfunction.

1.1 Types of hemodialysis access

Successful hemodialysis treatment requires access to the bloodstream to deliver a high enough blood flow to achieve an adequate dialysis dose. There are three primary types of hemodialysis vascular access to achieve this goal: (1) arteriovenous fistula, (2) arteriovenous graft, and (3) tunneled central venous catheter. Each type of access has unique advantages and individual problems.

1.1.1 Arteriovenous fistula

AVFs are the preferred vascular access for hemodialysis patients, because once mature and functional, they require fewer interventions to maintain patency and develop fewer infections compared to AVGs [9-13]. However, AVFs have higher rates of nonmaturation and longer maturation times compared to AVGs, which may lead to prolonged periods of CVC dialysis [9,14,15]. Recent reports from the United States have shown that up to 60% of AVFs never mature adequately to be successfully cannulated for dialysis [16] compared to 20-25 years ago where the nonmaturation rates in AVFs was approximately 10% [12].

1.1.2 Arteriovenous graft

Arteriovenous grafts (made from polytetrafluoroethylene, a synthetic fluoropolymer of tetrafluoroethylene) are advantageous because of short maturation time and relative ease to cannulation compared to AVFs [12,17-19]. Until recently, AVGs were the most common access used in hemodialysis patients in the Unites States [20]. However, the main disadvantages of AVGs are development of recurrent venous stenosis, requiring frequent interventions to maintain patency, and graft infection [19,21-24].

1.1.3 Tunneled central venous catheter

Tunneled central venous catheters have the advantage of immediate use, multiple sites for insertion, and the ability to provide access for hemodialysis for a period of months, permitting time for AVF or AVG maturation, in patients who require immediate hemodialysis [19,25-28]. However, the main disadvantages are the high risks of morbidity and mortality caused by infection [7,29-33], catheter thrombosis [19,34-37], and central venous stenosis [37-39].

2. Epidemiology and clinical significance of hemodialysis vascular access dysfunction

2.1 Epidemiology of hemodialysis vascular access

Due to reduced AVF use and increased AVG (70% in 1993 [40]) and catheter use in the United States from the mid-1980's-1990's, the National Kidney Foundation in 1997, in an effort to improve vascular access outcomes, published the first Kidney Disease Outcome Quality Initiative (K/DOQI) clinical practice guidelines for vascular access to optimize the care of vascular access in hemodialysis patients using evidenced and opinion-based guidelines [41]. Since these initial clinical practice guidelines have been published, we have seen the creation of the Fistula First Breakthrough Initiative (FFBI) [42-45] and two more revised K/DOQI clinical practice guidelines and performance measures for vascular access [19,46], which have clearly impacted and improved hemodialysis vascular access management. The most recent report from the 2009 United States Renal Data System (USRDS) has showed an AVF prevalence of 50% [47], a marked improvement since 2004 (39% AVF prevalence), 2000 (30% AVF prevalence), and 1998 (26% AVF prevalence)[48] in the United States. In contrast, AVF prevalence in Europe and Japan, reported from the Dialysis Outcomes and Practice Patterns Study (DOPPS) has been historically much higher, ranging from 57-91% [20].

While the K/DOQI guidelines and FFBI have clearly played an instrumental role in meeting the initial target goal of 50% AVF prevalence (new goal 66% [19,42]), the prevalence of CVC use continues to remain between 20-30% in the United States [42]. Furthermore, this trend of increased catheter use has also been observed in other countries, such as Spain, France, Belgium, Germany, and Italy [20]. This is likely due to an increase in the number of AVFs that have failed to mature for dialysis use in recent years [14,16].

2.2 Clinical significance and economic implications of hemodialysis vascular access dysfunction

When patients develop vascular access dysfunction, due to an immature AVF or thrombosed AVF or AVG, they are often consigned to CVC use for prolonged periods. Because dialysis with a catheter is associated with increased morbidity and mortality [49-55], CVC use has significant clinical implications such as increased risk of bacteremia which has been reported to occur at a frequency ranging from 2.5 to 5.5 episodes per 1000-catheter days [6,56], increased risk of 1-year mortality [49], and 60-70% higher risk of subsequent AVF failure [32,57]. The cost of treating one CVC-related bacteremia in the United States has been estimated to be as high as $45,000 per episode with an average of $22,000 per bacteremic episode [58].

3. Pathology and pathophysiologic mechanisms of hemodialysis vascular access dysfunction

3.1 Pathology of Hemodialysis Vascular Access Stenosis in AVF and AVG

Venous stenosis that occurs in both AVFs and AVGs is primarily due to neointimal hyperplasia. Venous stenosis in AVGs most frequently arises from the development of aggressive neointimal hyperplasia, characterized by (a) the presence of alpha smooth muscle actin positive cells myofibroblasts, and microvessels within the neointima, (b) an abundance of extracellular matrix components, (c) angiogenesis (neovascularization) within the neointima and adventitia, (d) a macrophage layer lining the perigraft region, and (e) an increased expression of mediators and inflammatory cytokines such as TGF-β, PDGF, and endothelin within the media, neointima and adventitia [59-64].

While the neointimal hyperplasia in AVFs is similar to AVGs in regards to pathogenesis, the venous stenosis that develops in AVFs is highly influenced by the capacity of the vein to vasodilitate and vascular injury from surgical technique [65]. In AVFs the two main etiologies of failure are an initial failure to mature (nonmaturation) and a subsequent (late) venous stenosis [4]. Similar to AVGs, venous neointimal hyperplasia in late AVF stenosis has been shown to be composed primarily of alpha smooth muscle actin positive cells, together with expression of mediators and cytokines such as TGF-β, PDGF, and endothelin within the media and intima of the vein [60,65]. However, recently, the lesion of AVF nonmaturation at 6 weeks after AVF creation has also been described to have significant neointimal hyperplasia [66].

3.2 Pathophysiologic mechanisms of neointimal hyperplasia formation in hemodialysis access dysfunction

The pathogenesis of venous neointimal hyperplasia in AVG stenosis and late AVF stenosis has been well described and is commonly divided into upstream and downstream events[4]. Upstream events are characterized as the initial events and insults that are responsible for endothelial and smooth muscle cell injury, which leads to a cascade of mediators (downstream events) that regulate oxidative stress, endothelial dysfunction, and inflammation (eventually resulting in venous neointimal hyperplasia). Upstream events that are believed to contribute to the pathogenesis of neointimal hyperplasia include [4,62,67-70]: (1) surgical trauma at the time of AV surgery, (2) hemodynamic shear stress at the vein-artery or vein-graft anastomosis, (3) bioincompatability of the AVG, (4) vessel injury due to dialysis needle punctures, (5) uremia resulting in endothelial dysfunction, and (6) repeated angioplasties causing further endothelial injury. Downstream events represent the response to endothelial (vascular) injury from the upstream events, resulting in the migration of smooth muscle cells from the media to the intima and eventually the development of neointimal hyperplasia [65].

The pathogenesis in AVFs that fail to mature (early failure) for dialysis, in contrast to AVG and late AVF failure, remains poorly understood. At a histological level early AVF failure is also characterized by aggressive neointimal hyperplasia in both animal and human models, seen as early as 1 month in animals [63,71] and 3 months in humans [64,66]. The underlying factors

(upstream events) which may contribute to early AVF failure, include [4,72-81]: (1) small diameter sizes in the vein and artery, (2) surgical injury at the time AV fistula placement, (3) previous venipunctures, (4) development of accessory veins after surgery, (5) hemodynamic shear stress at the AV anastomosis, (6) a genetic predisposition to vascular constriction and neointimal hyperplasia, and (7) pre-existing venous neointimal hyperplasia.
The subsequent sections will focus on the downstream events and three main mechanisms responsible for neointimal hyperplasia such as oxidative stress, inflammation, endothelial dysfunction, and alternative origins of neointimal-derived cells.

3.2.1 Oxidative stress

Many of the upstream mechanisms above (particularly hemodynamic shear stress and angioplasty injury) have been documented to result in an increase in the production of free radicals and its downstream products nitrotyrosine and latter (peroxynitrate). The latter is a potent upregulator of the matrix metalloproteinases (MMPs) [82,83]. MMPs are key enzymes that cause breakdown of extracellular matrix proteins such as collagen and elastin which facilitate the migration of vascular smooth muscle cells (VSMCs) in neointimal hyperplasia formation [84]. MMPs, paradoxically, have also been shown to facilitate a beneficial dilatation of the feeding artery (through degradation of the internal elastic laminae) in both rabbit and mouse AVF models [82,85]. Experimental studies of AVGs have demonstrated a differential upregulation of MMP-2 at the graft-vein anastomosis, with early expression (9 days) in the adventitia and a later expression (19 days) within the intima, supporting the concept of cellular migration from the adventitia to the intima [86]. Furthermore, linkages between hemodynamic shear stress and the expression of oxidative stress markers and cytokines have also been described in a porcine model of AVG stenosis [87]. Clinical studies of stenotic and thrombotic AVGs and AVFs have also demonstrated an upregulation of MMPs [88], and have documented the co-localization of oxidative stress markers with inflammatory cytokines such as transforming growth factor-beta (TGF-β), and platelet-derived growth factor (PDGF), within the neointima of both stenotic AVGs and AVFs [60].
Heme-oxygenase-1 (HO-1) is an important enzyme pathway which has been shown to confer protective effects in the vascular endothelium and other organ systems through its anti-inflammatory, antioxidant, or antiproliferative actions and properties [89]. Experimental studies in AVFs have described an increase in both the magnitude of arteriovenous stenosis and the frequency of thrombosis following the creation of AVFs in HO-1 knock out mice (increased baseline oxidative stress) as compared to wild type animals [90]. Furthermore, in the HO-1 knockout mice, there was significant induction of MMP-9 expression in the vein at 1 week compared to wild type mice, suggesting that MMP expression in vascular tissue and its deleterious effects with regard to promoting cellular migration may in part be inhibited by HO-1. Clinical studies have demonstrated a higher frequency of AVF failure in patients with heme-oxygenase-1 (HO-1) gene polymorphisms with long GT repeats (resulting in increased oxidative stress) [73].

3.2.2 Inflammation

ESRD is associated with a chronic inflammatory state, characterized by the elevation of circulating cytokines and chemokines [91]. This inflammation has been proposed to play an important role in the initiation and progression of atherosclerosis in ESRD, but may also play a significant role in vascular access stenosis. Support for this paradigm comes from recent work in which uremic mice developed a 2-3 fold greater magnitude of neointimal hyperplasia at the arteriovenous anastomosis as compared to non-uremic animals in a mouse model of AVF stenosis [92], and a recent study which showed marked upregulation of monocyte chemoattractant protein-1 (MCP-1) in the venous segment of AVF compared to rats deficient in the MCP-1 gene [93].

In clinical studies, possible linkages have described the presence of inflammatory cells (macrophages and lymphocytes), cytokines such as TGF-ß and insulin-like growth factor-1 (IGF-1) and the magnitude of neointimal hyperplasia and venous stenosis within stenotic AVFs [94].

Local bioincompatability to synthetic polytetrafluoroethylene (PTFE) material in AVGs could also result in local inflammation [95]. In vitro studies have demonstrated that conditioned media obtained after the interaction of peripheral blood mononuclear cells (PBMCs) with PTFE graft material resulted in a significant upregulation of smooth muscle cell proliferation as compared to control media [96]. This proliferative response has been shown to be attenuated by tumor necrosis-alpha (TNF-α) inhibitors [96]. Furthermore, the presence of macrophages that line PTFE graft material has been described in both experimental and clinical AVG stenosis with co-expression of inflammatory cytokines such as basic fibroblast growth factor (bFGF) [61,97].

3.2.3 Endothelial dysfunction

An intact and functional endothelium is essential for the vein to properly respond to acute changes in blood flow that occurs after creation of AVFs and AVGs [98]. Nitric oxide (NO) is an important mediator responsible for these transformations [99,100]. The presence of uremia in hemodialysis patients has been shown to exacerbate endothelial dysfunction, possibly through the pathways of inflammation and oxidative stress described above [101,102]. In the specific context of vascular access stenosis, endothelial dysfunction is likely to be responsible for the development of pre-existing venous neointimal hyperplasia [77-81], medial hypertrophy [77,81] and radial artery intima-media thickening [103-105] that is present even before the creation of AVFs in uremic patients. Pre-existing arterial intima-media thickness has been correlated with future AVF dysfunction [103]. Recently, pre-existing venous neointimal hyperplasia has been linked to poor AVF maturation in a small clinical study [77].

Asymmetrical dimethylarginine (ADMA) is an endogenous inhibitor of NO synthase and has been implicated as an important contributor to endothelial dysfunction in ESRD patients [106]. ADMA is not excreted in ESRD patients and its levels have been reported to be two to six times higher in this patient population as compared to non-uremic individuals [107]. In a recent clinical study in AVFs, patients with elevated ADMA levels at the time of percutaneous transluminal angioplasty of an initial AVF stenosis had a significantly increased risk of a recurrent AVF stenosis [108].

3.2.4 Alternative origins of neointimal cells

Although the traditional paradigm for the pathogenesis of neointimal hyperplasia has emphasized the migration of smooth muscle cells from the media to the intima, where they proliferate and contribute to the final volume of neointimal hyperplasia, a number of studies have reported that following coronary angioplasty or saphenous vein bypass grafting there is also a migration of cells (fibroblasts) from the adventitia, through the media, and into the intima, where these cells transform into "myofibroblasts" [109-111]. In dialysis access, a number of recent studies in AVGs have supported the concept of a migration of adventitial cells into the intima where they contribute to final neointimal volume [59,112]. In addition, recent data from several experimental AVF stenosis models have shown that smooth muscle cells in the neointima, may in part, originate from bone-marrow-derived cells that bind to the site of vascular injury and later differentiate into a smooth muscle cell phenotype in the neointima [82,113,114]. From a therapeutic standpoint, it is likely that better information about the true source of neointimal cells will allow for the development of novel therapeutic interventions targeting specific cell types.

3.3 Hemodynamic and vascular remodeling in hemodialysis access dysfunction

A number of experimental studies have shown that turbulent, low flow, low fluid sheer stress are involved in neointimal hyperplasia development [115-119]. High sheer stress has been associated with vascular dilatation through inhibition of smooth muscle cell proliferation and high levels of nitric oxide release, whereas low sheer stress has been associated with smooth muscle cell proliferation and lack of vasodilatation [120-123]. Poor hemodynamic profiles could be a risk factor for neointimal hyperplasia development and poor venous dilatation, and the degree of luminal stenosis is dependent upon both the magnitude of neointimal hyperplasia and the capacity for vasodilatation or vasocontriction. Therefore, a significant amount of neointimal hyperplasia and medial hypertrophy may not result in luminal stenosis in the presence of adequate vasodilatation, while a small amount of neointimal hyperplasia, but with poor vasodilatation, may result in severe venous stenosis [4,124]. Unfortunately, the factors that are responsible for vascular remodeling are unknown, but adventitial angiogenesis and scar formation are hypothesized to play a significant role[125,126]. Thus, the ideal therapy for vascular stenosis would be an intervention that would prevent vascular constriction (adverse remodeling) and neointimal hyperplasia[4]

4. Central venous dialysis catheters

CVC dysfunction and related-infection remains a common cause of morbidity, mortality, and high economic costs in treating chronic hemodialysis patients. This section will provide a brief overview of catheter dysfunction and catheter-related infections.

4.1 Catheter dysfunction

Catheter dysfunction can occur immediately after placement or in a catheter which has been previously functioning without difficulties, and most commonly manifests with low catheter blood flows during dialysis or negative arterial pressures on the dialysis machine [6]. In more severe cases catheter thrombosis is characterized by the inability to aspirate blood from the dialysis port [6]. Catheter dysfunction which occurs immediately after placement is most likely due to placement problems [6].

Installation of a thrombolytic agent for 30 to 60 minutes is a treatment for catheter dysfunction, followed by a second installation if necessary [6]. Recently published studies have reported varied success rate when treating catheter dysfunction with thrombolytics, ranging anywhere between 60-95% [26,28,35,127,128]. When thrombolytic therapy is unsuccessful in providing adequate blood flow and adequate dialysis, despite repeated installations, then catheter exchange needs to be performed. The current K/DOQI guidelines recommends treatment with thrombolytic agents in all catheters with a persistently low blood flow rate (<300 ml/min) [19].

The current standard of care to prevent catheter thrombosis is installation of an anticoagulant in both dialysis ports at the completion of each dialysis session. In the United States, heparin is most commonly used, while in Europe citrate is the more common anticoagulant [6]. The studies to-date have shown similar efficacy when comparing citrate to heparin for prophylaxis of catheter thrombosis, but with fewer complications of systemic bleeding with citrate [129-132]. A recent multicenter, randomized-controlled trial has reported that use of a thrombolytic, tissue plasminogen activator as a locking solution compared to heparin had reduced incidence of catheter dysfunction [34].

4.2 Catheter-related bacteremia

Currently, a precise definition for diagnosis catheter-related bacteremia is lacking. More rigorous definitions require a positive blood culture obtained from the catheter and a peripheral vein with the quantitative colony count being at minimum four-fold higher from the catheter sample [133]. However, recently, the Infectious Disease Society of America has recognized the challenges in obtaining peripheral blood cultures from hemodialysis patients (e.g. priority for preserving veins and difficult cannulations) and has considered a definition of "possible" catheter-related bacteremia as positive blood culture obtained from the catheter in a symptomatic patient [134].

The two main pathways where organisms can gain entry into the blood stream to initiate catheter-related bacteremia are intraluminal and extraluminal [135]. Organisms gain entrance through the bloodstream extraluminally through contact between the skin surface organisms and the external surface of the catheter at the time of catheter placement or following catheter placement before healing of the exit site or endothelialization of the subcutaneous tunnel [7]. Subsequently, the organisms colonize or migrate through the intracutaneous exterior tract of the catheter to the tip, allowing for hematagenous dispersion of the organisms and leading to catheter-related bacteremia [7]. Intraluminal-derived infections results from the transfer of organisms from hand contact with the catheter, leading to contamination of the internal catheter surfaces [7]. Infection from the extraluminal pathway most commonly occurs immediately after catheter insertion, while infections from the intraluminal pathway occurs throughout the life of the catheter [7]. Irrespective of the route of bacterial entry, the bacteria will either adhere to the CVC or become incorporated into a fibrin sheath. Adherence of the bacterial organisms to the CVC initiates a common pathway of biofilm production. A mature biofilm is a self-sustaining colony of microorganism, guarded by an exopolysaccharide matrix, that is stimulated and secreted by the organism and very difficult to eradicate [7,136-140].

Catheter-related bacteremia can result in devastating complications such as endocarditis, osteomyelitis, thrombophlebitis, septic arthritis, spinal epidural abscess, and large atrial thrombi [30,31,141-149]. The majority of isolated organisms from catheter-related bacteremia are gram-positive organisms (52-84%) with *Staph Aureus* responsible for the majority of these organisms [7,30,31,143,150,151]. Gram-negative are isolated in 27-36% of episodes and fungal isolated are relatively uncommon (<10%) [141-143,149,152]. Therefore, it is important to identify catheter-related bacteremia early so treatment can be initiated immediately.

4.2.1 Treatment of catheter-related bacteremia

Initial empiric antibiotic treatment should include broad-spectrum coverage for gram-positive and gram-negative organisms using knowledge of the common organisms and sensitivity patterns that are grown at the dialysis center. Due to the high prevalence of methicillin-resistant *Staph Aureus* (MRSA), empiric therapy should include coverage for MRSA. When the specific organism and antibiotic sensitivities are identified, it is important to narrow the antibiotic therapy to prevent the development of drug resistant organisms. While the exact duration of antibiotic treatment for catheter-related bacteremia is uncertain, the Infectious Disease society of America recommends a 2 week course of antibiotics [153], while the K/DOQI guidelines recommends a 3 week course of antibiotics [19]. Other therapies, which have been used in conjunction with systemic antibiotics, to treat catheter-related bacteremia are antibiotic catheter locks. A number of studies have shown that antibiotic locks (which may treat the biofilm layer) used in conjunction with systemic antibiotics, in tunneled dialysis catheters, have documented a 70% cure rate [30,145,154-156].

Recent studies have evaluated pharmacologic therapies to prevent catheter-related bacteremia. Routine application of topical antibiotic ointments at the CVC exit such as mupirocin, povidine-iodine, and polysporin triple ointment has been associated with a 73-93% reduction in the risk of catheter-related bacteremia [7,151,157-159]. Prophylactic antibiotic catheter locks have also recently been evaluated. A marked reduction in catheter-related bacteremia has been reported, ranging from 51-99%, with use of a prophylactic antibiotic catheter locking solution [7,160-164]. However, of concern, a recent study has shown emergence of gentamicin-resistant organisms after 6 months when using a gentamicin-heparin prophylactic catheter lock [165].

The above strategies for treatment of catheter-related bacteremia apply to patients who are clinically stable. However, catheter removal, in addition to antibiotic therapy, should be the treatment of choice when patients: (1) are clinically unstable, (2) have persistent fever for 48 hours, (3) have evidence of tunnel infection, or (4) develop metastatic infectious complications [7].

5. Translating science to therapies in hemodialysis vascular access dysfunction: from the bench to bedside

There are currently few if any effective therapies to treat hemodialysis vascular access stenosis and neointimal hyperplasia. However, the knowledge obtained in recent years regarding the pathology and pathogenesis of vascular access access dysfunction has provided a framework for development of therapies that target neointimal hyperplasia and vascular stenosis. The purpose of the next section is to (1) describe current therapies for AVF and AVG stenosis and (2) novel therapies using localized delivery systems for AVF and AVG.

5.1 Systemic therapies

Systemic therapies, such as dipyridamole, angiotensin-converting enzyme inhibitors, aspirin, and fish oil, from small clinical trials and observational studies have been shown to have the potential to block smooth muscle cell proliferation and migration and to prevent thrombosis in AVFs and AVGs [166-170]. Most recently, two large randomized controlled trials, sponsored by the National Institutes of Health, evaluating anti-platelet agents in AVG and AVF to prevent neointimal hyperplasia were published [16,171]. In the AVG study, dipyridamole and aspirin, modestly reduced the risk of stenosis and improved primary unassisted patency [171]. In the AVF study clopidogrel reduced frequency of early thrombosis but did not improve AVF suitability defined as cannulation with two needles, minimum dialysis blood flow of 300ml/min, successful use 8/12 dialysis sessions, and use after 120 days from creation [16]. While these two studies have shown some promising results, the clinical significance of these drugs used as standard treatment for hemodialysis access stenosis remains questionable.

Fish oil has been shown to prevent AVG stenosis and thrombosis in one randomized, controlled trial [172]. Currently, another study evaluating fish oil and AVG stenosis and thrombosis is ongoing [173]. Other systemic agents, though not tested in randomized clinical trials, which have shown potential anti-proliferative effects targeting neointimal hyperplasia in CVD or PVD models, include peroxisome proliferation-activated receptor γ agonist [174-176], sirolimus [177], and imatinib mesylate [176,178,179].

5.2 Radiation therapy

Radiation therapy has been hypothesized to be a potential therapy to treat vascular stenosis due to its antiproliferative effects and potential beneficial effects of vascular remodeling[180-183]. In experimental models, both external beam and endovascular radiation therapy has proven effective to reduce neointimal hyperplasia in AVF and AVG [184,185]. However, in clinical studies, a recent randomized-controlled trial of in AVGs 25 patients showed that 42% of the radiated AVGs achieved the target lesion primary patency end point at 6 months as compared to 0% of the control group ($p = 0.015$), but this did not translate into an improvement in secondary patency at either 6 or 12 months [186].

5.3 Far infrared therapy

Infrared radiation is an invisible electromagnetic wave with a longer wavelength than that of visible light. In experimental models, far infrared therapy has been shown to improve skin blood flow and endothelial function in cardiovascular disease [187-189]. The rationale for far infrared therapy to treat dialysis vascular access stenosis is that the dialysis vascular access in patients are located at a superficial site and improving access flow may improve vascular access performance. In the lone clinical study of far infrared in dialysis access in AVFs, patients who received far infrared therapy had improved access flows and longer unassisted patencies [190].

5.4 Local drug delivery systems for hemodialysis access

The rationale behind local delivery of drugs treat hemodialysis vascular access stenosis is that (1) AVFs and AVGs could be the ideal clinical model for the use of perivascular therapies since these can be easily applied at the time of surgery, (2) perivascular therapies preferentially target the "active" adventitia, (3) studies have demonstrated that lipophilic molecules when placed over the adventitia rapidly diffuse through all the layers of the vessel wall, and (4) small amounts of otherwise toxic drugs can be safely delivered to the site of stenosis using the perivascular approach resulting in high local concentrations with minimal systemic toxicity [4]. The subsequent section will discuss local therapies to treat hemodialysis vascular access stenosis from experimental models and clinical studies.

5.4.1 Drug eluting paclitaxel perivascular wraps

Experimental studies have previously demonstrated the efficacy of paclitaxel eluting wraps in AVG stenosis likely due to anti-proliferative effects [191-193]. In 2007, a large multi-center randomized-controlled study, evaluating the use of paclitaxel-eluting mesh wraps, Vascular

Wrap™, (Angiotech Pharmaceuticals, Inc.; Vancouver, British Columbia, Canada), was initiated to study the effectiveness and safety of this therapy on primary AVG patency compared to a standard AVG. However, this study was recently suspended in 2009 following a data safety monitoring review, due to an imbalance in the incidence of infections in one of the arms (either control or treatment). An alternative approach is the use of sirolimus eluting COLL-R® wraps (Covalon Technologies Ltd: Mississauga, Ontario, Canada). An initial Phase II study demonstrated primary unassisted AVG patency of 75% and 38% at 1 and 2 years respectively with these wraps [194].

5.4.2 Endothelial cell loaded gel foam wraps

The rationale behind the use of these wraps is that the endothelial cell (in addition to lining blood vessels) is also a "bioreactor" which produces a large number of beneficial mediators that reduces thrombosis, inflammation, stenosis, and increases lumen diameter. Initial experimental studies have documented a beneficial effect of endothelial cell loaded gel-foam wraps in porcine models of AV fistula and graft stenosis [195-198]. A recent Phase II study ("V-HEALTH") was able to demonstrate technical feasibility and safety in hemodialysis patients who received a "Vascugel®" wrap loaded with treated human aortic endothelial cells at the time of AVF or AVG placement [97]. A phase III multi-center randomized-controlled study using the Vascugel® (Pervasis Therapeutics, Inc., Cambridge, MA) wraps in human AVGs is currently being designed.

5.4.3 Vascular Endothelial Growth Factor D (VEGF-D) gene therapy

In animal models of angioplasty induced restenosis, the delivery of adenoviral particles encoding for vascular-endothelial growth factor C to the site of vascular injury has been shown to trigger the release of nitric oxide and prostacyclin and reduce neointimal hyperplasia [199]. Preliminary studies on the use of VEGF-D gene therapy (using a packaged adenoviral vector and a biodegradable local delivery device (collar) made of collagen wrapped at the venous anastomosis at the time of surgery), "Trinam®" (Ark Therapeutics; London, UK), in patients receiving AVGs, have been able to document technical feasibility and safety. A phase III study using this technology was initiated in 2009 but terminated in 2010 due to poor enrollment.

5.4.4 Recombinant elastase PRT-201

PRT-201 (Proteon Therapeutics; Waltham, MA) is a recombinant pancreatic elastase topically applied at the outflow vein at the time of surgery access creation which has been shown to result in both arterial and venous dilation and an increase in AVF blood flow in experimental models [200]. The clinical benefit of this approach is the potential ability to enhance AVF maturation (through rapid vascular dilation) and prevent venous stenosis in AVGs. A phase II study using this novel technology is ongoing in the United States evaluating this therapy and whether or not it improves primary patency and cumulative survival in AVG and AVF, as well as safety.

5.5 Endovascular stent therapy

Endovascular vascular therapies (angioplasty or angioplasty with stent placement) remains the only true intervention available to treat vascular stenosis. The main advantage of stent therapy after angioplasty is a reduction in adverse remodeling. In dialysis access, placement

of bare metal stents after angioplasty compared to angioplasty [201] alone has been shown to improve primary patency [202,203]. However, bare-metal stents have yielded poor results due to aggressive development of in-stent restenosis. In experimental models of dialysis access in AVGs, drug-eluting stents have shown to reduce neointimal hyperplasia and improve luminal stenosis compared to bare-metal stents [204]. However, there are no clinical studies evaluating drug-eluting stents in dialysis access to date.
Stent grafts (covered stents constructed from the same material of AVGs) have received recent attention as a therapy for prevention of restenosis due to its ability to prevent elastic recoil and inability of the neointimal cells to penetrate the covered barrier. A recently published multicenter, randomized controlled, clinical trial showed stent grafts (Bard Peripheral Vascular, Tempe, AZ), placed after angioplasty, to treat venous stenosis had better primary unassisted patency compared to angioplasty alone [205]. This is the only treatment to date that has shown to be effective to treat vascular access stenosis in a large, randomized, clinical trial.

5.6 Improving hemodynamics

Hemodynamic sheer stresses play a significant role in development of neointimal hyperplasia [87,112,206,207]. Therefore, altering the sheer stress pattern to prevent turbulent, low-flow, and low-sheer stresses could reduce the development of neointimal hyperplasia. Previous clinical data to date to support such an intervention comes from several studies evaluating cuffed AVG grafts ("Venaflo"; Bard Vascular, Tempe Arizona) [208-210]. In a recent randomized control trial evaluating cuffed vs non-cuffed AVG, cuffed AVGs showed better primary patency and cumulative survival [211]. Finally, results from a newly developed anastomotic implant device, "OptiflowTM" (Bioconnect Systems; Ambler, PA), to connect the artery and vein in AVFs and improve hemodynamics by providing a symmetric flow pattern, have shown a primary patency of 83% at 90 days [212]. This primary patency rate was higher compared to other similarly published studies [213].

6. Future perspectives: new frontiers in research

In the last decade our knowledge of vascular access dysfunction has significantly evolved. We now understand that the most common pathologic lesion seen in AVF and AVG dysfunction is aggressive venous neointimal hyperplasia, and biofilms and fibrin sheaths play a major role in CVC infection and dysfunction. In order to advance the field further, we need to further our current understanding of both the clinical and experimental pathways that result in venous neointimal hyperplasia and mechanisms that lead to biofilm and fibrin sheath production in CVCs by using the advanced technologies and tools in cellular and molecular biology, bioengineering, genomics, proteomics, and vascular imaging (ultrasound, computed tomography, and magnetic resonance imaging) [65,124,214]. Finally, small and large animal models of AVF and AVG, which a number of investigators in this field have already developed [61,93,207,215-217], will play an essential role in "translating" our knowledge of pathophysiologic mechanisms in vascular access dysfunction to novel therapies for patients.

7. Conclusion

The magnitude and costs of dialysis access dysfunction is clearly evident, and will only become magnified in the coming years as the prevalent dialysis population continues to increase. Only by launching a "translational" research initiative ("from animal to human") can recent advances in the understanding of the mechanisms of neointimal hyperplasia formation and vascular stenosis and catheter dysfunction be translated to the development of novel effective therapies for patients.

8. References

Collins AJ, Foley RN, Gilbertson DT, Chen SC. The state of chronic kidney disease, ESRD, and morbidity and mortality in the first year of dialysis. Clin J Am Soc Nephrol 2009;4 Suppl 1:S5-11.

Feldman HI, Kobrin S, Wasserstein A. Hemodialysis vascular access morbidity. J Am Soc Nephrol 1996;7:523-35.

Dhingra RK, Young EW, Hulbert-Shearon TE, Leavey SF, Port FK. Type of vascular access and mortality in U.S. hemodialysis patients. Kidney Int 2001;60:1443-51.

Roy-Chaudhury P, Sukhatme VP, Cheung AK. Hemodialysis vascular access dysfunction: a cellular and molecular viewpoint. J Am Soc Nephrol 2006;17:1112-27.

Roy-Chaudhury P, Kelly BS, Melhem M, et al. Vascular access in hemodialysis: issues, management, and emerging concepts. Cardiol Clin 2005;23:249-73.

Allon M. Current management of vascular access. Clin J Am Soc Nephrol 2007;2:786-800. Lok CE, Mokrzycki MH. Prevention and management of catheter-related infection in hemodialysis patients. Kidney Int 2011;79:587-98.

Moist LM, Trpeski L, Na Y, Lok CE. Increased hemodialysis catheter use in Canada and associated mortality risk: data from the Canadian Organ Replacement Registry 2001-2004. Clin J Am Soc Nephrol 2008;3:1726-32.

Oliver MJ, McCann RL, Indridason OS, Butterly DW, Schwab SJ. Comparison of transposed brachiobasilic fistulas to upper arm grafts and brachiocephalic fistulas. Kidney Int 2001;60:1532-9.

Palder SB, Kirkman RL, Whittemore AD, Hakim RM, Lazarus JM, Tilney NL. Vascular access for hemodialysis. Patency rates and results of revision. Annals of surgery 1985;202:235-9.

Allon M. Current management of vascular access. Clinical journal of the American Society of Nephrology : CJASN 2007;2:786-800.

Allon M, Robbin ML. Increasing arteriovenous fistulas in hemodialysis patients: problems and solutions. Kidney Int 2002;62:1109-24.

Schwab SJ, Harrington JT, Singh A, et al. Vascular access for hemodialysis. Kidney international 1999;55:2078-90.

Lok CE, Allon M, Moist L, Oliver MJ, Shah H, Zimmerman D. Risk equation determining unsuccessful cannulation events and failure to maturation in arteriovenous fistulas (REDUCE FTM I). J Am Soc Nephrol 2006;17:3204-12.

Lee T, Barker J, Allon M. Comparison of survival of upper arm arteriovenous fistulas and grafts after failed forearm fistula. J Am Soc Nephrol 2007;18:1936-41.

Dember LM, Beck GJ, Allon M, et al. Effect of Clopidogrel on Early Failure of Arteriovenous Fistulas for Hemodialysis: A Randomized Controlled Trial. JAMA 2008;299:2164-71.

Raju S. PTFE grafts for hemodialysis access. Techniques for insertion and management of complications. Annals of surgery 1987;206:666-73.

Fan PY, Schwab SJ. Vascular access: concepts for the 1990s. Journal of the American Society of Nephrology : JASN 1992;3:1-11.

Clinical Practice Guidelines for Vascular Access. Am J Kidney Dis 2006;48:S176-S273. Ethier J, Mendelssohn DC, Elder SJ, et al. Vascular access use and outcomes: an international perspective from the Dialysis Outcomes and Practice Patterns Study. Nephrol Dial Transplant 2008;23:3219-26.

Maya ID, Weatherspoon J, Young CJ, Barker J, Allon M. Increased risk of infection associated with polyurethane dialysis grafts. Semin Dial 2007;20:616-20.

Schwab SJ. Reducing the risk of hemodialysis access. American journal of kidney diseases : the official journal of the National Kidney Foundation 1999;34:362-3.

Akoh JA, Patel N. Infection of hemodialysis arteriovenous grafts. The journal of vascular access 2010;11:155-8.

Schwab SJ, Oliver MJ, Suhocki P, McCann R. Hemodialysis arteriovenous access: detection of stenosis and response to treatment by vascular access blood flow. Kidney Int 2001;59:358-62.

Fan PY. Acute vascular access: new advances. Advances in renal replacement therapy 1994;1:90-8.

Schwab SJ, Buller GL, McCann RL, Bollinger RR, Stickel DL. Prospective evaluation of a Dacron cuffed hemodialysis catheter for prolonged use. American journal of kidney diseases : the official journal of the National Kidney Foundation 1988;11:166-9.

Moss AH, McLaughlin MM, Lempert KD, Holley JL. Use of a silicone catheter with a Dacron cuff for dialysis short-term vascular access. American journal of kidney diseases : the official journal of the National Kidney Foundation 1988;12:492-8.

Moss AH, Vasilakis C, Holley JL, Foulks CJ, Pillai K, McDowell DE. Use of a silicone dual-lumen catheter with a Dacron cuff as a long-term vascular access for hemodialysis patients. American journal of kidney diseases : the official journal of the National Kidney Foundation 1990;16:211-5.

Allon M. Dialysis catheter-related bacteremia: treatment and prophylaxis. Am J Kidney Dis 2004;44:779-91.

Krishnasami Z, Carlton D, Bimbo L, et al. Management of hemodialysis catheter-related bacteremia with an adjunctive antibiotic lock solution. Kidney Int 2002;61:1136-42.

Tanriover B, Carlton D, Saddekni S, et al. Bacteremia associated with tunneled dialysis catheters: comparison of two treatment strategies. Kidney Int 2000;57:2151-5.

Lee T, Barker J, Allon M. Tunneled catheters in hemodialysis patients: reasons and subsequent outcomes. Am J Kidney Dis 2005;46:501-8.

Allon M. Treatment guidelines for dialysis catheter-related bacteremia: an update. Am J Kidney Dis 2009;54:13-7.

Hemmelgarn BR, Moist LM, Lok CE, et al. Prevention of dialysis catheter malfunction with recombinant tissue plasminogen activator. N Engl J Med 2011;364:303-12.

Suhocki PV, Conlon PJ, Jr., Knelson MH, Harland R, Schwab SJ. Silastic cuffed catheters for hemodialysis vascular access: thrombolytic and mechanical correction of malfunction. American journal of kidney diseases : the official journal of the National Kidney Foundation 1996;28:379-86.

Crain MR, Mewissen MW, Ostrowski GJ, Paz-Fumagalli R, Beres RA, Wertz RA. Fibrin sleeve stripping for salvage of failing hemodialysis catheters: technique and initial results. Radiology 1996;198:41-4.
Caruana RJ, Raja RM, Zeit RM, Goldstein SJ, Kramer MS. Thrombotic complications of indwelling central catheters used for chronic hemodialysis. American journal of kidney diseases : the official journal of the National Kidney Foundation 1987;9:497- 501.
Maya ID, Saddekni S, Allon M. Treatment of refractory central vein stenosis in hemodialysis patients with stents. Semin Dial 2007;20:78-82.
Schwab SJ, Quarles LD, Middleton JP, Cohan RH, Saeed M, Dennis VW. Hemodialysis-associated subclavian vein stenosis. Kidney international 1988;33:1156-9.
Tokars JI, Miller ER, Alter MJ, Arduino MJ. National surveillance of dialysis-associated diseases in the United States, 1997. Semin Dial 2000;13:75-85.
NKF-DOQI clinical practice guidelines for vascular access. National Kidney Foundation-Dialysis Outcomes Quality Initiative. Am J Kidney Dis 1997;30:S150-91.
Fistula First National Access Improvements Initiative. Available at: http://www.fistulafirst.org/. Accessed January 23, 2011.
Gold JA, Hoffman K. Fistula First: the National Vascular Access Improvement Initiative. Wmj 2006;105:71-3.
Lok CE. Fistula first initiative: advantages and pitfalls. Clin J Am Soc Nephrol 2007;2:1043-53.
Peters VJ, Clemons G, Augustine B. "Fistula First" as a CMS breakthrough initiative: improving vascular access through collaboration. Nephrol Nurs J 2005;32:686-7.
National Kidney Foundation: DOQI Clinical Practice Guidelines for Vascular Access: Update 2000. Am J Kidney Dis 2001;37:S137-S81.
U.S. Renal Data System, USRDS 2009 Annual Data Report: Atlas of CKD and ESRD in the United States, National Institutes of Health, National Institute of Diabetes and Digestive and Kidney Diseases, Bethesda, MD, 2009.
Kinney R. 2005 Annual Report: ESRD Clinical Performance Measures Project. American Journal of Kidney Diseases 2006;48:S1-S105.
Xue JL, Dahl D, Ebben JP, Collins AJ. The association of initial hemodialysis access type with mortality outcomes in elderly Medicare ESRD patients. Am J Kidney Dis 2003;42:1013-9.
Oliver MJ, Rothwell DM, Fung K, Hux JE, Lok CE. Late creation of vascular access for hemodialysis and increased risk of sepsis. J Am Soc Nephrol 2004;15:1936-42.
Allon M, Daugirdas J, Depner TA, Greene T, Ornt D, Schwab SJ. Effect of change in vascular access on patient mortality in hemodialysis patients. Am J Kidney Dis 2006;47:469-77.
Lacson E, Jr., Wang W, Hakim RM, Teng M, Lazarus JM. Associates of mortality and hospitalization in hemodialysis: potentially actionable laboratory variables and vascular access. Am J Kidney Dis 2009;53:79-90.
Foley RN, Chen SC, Collins AJ. Hemodialysis access at initiation in the United States, 2005 to 2007: still "catheter first". Hemodial Int 2009;13:533-42.
Astor BC, Eustace JA, Powe NR, Klag MJ, Fink NE, Coresh J. Type of vascular access and survival among incident hemodialysis patients: the Choices for Healthy Outcomes in Caring for ESRD (CHOICE) Study. J Am Soc Nephrol 2005;16:1449-55.

Bradbury BD, Fissell RB, Albert JM, et al. Predictors of early mortality among incident US hemodialysis patients in the Dialysis Outcomes and Practice Patterns Study (DOPPS). Clin J Am Soc Nephrol 2007;2:89-99.

Allon M. Prophylaxis against dialysis catheter-related bacteremia: a glimmer of hope. Am J Kidney Dis 2008;51:165-8.

Rayner HC, Pisoni RL, Gillespie BW, et al. Creation, cannulation and survival of arteriovenous fistulae: data from the Dialysis Outcomes and Practice Patterns Study. Kidney Int 2003;63:323-30.

Reed SD, Friedman JY, Engemann JJ, et al. Costs and outcomes among hemodialysis-dependent patients with methicillin-resistant or methicillin-susceptible Staphylococcus aureus bacteremia. Infection control and hospital epidemiology : the official journal of the Society of Hospital Epidemiologists of America 2005;26:175-83.

Roy-Chaudhury P, McKee, L., Miller, M., Reaves, A., Armstrong, J., Duncan, H., Munda, R., Kelly, B., Heffelfinger, S. Adventitial fibroblasts contribute to venous neointimal hyperplasia in PTFE grafts [Abstract]. J Am Soc Nephrol 2001;12:301A.

Weiss MF, Scivittaro V, Anderson JM. Oxidative stress and increased expression of growth factors in lesions of failed hemodialysis access. Am J Kidney Dis 2001;37:970-80.

Kelly BS, Heffelfinger SC, Whiting JF, et al. Aggressive venous neointimal hyperplasia in a pig model of arteriovenous graft stenosis. Kidney Int 2002;62:2272-80.

Roy-Chaudhury P, Kelly BS, Miller MA, et al. Venous neointimal hyperplasia in polytetrafluoroethylene dialysis grafts. Kidney Int 2001;59:2325-34.

Wang Y, Krishnamoorthy M, Banerjee R, et al. Venous stenosis in a pig arteriovenous fistula model--anatomy, mechanisms and cellular phenotypes. Nephrol Dial Transplant 2008;23:525-33.

Roy-Chaudhury P, Wang Y, Krishnamoorthy M, et al. Cellular phenotypes in human stenotic lesions from haemodialysis vascular access. Nephrol Dial Transplant 2009;24:2786-91.

Lee T, Roy-Chaudhury P. Advances and new frontiers in the pathophysiology of venous neointimal hyperplasia and dialysis access stenosis. Adv Chronic Kidney Dis 2009;16:329-38.

Roy-Chaudhury P, Arend L, Zhang J, et al. Neointimal hyperplasia in early arteriovenous fistula failure. Am J Kidney Dis 2007;50:782-90.

Ene-Iordache B, Mosconi L, Antiga L, et al. Radial artery remodeling in response to shear stress increase within arteriovenous fistula for hemodialysis access. Endothelium 2003;10:95-102.

Paszkowiak JJ, Dardik A. Arterial wall shear stress: observations from the bench to the bedside. Vascular and endovascular surgery 2003;37:47-57.

Huynh TN, Chacko BK, Teng X, et al. Effects of venous needle turbulence during ex vivo hemodialysis on endothelial morphology and nitric oxide formation. Journal of biomechanics 2007;40:2158-66.

Chang CJ, Ko PJ, Hsu LA, et al. Highly increased cell proliferation activity in the restenotic hemodialysis vascular access after percutaneous transluminal angioplasty: implication in prevention of restenosis. Am J Kidney Dis 2004;43:74-84.

Lin T, Horsfield C, Robson MG. Arteriovenous fistula in the rat tail: a new model of hemodialysis access dysfunction. Kidney Int 2008;74:528-31.
Roy-Chaudhury P, Melhem M, Husted T, Kelly BS. Solutions for hemodialysis vascular access dysfunction: thinking out of the box!! J Vasc Access 2005;6:3-8.
Lin CC, Yang WC, Lin SJ, et al. Length polymorphism in heme oxygenase-1 is associated with arteriovenous fistula patency in hemodialysis patients. Kidney Int 2006;69:165-72.
Heine GH, Ulrich C, Kohler H, Girndt M. Is AV fistula patency associated with angiotensin-converting enzyme (ACE) polymorphism and ACE inhibitor intake? Am J Nephrol 2004;24:461-8.
Heine GH, Ulrich C, Sester U, Sester M, Kohler H, Girndt M. Transforming growth factor beta1 genotype polymorphisms determine AV fistula patency in hemodialysis patients. Kidney Int 2003;64:1101-7.
Girndt M, Heine GH, Ulrich C, Kohler H. Gene polymorphism association studies in dialysis: vascular access. Semin Dial 2007;20:63-7.
Lee T, Chauhan V, Krishnamoorthy M, et al. Severe venous neointimal hyperplasia prior to dialysis access surgery. Nephrology, dialysis, transplantation : official publication of the European Dialysis and Transplant Association - European Renal Association 2011.
Wali MA, Eid RA, Al-Homrany MA. Smooth muscle changes in the cephalic vein of renal failure patients before use as an arteriovenous fistula (AVF). J Smooth Muscle Res 2002;38:75-85.
Wali MA, Eid RA, Dewan M, Al-Homrany MA. Intimal changes in the cephalic vein of renal failure patients before arterio-venous fistula (AVF) construction. J Smooth Muscle Res 2003;39:95-105.
Wali MA, Eid RA, Dewan M, Al-Homrany MA. Pre-existing histopathological changes in the cephalic vein of renal failure patients before arterio-venous fistula (AVF) construction. Ann Thorac Cardiovasc Surg 2006;12:341-8.
Feinfeld DA, Batista R, Mir R, Babich D. Changes in venous histology in chronic hemodialysis patients. Am J Kidney Dis 1999;34:702-5.
Castier Y, Lehoux S, Hu Y, Foteinos G, Tedgui A, Xu Q. Characterization of neointima lesions associated with arteriovenous fistulas in a mouse model. Kidney Int 2006;70:315-20.
Dixon BS. Why don't fistulas mature? Kidney Int 2006;70:1413-22.
Rotmans JI, Velema E, Verhagen HJ, et al. Matrix metalloproteinase inhibition reduces intimal hyperplasia in a porcine arteriovenous-graft model. J Vasc Surg 2004;39:432-9.
Tronc F, Mallat Z, Lehoux S, Wassef M, Esposito B, Tedgui A. Role of matrix metalloproteinases in blood flow-induced arterial enlargement: interaction with NO. Arterioscler Thromb Vasc Biol 2000;20:E120-6.
Misra S, Doherty MG, Woodrum D, et al. Adventitial remodeling with increased matrix metalloproteinase-2 activity in a porcine arteriovenous polytetrafluoroethylene grafts. Kidney Int 2005;68:2890-900.
Misra S, Fu AA, Puggioni A, et al. Increased shear stress with upregulation of VEGF-A and its receptors and MMP-2, MMP-9, and TIMP-1 in venous stenosis of hemodialysis grafts. Am J Physiol Heart Circ Physiol 2008;294:H2219-30.
Misra S, Fu AA, Rajan DK, et al. Expression of hypoxia inducible factor-1 alpha,

macrophage migration inhibition factor, matrix metalloproteinase-2 and -9, and their inhibitors in hemodialysis grafts and arteriovenous fistulas. J Vasc Interv Radiol 2008;19:252-9.

Nath KA. Heme oxygenase-1: a provenance for cytoprotective pathways in the kidney and other tissues. Kidney Int 2006;70:432-43.

Juncos JP, Tracz MJ, Croatt AJ, et al. Genetic deficiency of heme oxygenase-1 impairs functionality and form of an arteriovenous fistula in the mouse. Kidney Int 2008;74:47-51.

Sezer S, Ozdemir FN, Arat Z, Turan M, Haberal M. Triad of malnutrition, inflammation, and atherosclerosis in hemodialysis patients. Nephron 2002;91:456- 62.

Kokubo T, Ishikawa N, Uchida H, et al. CKD accelerates development of neointimal hyperplasia in arteriovenous fistulas. J Am Soc Nephrol 2009;20:1236-45.

Juncos JP, Grande JP, Kang L, et al. MCP-1 contributes to arteriovenous fistula failure. Journal of the American Society of Nephrology : JASN 2011;22:43-8.

Stracke S, Konner K, Kostlin I, et al. Increased expression of TGF-beta1 and IGF-I in inflammatory stenotic lesions of hemodialysis fistulas. Kidney Int 2002;61:1011-9.

Li L, Terry CM, Shiu Y-TE, Cheung AK. Neointimal hyperplasia associated with synthetic hemodialysis grafts. Kidney Int 2008;74:1247-61.

Mattana J, Effiong C, Kapasi A, Singhal PC. Leukocyte-polytetrafluoroethylene interaction enhances proliferation of vascular smooth muscle cells via tumor necrosis factor-alpha secretion. Kidney Int 1997;52:1478-85.

Conte MS, Nugent HM, Gaccione P, Guleria I, Roy-Chaudhury P, Lawson JH. Multicenter phase I/II trial of the safety of allogeneic endothelial cell implants after the creation of arteriovenous access for hemodialysis use: the V-HEALTH study. J Vasc Surg 2009;50:1359-68 e1.

Shuhaiber JH, Evans AN, Massad MG, Geha AS. Mechanisms and future directions for prevention of vein graft failure in coronary bypass surgery. European journal of cardio-thoracic surgery : official journal of the European Association for Cardio- thoracic Surgery 2002;22:387-96.

Langille BL, O'Donnell F. Reductions in arterial diameter produced by chronic decreases in blood flow are endothelium-dependent. Science 1986;231:405-7.

Ignarro LJ, Buga GM, Wood KS, Byrns RE, Chaudhuri G. Endothelium-derived relaxing factor produced and released from artery and vein is nitric oxide. Proceedings of the National Academy of Sciences of the United States of America 1987;84:9265-9.

Bolton CH, Downs LG, Victory JG, et al. Endothelial dysfunction in chronic renal failure: roles of lipoprotein oxidation and pro-inflammatory cytokines. Nephrol Dial Transplant 2001;16:1189-97.

Ghiadoni L, Cupisti A, Huang Y, et al. Endothelial dysfunction and oxidative stress in chronic renal failure. J Nephrol 2004;17:512-9.

Kim YO, Choi YJ, Kim JI, et al. The impact of intima-media thickness of radial artery on early failure of radiocephalic arteriovenous fistula in hemodialysis patients. J Korean Med Sci 2006;21:284-9.

Kim YO, Song HC, Yoon SA, et al. Preexisting intimal hyperplasia of radial artery is associated with early failure of radiocephalic arteriovenous fistula in hemodialysis patients. Am J Kidney Dis 2003;41:422-8.

Ku YM, Kim YO, Kim JI, et al. Ultrasonographic measurement of intima-media thickness of radial artery in pre-dialysis uraemic patients: comparison with histological examination. Nephrol Dial Transplant 2006;21:715-20.
Zoccali C. Endothelial damage, asymmetric dimethylarginine and cardiovascular risk in end-stage renal disease. Blood Purif 2002;20:469-72.
Cooke JP. Does ADMA cause endothelial dysfunction? Arterioscler Thromb Vasc Biol 2000;20:2032-7.
Wu CC, Wen SC, Yang CW, Pu SY, Tsai KC, Chen JW. Plasma ADMA predicts restenosis of arteriovenous fistula. J Am Soc Nephrol 2009;20:213-22.
Scott NA, Cipolla GD, Ross CE, et al. Identification of a potential role for the adventitia in vascular lesion formation after balloon overstretch injury of porcine coronary arteries. Circulation 1996;93:2178-87.
Shi Y, O'Brien JE, Fard A, Mannion JD, Wang D, Zalewski A. Adventitial myofibroblasts contribute to neointimal formation in injured porcine coronary arteries. Circulation 1996;94:1655-64.
Shi Y, O'Brien JE, Jr., Mannion JD, et al. Remodeling of autologous saphenous vein grafts. The role of perivascular myofibroblasts. Circulation 1997;95:2684-93.
Li L, Terry CM, Blumenthal DK, et al. Cellular and morphological changes during neointimal hyperplasia development in a porcine arteriovenous graft model. Nephrol Dial Transplant 2007;22:3139-46.
Caplice NM, Wang S, Tracz M, et al. Neoangiogenesis and the presence of progenitor cells in the venous limb of an arteriovenous fistula in the rat. Am J Physiol Renal Physiol 2007;293:F470-5.
Diao Y, Guthrie S, Xia SL, et al. Long-term engraftment of bone marrow-derived cells in the intimal hyperplasia lesion of autologous vein grafts. Am J Pathol 2008;172:839-48.
Haruguchi H, Teraoka S. Intimal hyperplasia and hemodynamic factors in arterial bypass and arteriovenous grafts: a review. Journal of artificial organs : the official journal of the Japanese Society for Artificial Organs 2003;6:227-35.
Sivanesan S, How TV, Black RA, Bakran A. Flow patterns in the radiocephalic arteriovenous fistula: an in vitro study. Journal of biomechanics 1999;32:915-25.
Krishnamoorthy MK, Banerjee RK, Wang Y, et al. Hemodynamic wall shear stress profiles influence the magnitude and pattern of stenosis in a pig AV fistula. Kidney Int 2008;74:1410-9.
Paszkowiak JJ, Dardik A. Arterial wall shear stress: observations from the bench to the bedside. Vasc Endovascular Surg 2003;37:47-57.
Corpataux JM, Haesler E, Silacci P, Ris HB, Hayoz D. Low-pressure environment and remodelling of the forearm vein in Brescia-Cimino haemodialysis access. Nephrol Dial Transplant 2002;17:1057-62.
Mondy JS, Lindner V, Miyashiro JK, Berk BC, Dean RH, Geary RL. Platelet-derived growth factor ligand and receptor expression in response to altered blood flow in vivo. Circulation research 1997;81:320-7.
Sterpetti AV, Cucina A, Santoro L, Cardillo B, Cavallaro A. Modulation of arterial smooth muscle cell growth by haemodynamic forces. Eur J Vasc Surg 1992;6:16-20.
Kraiss LW, Geary RL, Mattsson EJ, Vergel S, Au YP, Clowes AW. Acute reductions in blood flow and shear stress induce platelet-derived growth factor-A expression in baboon prosthetic grafts. Circulation research 1996;79:45-53.

Ueba H, Kawakami M, Yaginuma T. Shear stress as an inhibitor of vascular smooth muscle cell proliferation. Role of transforming growth factor-beta 1 and tissue-type plasminogen activator. Arteriosclerosis, thrombosis, and vascular biology 1997;17:1512-6.

Roy-Chaudhury P, Lee TC. Vascular stenosis: biology and interventions. Curr Opin Nephrol Hypertens 2007;16:516-22.

O'Brien JE, Jr., Shi Y, Fard A, Bauer T, Zalewski A, Mannion JD. Wound healing around and within saphenous vein bypass grafts. The Journal of thoracic and cardiovascular surgery 1997;114:38-45.

Kwon HM, Sangiorgi G, Ritman EL, et al. Enhanced coronary vasa vasorum neovascularization in experimental hypercholesterolemia. J Clin Invest 1998;101:1551-6.

Daeihagh P, Jordan J, Chen J, Rocco M. Efficacy of tissue plasminogen activator administration on patency of hemodialysis access catheters. American journal of kidney diseases : the official journal of the National Kidney Foundation 2000;36:75- 9.

Lund GB, Trerotola SO, Scheel PF, Jr., et al. Outcome of tunneled hemodialysis catheters placed by radiologists. Radiology 1996;198:467-72.

Grudzinski L, Quinan P, Kwok S, Pierratos A. Sodium citrate 4% locking solution for central venous dialysis catheters--an effective, more cost-efficient alternative to heparin. Nephrology, dialysis, transplantation : official publication of the European Dialysis and Transplant Association - European Renal Association 2007;22:471-6.

Lok CE, Appleton D, Bhola C, Khoo B, Richardson RM. Trisodium citrate 4%--an alternative to heparin capping of haemodialysis catheters. Nephrology, dialysis, transplantation : official publication of the European Dialysis and Transplant Association - European Renal Association 2007;22:477-83.

Dogra GK, Herson H, Hutchison B, et al. Prevention of tunneled hemodialysis catheter-related infections using catheter-restricted filling with gentamicin and citrate: a randomized controlled study. J Am Soc Nephrol 2002;13:2133-9.

Weijmer MC, van den Dorpel MA, Van de Ven PJ, et al. Randomized, clinical trial comparison of trisodium citrate 30% and heparin as catheter-locking solution in hemodialysis patients. Journal of the American Society of Nephrology : JASN 2005;16:2769-77.

Mermel LA, Farr BM, Sherertz RJ, et al. Guidelines for the management of intravascular catheter-related infections. Clinical infectious diseases : an official publication of the Infectious Diseases Society of America 2001;32:1249-72.

Mermel LA, Allon M, Bouza E, et al. Clinical practice guidelines for the diagnosis and management of intravascular catheter-related infection: 2009 Update by the Infectious Diseases Society of America. Clinical infectious diseases : an official publication of the Infectious Diseases Society of America 2009;49:1-45.

Cheesbrough JS, Finch RG, Burden RP. A prospective study of the mechanisms of infection associated with hemodialysis catheters. The Journal of infectious diseases 1986;154:579-89.

Costerton JW. In response to: In vivo efficacy of silver-coated (Sil-zone) infection- resistant polyester fabric against a biofilm-producing bacteria, Staphylococcus epidermidis. J Heart Valve Disease; 1998;7:524-530. J Heart Valve Dis 1999;8:346-8.

Costerton JW. Introduction to biofilm. Int J Antimicrob Agents 1999;11:217-21; discussion 37-9.
Costerton JW, Stewart PS, Greenberg EP. Bacterial biofilms: a common cause of persistent infections. Science 1999;284:1318-22.
Donlan RM, Costerton JW. Biofilms: survival mechanisms of clinically relevant microorganisms. Clin Microbiol Rev 2002;15:167-93.
Hoyle BD, Alcantara J, Costerton JW. Pseudomonas aeruginosa biofilm as a diffusion barrier to piperacillin. Antimicrobial agents and chemotherapy 1992;36:2054-6.
Mokrzycki MH, Zhang M, Cohen H, Golestaneh L, Laut JM, Rosenberg SO. Tunnelled haemodialysis catheter bacteraemia: risk factors for bacteraemia recurrence, infectious complications and mortality. Nephrology, dialysis, transplantation : official publication of the European Dialysis and Transplant Association - European Renal Association 2006;21:1024-31.
Beathard GA. Management of bacteremia associated with tunneled-cuffed hemodialysis catheters. Journal of the American Society of Nephrology : JASN 1999;10:1045-9.
Marr KA, Sexton DJ, Conlon PJ, Corey GR, Schwab SJ, Kirkland KB. Catheter-related bacteremia and outcome of attempted catheter salvage in patients undergoing hemodialysis. Annals of internal medicine 1997;127:275-80.
Negulescu O, Coco M, Croll J, Mokrzycki MH. Large atrial thrombus formation associated with tunneled cuffed hemodialysis catheters. Clinical nephrology 2003;59:40-6.
Poole CV, Carlton D, Bimbo L, Allon M. Treatment of catheter-related bacteraemia with an antibiotic lock protocol: effect of bacterial pathogen. Nephrol Dial Transplant 2004;19:1237-44.
Kovalik EC, Raymond JR, Albers FJ, et al. A clustering of epidural abscesses in chronic hemodialysis patients: risks of salvaging access catheters in cases of infection. Journal of the American Society of Nephrology : JASN 1996;7:2264-7.
Ghani MK, Boccalandro F, Denktas AE, Barasch E. Right atrial thrombus formation associated with central venous catheters utilization in hemodialysis patients. Intensive Care Med 2003;29:1829-32.
Obrador GT, Levenson DJ. Spinal epidural abscess in hemodialysis patients: report of three cases and review of the literature. American journal of kidney diseases : the official journal of the National Kidney Foundation 1996;27:75-83.
Hemmelgarn BR, Moist LM, Lok CE, et al. Prevention of dialysis catheter malfunction with recombinant tissue plasminogen activator. The New England journal of medicine 2011;364:303-12.
Saad TF. Bacteremia associated with tunneled, cuffed hemodialysis catheters. American journal of kidney diseases : the official journal of the National Kidney Foundation 1999;34:1114-24.
Lok CE, Stanley KE, Hux JE, Richardson R, Tobe SW, Conly J. Hemodialysis infection prevention with polysporin ointment. J Am Soc Nephrol 2003;14:169-79.
Zhang J, Melhem M, Kassing W, et al. In vitro paclitaxel and radiation effects on the cell types responsible for vascular stenosis: a preliminary analysis. Blood Purif 2007;25:155-60.
Mermel LA, Farr BM, Sherertz RJ, et al. Guidelines for the management of intravascular catheter-related infections. Clin Infect Dis 2001;32:1249-72.

Capdevila JA, Segarra A, Planes AM, et al. Successful treatment of haemodialysis catheter-related sepsis without catheter removal. Nephrology, dialysis, transplantation : official publication of the European Dialysis and Transplant Association - European Renal Association 1993;8:231-4.

Fernandez-Hidalgo N, Almirante B, Calleja R, et al. Antibiotic-lock therapy for long-term intravascular catheter-related bacteraemia: results of an open, non-comparative study. J Antimicrob Chemother 2006;57:1172-80.

Vardhan A, Davies J, Daryanani I, Crowe A, McClelland P. Treatment of haemodialysis catheter-related infections. Nephrology, dialysis, transplantation : official publication of the European Dialysis and Transplant Association - European Renal Association 2002;17:1149-50.

Levin A, Mason AJ, Jindal KK, Fong IW, Goldstein MB. Prevention of hemodialysis subclavian vein catheter infections by topical povidone-iodine. Kidney international 1991;40:934-8.

Sesso R, Barbosa D, Leme IL, et al. Staphylococcus aureus prophylaxis in hemodialysis patients using central venous catheter: effect of mupirocin ointment. Journal of the American Society of Nephrology : JASN 1998;9:1085-92.

Johnson LB, Jose J, Yousif F, Pawlak J, Saravolatz LD. Prevalence of colonization with community-associated methicillin-resistant Staphylococcus aureus among end- stage renal disease patients and healthcare workers. Infection control and hospital epidemiology : the official journal of the Society of Hospital Epidemiologists of America 2009;30:4-8.

James MT, Conley J, Tonelli M, Manns BJ, MacRae J, Hemmelgarn BR. Meta-analysis: antibiotics for prophylaxis against hemodialysis catheter-related infections. Annals of internal medicine 2008;148:596-605.

Yahav D, Rozen-Zvi B, Gafter-Gvili A, Leibovici L, Gafter U, Paul M. Antimicrobial lock solutions for the prevention of infections associated with intravascular catheters in patients undergoing hemodialysis: systematic review and meta-analysis of randomized, controlled trials. Clinical infectious diseases : an official publication of the Infectious Diseases Society of America 2008;47:83-93.

Jaffer Y, Selby NM, Taal MW, Fluck RJ, McIntyre CW. A meta-analysis of hemodialysis catheter locking solutions in the prevention of catheter-related infection. American journal of kidney diseases : the official journal of the National Kidney Foundation 2008;51:233-41.

Snaterse M, Ruger W, Scholte Op Reimer WJ, Lucas C. Antibiotic-based catheter lock solutions for prevention of catheter-related bloodstream infection: a systematic review of randomised controlled trials. The Journal of hospital infection 2010;75:1- 11.

Pervez A, Ahmed M, Ram S, et al. Antibiotic lock technique for prevention of cuffed tunnel catheter associated bacteremia. The journal of vascular access 2002;3:108-13.

Landry DL, Braden GL, Gobeille SL, Haessler SD, Vaidya CK, Sweet SJ. Emergence of gentamicin-resistant bacteremia in hemodialysis patients receiving gentamicin lock catheter prophylaxis. Clinical journal of the American Society of Nephrology : CJASN 2010;5:1799-804.

Diskin CJ, Stokes TJ, Jr., Pennell AT. Pharmacologic intervention to prevent hemodialysis vascular access thrombosis. Nephron 1993;64:1-26.

Sreedhara R, Himmelfarb J, Lazarus JM, Hakim RM. Anti-platelet therapy in graft thrombosis: results of a prospective, randomized, double-blind study. Kidney Int 1994;45:1477-83.
Schmitz PG, McCloud LK, Reikes ST, Leonard CL, Gellens ME. Prophylaxis of hemodialysis graft thrombosis with fish oil: double-blind, randomized, prospective trial. Journal of the American Society of Nephrology : JASN 2002;13:184-90.
Gradzki R, Dhingra RK, Port FK, Roys E, Weitzel WF, Messana JM. Use of ACE inhibitors is associated with prolonged survival of arteriovenous grafts. American journal of kidney diseases : the official journal of the National Kidney Foundation 2001;38:1240-4.
Saran R, Dykstra DM, Wolfe RA, Gillespie B, Held PJ, Young EW. Association between vascular access failure and the use of specific drugs: the Dialysis Outcomes and Practice Patterns Study (DOPPS). Am J Kidney Dis 2002;40:1255-63.
Dixon BS, Beck GJ, Vazquez MA, et al. Effect of dipyridamole plus aspirin on hemodialysis graft patency. N Engl J Med 2009;360:2191-201.
Schmitz PG, McCloud LK, Reikes ST, Leonard CL, Gellens ME. Prophylaxis of hemodialysis graft thrombosis with fish oil: double-blind, randomized, prospective trial. J Am Soc Nephrol 2002;13:184-90.
Lok CE, Allon M, Donnelly S, et al. Design of the fish oil inhibition of stenosis in hemodialysis grafts (FISH) study. Clin Trials 2007;4:357-67.
Murthy SN, Obregon DF, Chattergoon NN, et al. Rosiglitazone reduces serum homocysteine levels, smooth muscle proliferation, and intimal hyperplasia in Sprague-Dawley rats fed a high methionine diet. Metabolism 2005;54:645-52.
Takagi T, Yamamuro A, Tamita K, Katayama M, Morioka S. Thiazolidinedione treatment attenuates diffuse neointimal hyperplasia in restenotic lesions after coronary stent implantation in type 2 diabetic patients: an intravascular ultrasound study. J Cardiol 2005;45:139-47.
Davies MG, Owens EL, Mason DP, et al. Effect of platelet-derived growth factor receptor-alpha and -beta blockade on flow-induced neointimal formation in endothelialized baboon vascular grafts. Circ Res 2000;86:779-86.
Hausleiter J, Kastrati A, Mehilli J, et al. Randomized, double-blind, placebo-controlled trial of oral sirolimus for restenosis prevention in patients with in-stent restenosis: the Oral Sirolimus to Inhibit Recurrent In-stent Stenosis (OSIRIS) trial. Circulation 2004;110:790-5.
Rutherford C, Martin W, Salame M, Carrier M, Anggard E, Ferns G. Substantial inhibition of neo-intimal response to balloon injury in the rat carotid artery using a combination of antibodies to platelet-derived growth factor-BB and basic fibroblast growth factor. Atherosclerosis 1997;130:45-51.
Leppanen O, Rutanen J, Hiltunen MO, et al. Oral imatinib mesylate (STI571/gleevec) improves the efficacy of local intravascular vascular endothelial growth factor-C gene transfer in reducing neointimal growth in hypercholesterolemic rabbits. Circulation 2004;109:1140-6.
Fareh J, Martel R, Kermani P, Leclerc G. Cellular effects of beta-particle delivery on vascular smooth muscle cells and endothelial cells: a dose-response study. Circulation 1999;99:1477-84.
Rubin P, Williams JP, Riggs PN, et al. Cellular and molecular mechanisms of radiation

inhibition of restenosis. Part I: role of the macrophage and platelet-derived growth factor. International journal of radiation oncology, biology, physics 1998;40:929-41.

Sabate M, Serruys PW, van der Giessen WJ, et al. Geometric vascular remodeling after balloon angioplasty and beta-radiation therapy: A three-dimensional intravascular ultrasound study. Circulation 1999;100:1182-8.

Mayberg MR, Luo Z, London S, Gajdusek C, Rasey JS. Radiation inhibition of intimal hyperplasia after arterial injury. Radiat Res 1995;142:212-20.

Kelly BS, Narayana A, Heffelfinger SC, et al. External beam radiation attenuates venous neointimal hyperplasia in a pig model of arteriovenous polytetrafluoroethylene (PTFE) graft stenosis. International journal of radiation oncology, biology, physics 2002;54:263-9.

Sun S, Beitler JJ, Ohki T, et al. Inhibitory effect of brachytherapy on intimal hyperplasia in arteriovenous fistula. The Journal of surgical research 2003;115:200-8.

Misra S, Bonan R, Pflederer T, Roy-Chaudhury P. BRAVO I: A pilot study of vascular brachytherapy in polytetrafluoroethylene dialysis access grafts. Kidney Int 2006;70:2006-13.

Yu SY, Chiu JH, Yang SD, Hsu YC, Lui WY, Wu CW. Biological effect of far-infrared therapy on increasing skin microcirculation in rats. Photodermatology, Photoimmunology & Photomedicine 2006;22:78-86.

Akasaki Y, Miyata M, Eto H, et al. Repeated thermal therapy up-regulates endothelial nitric oxide synthase and augments angiogenesis in a mouse model of hindlimb ischemia. Circulation journal : official journal of the Japanese Circulation Society 2006;70:463-70.

Ikeda Y, Biro S, Kamogawa Y, et al. Repeated thermal therapy upregulates arterial endothelial nitric oxide synthase expression in Syrian golden hamsters. Jpn Circ J 2001;65:434-8.

Lin CC, Chang CF, Lai MY, Chen TW, Lee PC, Yang WC. Far-infrared therapy: a novel treatment to improve access blood flow and unassisted patency of arteriovenous fistula in hemodialysis patients. J Am Soc Nephrol 2007;18:985-92.

Kelly B, Melhem M, Zhang J, et al. Perivascular paclitaxel wraps block arteriovenous graft stenosis in a pig model. Nephrol Dial Transplant 2006;21:2425-31.

Melhem M, Kelly B, Zhang J, et al. Development of a local perivascular paclitaxel delivery system for hemodialysis vascular access dysfunction: polymer preparation and in vitro activity. Blood Purif 2006;24:289-98.

Masaki T, Rathi R, Zentner G, et al. Inhibition of neointimal hyperplasia in vascular grafts by sustained perivascular delivery of paclitaxel. Kidney international 2004;66:2061-9.

Paulson WD, Kipshidze N, Kipiani K, et al. Safety and Efficacy of Locally Eluted Sirolimus for Prolonging AV Graft Patency (PTFE Graft Plus Coll-R) First in Man Experience. Journal of the American Society of Nephrology 2008:252A.

Nugent HM, Edelman ER. Endothelial implants provide long-term control of vascular repair in a porcine model of arterial injury. J Surg Res 2001;99:228-34.

Nugent HM, Groothuis A, Seifert P, et al. Perivascular endothelial implants inhibit intimal hyperplasia in a model of arteriovenous fistulae: a safety and efficacy study in the pig. J Vasc Res 2002;39:524-33.

Nugent HM, Rogers C, Edelman ER. Endothelial implants inhibit intimal hyperplasia after porcine angioplasty. Circ Res 1999;84:384-91.

Nugent HM, Sjin RT, White D, et al. Adventitial endothelial implants reduce matrix metalloproteinase-2 expression and increase luminal diameter in porcine arteriovenous grafts. J Vasc Surg 2007;46:548-56.

Hiltunen MO, Laitinen M, Turunen MP, et al. Intravascular adenovirus-mediated VEGF-C gene transfer reduces neointima formation in balloon-denuded rabbit aorta. Circulation 2000;102:2262-8.

Burke SK, LaRochelle A, Mendenhall HV. Local Application of Recombinant Human Type I Pancreatic Elastase (PRT-201) to an Arteriovenous Fistula (AVF) Increase AVF Blood Flow in a Rabbit Model. Journal of the American Society of Nephrology 2008:252A.

Haskal ZJ, Trerotola S, Dolmatch B, et al. Stent graft versus balloon angioplasty for failing dialysis-access grafts. The New England journal of medicine 2010;362:494- 503.

Maya ID, Allon M. Outcomes of thrombosed arteriovenous grafts: comparison of stents vs angioplasty. Kidney Int 2006;69:934-7.

Chan MR, Bedi S, Sanchez RJ, et al. Stent placement versus angioplasty improves patency of arteriovenous grafts and blood flow of arteriovenous fistulae. Clin J Am Soc Nephrol 2008;3:699-705.

Rotmans JI, Pattynama PM, Verhagen HJ, et al. Sirolimus-eluting stents to abolish intimal hyperplasia and improve flow in porcine arteriovenous grafts: a 4-week follow-up study. Circulation 2005;111:1537-42.

Haskal ZJ, Trerotola S, Dolmatch B, et al. Stent graft versus balloon angioplasty for failing dialysis-access grafts. N Engl J Med 2010;362:494-503.

Krishnamoorthy MK, Banerjee RK, Wang Y, et al. Hemodynamic wall shear stress profiles influence the magnitude and pattern of stenosis in a pig AV fistula. Kidney Int 2008.

Misra S, Woodrum DA, Homburger J, et al. Assessment of Wall Shear Stress Changes in Arteries and Veins of Arteriovenous Polytetrafluoroethylene Grafts Using Magnetic Resonance Imaging. Cardiovasc Intervent Radiol 2006.

Nyberg SL, Hughes CB, Valenzuela YM, et al. Preliminary experience with a cuffed ePTFE graft for hemodialysis vascular access. Asaio J 2001;47:333-7.

Tsoulfas G, Hertl M, Ko DS, et al. Long-term outcome of a cuffed expanded PTFE graft for hemodialysis vascular access. World journal of surgery 2008;32:1827-31.

Sorom AJ, Hughes CB, McCarthy JT, et al. Prospective, randomized evaluation of a cuffed expanded polytetrafluoroethylene graft for hemodialysis vascular access. Surgery 2002;132:135-40.

Ko PJ, Liu YH, Hung YN, Hsieh HC. Patency rates of cuffed and noncuffed extended polytetrafluoroethylene grafts in dialysis access: a prospective, randomized study. World journal of surgery 2009;33:846-51.

Roy-Chaudhury P, Wang Y, Krishnamoorthy M, Dakin A. Optiflow: A Novel Anastomotic Conduit for Reducing AV Fistula Dysfunction. J Am Soc Nephrol 2008;19:253A.

Falk A. Maintenance and salvage of arteriovenous fistulas. J Vasc Interv Radiol 2006;17:807-13.

Yevzlin AS, Chan MR, Becker YT, Roy-Chaudhury P, Lee T, Becker BN. "Venopathy" at work: recasting neointimal hyperplasia in a new light. Transl Res 2010;156:216-25.

11

Nontraditional Anti-Infectious Agents in Hemodialysis

Martin Sedlacek
Dartmouth Hitchcock Medical Center, One Medical Center Drive
Lebanon

1. Introduction

The distinction between antibiotic and non antibiotic medications is in fact quite arbitrary as drugs against bacteria can have unpredictable side effects in man and drugs developed for use in humans can affect microbes. It would be extremely surprising if it was otherwise, as eukaryotes and prokaryotes are related by evolution and share conserved molecular mechanisms. Many antibiotic and non antibiotic medications have closely related chemistries and share the same historic roots.

For example, both antimicrobial activity and an affinity for brain tissue of the phenothiazine compound methylene blue were described by Paul Ehrlich in the 19th century. Early uses of phenothiazines included treatment of urinary tract infection and postoperative analgesia. As a positive effect on psychotic patients was discovered, phenothiazines became with the development of chlorpromazine an important tool in psychiatry (Williams, 1995). With the discovery of penicillin the antimicrobial activities of phenothiazines and other earlier compounds fell into the background, but with the emergent problem of antibiotic resistance in more recent years there was new interest. Phenothiazines have activity against multidrug resistant *Staphylococcus aureus* and *Enterococcus faecalis*, presumably through the inhibition of bacterial efflux pumps (Kristiansen J.E. et al., 2007).

As a routine, antibiotic medications are tested for their effects on the eukaryotic host as these constitute potential side effects. While the ideal antibiotic would have no side effects at all, the discovery of unexpected side effects has lead to important drug developments. For instance, the clinical observation of a hypoglycemic effect of sulfonamide antibiotics led to the development of sulfonylureas for the treatment of diabetes. Likewise the observation that Sulfanilamide causes hens to lay eggs without shells because of alkaline diuresis led to the development of acetazolamide and ultimately the thiazide diuretics. The initial observation derived from the similarity between the sulfonamide ion and the bicarbonate ion. The antiviral amantadine was found to be useful in the treatment of Parkinson's disease and motility agents to treat gastroparesis are derived from the observation of the bothersome gastrointestinal side effects of erythromycin. As described below, even Lipitor, the "best selling drug in the world" with $11 Billion of annual sales according to Forbes magazine, was developed from a compound initially discovered as an antibiotic originating from a fungal broth.

On the other hand side, the efforts to look into the unintended effects on microbes of non antibiotic medications have been less systematic. Non antibiotic medications can affect microbes in various ways: Compounds may have direct anti microbial effects in vitro, similar to traditional antibiotics. However, to be clinically useful the drug level to achieve minimum inhibitory concentration has to be within a range that is achievable and tolerable in humans. Compounds can exert an antimicrobial effect by inhibition of bacterial pumps. A well known example is the potentiation of antibiotic treatment against *Helicobacter pylori* through omeprazole. Many psychotropic medications including the phenothiazines fall into this category. Aspirin appears to modulate the expression of genes that are important for Staphylococcal virulence and the statins appear to have immune modulatory effects. Both medications are discussed in more detail below.

This chapter deals with the anti microbial effects of medications that are not traditionally regarded as antibiotics with regards to dialysis.

2. A combination of unfortunate events: infection in dialysis

The current epidemic of obesity and, as a complication, diabetic nephropathy associated to type 2 diabetes mellitus has fueled the spectacular growth of hemodialysis into an industry that is dominated by a handful of large companies. Infection is a leading cause of morbidity and mortality in dialysis patients and the annual mortality rate caused by sepsis is several hundred folds higher in patients with end stage renal disease than in the general population (Laupland et al., 2004). The incidence of bacteremia has increased in hemodialysis patients over the years, mainly because of increased rates of serious *Staphylococcus aureus* infection in this population (Foley at al., 2004). *S. aureus* has its name from a gold coloured caroten virulence factor called staphyloxanthin which allows the bacteria to survive oxidative bursts of neutrophils (Liu G.Y. & Nizet V., 2009). *S.aureus* produces a battery of surface proteins, enzymes and toxins which enable the bacteria to both persist in intracellular locations and in biofilms for long periods of time, and to rapidly disseminate in the host in an opportunistic fashion which makes it one of the most dangerous and pathogenic bacteria in humans.

The use of dialysis catheters is a major risk factor for developing *S.aureus* infection because of disruption of the normal skin barrier, thus forming a gateway for bacterial entry into the blood stream (Vandecasteele S.J. et al., 2009). Despite Kidney Disease Outcomes Quality Initiative clinical practice guidelines recommending the use of auto logos arterio-venous fistulae as dialysis access and other efforts, the overall prevalence of hemodialysis catheter use has been increasing, approaching 30% in the United States (Rayner et al., 2004). Humans are the main natural reservoir for *S.aureus* which can colonize skin, gastrointestinal and urogenital tracts. The most frequent site of colonization is the anterior nose and longitudinal studies have shown that there are three types of *S.aureus* nasal carriage in healthy adults: fifty percent are persistent non carriers, thirty percent are intermittent carriers and twenty percent are persistent carriers (VandenBergh et al., 1999). Hands are the main vector of transmission and in the majority of cases the same strain that is found in the bloodstream is also found on the hands and in the nose (von Eiff C. et al., 2001). It follows that rigorous hand washing is extremely important to prevent infection in the dialysis units as it is elsewhere in the medical setting. The majority of *S.aureus* infections has its source in the endogenous reservoir in the nose of the same person and can thus be considered an "autoinfection" (Boelart et al., 1995 as quoted in Vandecasteele et al., 2009). Consistent with this view is that in prospective studies the interval between catheter placement and staphylococcemia can be very short, with 23% of episodes occurring less than one week after catheter insertion (Little M.A. et al., 2001). *S.aureus* bacteremia is associated frequently with metastatic infection such as endocarditis, osteoarticular infection, septic pulmonary embolism and epidural abscess and carries a mortality that is higher than with other pathogens. While the original observation by Fleming that led to the discovery of penicillin involved the accidental overgrowth of an *S.aureus* culture with fungus, staphylococcal resistance to penicillin has since become very frequent both in community and hospital acquired infections. A recent study in the US found that methicillin resistant *S.aureus* accounted for 65% of isolates from the nose in hospitalized dialysis patients (Johnson L.B. et al., 2009). As with methicillin sensive *S.aureus*, colonization seems to precede clinical infection. A scheme of three times a week nasal mupirocin ointment can decrease nasal carriage but is cumbersome, the rate of recurrence is high and rapid development of resistance has been observed (Vandecasteele et al., 2009).

3. Salicylic acid

Salicylic acid, the active ingredient of willow bark, is one of the oldest medicines still in use, in the buffered form of aspirin. The beneficial effect on fever, pain and inflammation were already described by Hippocrates. Fallen out of favour because of other non steroidal anti inflammatory drugs with more favorable side effects profiles aspirin has made a spectacular come back fifty years ago as the antiplatelet effects of aspirin were discovered. Since then aspirin has found widespread therapeutic use in the treatment of cardiovascular disease. Chronic treatment with Aspirin may prevent colorectal cancer, presumably by inhibition of cyclooxygenase 2 (COX-2) which is expressed in large amounts in adenocarcinoma (Ruder E.H. et al., 2011). Salicylic acid is ubiquitous in plants as a phytohormone. It is part of the innate immune system of plants, involved in local resistance to pathogens and in systemic acquired resistance (SAR), where a pathogenic attack one part of a plant induces resistance in other parts. Depending on the amount of fruit and vegetables in the diet humans have detectable serum levels of salicylic acid. It has been hypothesized that diet derived salicylic acid could in part account for the observed link between diet and colorectal cancer (Paterson J.R.& Lawrence J.R., 2001) and this might possibly apply to the relation between diet and cardiovascular disease as well. Salicylic acid is used as a food preservative and an antiseptic in toothpaste. Aspirin is thus not only one of the oldest but also one of the most versatile and successful drugs known.

3.1 Laboratory evidence for an anti staphylococcal effect of salicylic acid

Early studies in the rabbit endocarditis model showed that platelets provide a nidus for bacteria and that aspirin can decrease vegetation size (Pujadas et al., 1988). The observation was made that aspirin can reduce not only the weight of vegetations in a rabbit model of *S.aureus* endocarditis but also bacterial density although neither aspirin nor salicylic acid have known antibacterial effects at the low concentrations employed (Nicolau D.P. et al., 1993). This benefit was seen if aspirin was given together with antibiotics but also if aspirin was provided prior to the infectious challenge with which endocarditis was induced (Nicolau D.P. et al., 1995). Even more puzzling in this study was that vegetation weight and bacterial density were higher if higher doses of aspirin were administered while the optimum beneficial effect was seen at a lower dose, suggesting that serum levels may be very important. Subsequently this observation has been called the "Goldilocks effect" in which too little and too much aspirin may cause paradoxically diminished effects on outcome parameters in the infectious endocarditis model (Eisen et al., 2008). The beneficial effects of aspirin in the rabbit model of endocarditis have been recapitulated with salicylic acid, its major biometabolite (Kupferwasser et al., 1999). As salicylic acid has no anti-platelet properties, this indicates that platelet independent mechanisms are likely to have a more significant role in the action of aspirin on *S.aureus* endocarditis that the platelet dependant effects. Further experimental work in vivo in animal models of infectious *S.aureus* endocarditis showed that aspirin reduced a multitude of measurable parameters of the severity of the infection and metastasis such as vegetation weight and the bacterial density in vegetations and the number of renal emboli and these effects were dose dependant, more pronounced at lower rather than higher doses (Kupferwasser et al., 1999). In vitro studies showed that salicylic acid inhibits the expression of two key virulence genes in *S. aureus* that are involved in endovascular pathogenesis: alpha-toxin [hla] and fibronectin-binding adhesion [fnbA], through activation of genetic pathways involving the major stress response operon, sigma factor B (Kupferwasser et al., 2003). These aspirin mediated effects on sigma factor B were observed at serum concentrations that are achieved by usual clinical dosages of aspirin in humans (Kupferwasser et al., 2003). On the other hand side, it has been shown that the presence of salicylic acid decreases expression of capsular polysaccharides. It has been hypothesized that the loss of these capsular virulence factors could lead to an increased capacity of *S.aureus* to invade epithelial cells and that chronic treatment with aspirin could potentially lead to more persistent or recurrent infection (Alvarez C.P. et al., 2010).

In conclusion a significant body of in vitro and in vivo evidence indicates that aspirin may have the potential to be useful in the treatment of *S.aureus* infection by down modulating key regulator and structural genes resulting in the abrogation of virulent phenotypes but it has to be noted that important questions remain.

3.2 Clinical evidence for a beneficial effect of aspirin in *S.aureus* endocarditis

The earliest clinical observations of a potential salutatory role of aspirin come from the study of bacterial endocarditis. In a small retrospective study a decreased rate of embolic events was found in patients with native valve endocarditis who were on long term aspirin treatment (11% versus 47%), although the number of patients treated with aspirin was too small to be conclusive (Schunemann S. et al., 1997). A small preliminary prospective observational study conducted in 9 patients found adjunctive treatment of established endocarditis with aspirin beneficial (Taha et al., 1992).

Subsequently, a Canadian prospective multicenter study in 115 patients with endocarditis showed no benefit of the adjunctive treatment with a 325mg dose of aspirin (Chan et al., 2003). Despite its prospective design this study was criticized as patients on chronic aspirin treatment were excluded from this study although the greatest benefit might be expected in this population. Moreover, Aspirin was added only after an average of 35 days after onset of symptoms. Only 14 patients (25%) in the Aspirin treatment group had *Staphylococcus aureus* endocarditis while the majority had streptococcal endocarditis. As the putative mechanism of action of aspirin involves the inhibition of *S.aureus* virulence factors, the benefit of aspirin is likely greatest if it is used before infection occurs. The benefit of aspirin is also very likely to be limited to *S.aureus* as the mechanism seems to be specific to this pathogen. The same authors presented a post hoc analysis of their data in 2008, comparing 84 patients who had been excluded from their previous study because of long term aspirin treatment with 54 patients in the placebo arm and again found no significant clinical differences in the outcome between both groups (Chan et al., 2008). Only 29% of patients, 16 and 24 patients respectively, in both arms had *S.aureus* endocarditis and thus the same concern that the study was underpowered to detect a difference was voiced for this study as well (Eisen D.P. & Bayer A.S., 2008).

A retrospective single center cohort study of 600 patients with infectious endocarditis, who were treated over a 18 year period at the Mayo Clinic, found that the odds of suffering symptomatic embolic events was decreased by 64% in patients who were treated with antiplatelet agents for at least 6 months prior to the diagnosis: Aspirin was the antiplatelet agent in 98% of cases and an 81mg daily dose was used in the majority of patients (Anavekar et al., 2007).

Eisen et al. used the International Collaboration on Endocarditis –Prospective Cohort Study (ICE-PCS) database to assess the influence of aspirin usage at the time of diagnosis on the outcome of definitive *S.aureus* endocarditis. A cohort of 670 patients had both information on prior aspirin use and *S.aureus* endocarditis. Aspirin use at the time of diagnosis in 132 patients was a predictor for a decreased risk of acute valve surgery, independent of methicillin resistance status. A statistically significant decrease in embolic events in aspirin users was found in a univariate analysis that became a trend in multivariate analysis. A comparison of groups with and without aspirin use among patients with Streptococcal endocarditis was made and no association of aspirin with improved outcomes was found (Eisen et al., 2009).

Thus the data on aspirin use in *S.aureus* endocarditis suggests that aspirin likely does alter the course of illness. The non dependence of the effect on methicillin resistance status and the absence of an observed effect of aspirin on other pathogens are consistent with the proposed specific mechanism of aspirin on staphylococcal virulence factors. It is also noteworthy that Staphylococcal endocarditis is rather difficult to study in adequate numbers as the population incidence is fortunately low.

3.3 Aspirin and *S.aureus* nasal carriage

Karabay et al. investigated the prevalence of *S.aureus* nasal carriage in an outpatient cardiology clinic. Of a total of 346 patients 199 were chronic aspirin user while 147 patients were not. The prevalence of *S.aureus* nasal carriage was 5% on patient treated chronically with aspirin versus 16% in those that did not take aspirin. Only aspirin was found to be associated with a decreased rate of nasal carriage in a multivariate analysis (Karabay et al., 2006). These findings are of obvious significance to hemodialysis patients as nasal colonization is considered the initiating event that leads to catheter associated staphylococcal bacteremia. If confirmed, aspirin could decrease nasal carriage at a fraction of the cost and effort of mupirocin ointment. Given the fact that aspirin is a very old drug the findings of Karabay et al. have another potential significance: If a clinical effect of aspirin on *S.aureus* can still be detected after decades of over-the-counter use it would be unlikely that *S.aureus* would develop resistance to this effect in the future. It is clear that the important findings of Karabay et al. merit further investigation both in hemodialysis and in the general population.

3.4 A potential beneficial effect of aspirin in hemodialysis patients

Patient undergoing hemodialysis treatments suffer staphylococcal infections with increased frequency because of a high prevalence of tunneled or non tunneled dialysis catheters. The hemodialysis setting is thus well suited to study the potential beneficial clinical anti staphylococcal effects of aspirin.

We conducted a single center retrospective study in 872 patients with tunneled catheters who dialyzed over a ten year time period from 1995 to 2005. During this time period our patients had 1853 tunneled dialysis catheters placed and accumulated more than 476 patient-catheter-years and had 4722 blood cultures performed. Temporary dialysis catheters were excluded because of the high variability in the circumstances of placement of temporay catheters and also greater difficulty in tracking them retrospectively. The overall incidence of bacteremia was 7.2 episodes per 100 patient-catheter-months and the incidence of *S.aureus* bacteremia was 2.1 episodes per 100 patient-catheter-months. The incidence of *S.aureus* endocarditis was 0.16 episodes per 100 patient-catheter-months. These numbers are within the range reported in the literature. Blood cultures were obtained at the discretion of the treating physician if infection was suspected. Tunneled catheters that were a suspected source of infection were usually removed and negative cultures were required before insertion of a new tunneled catheter. All tunneled catheters were placed and removed by the same interventional radiology service. Suspected infection was the principal reason for tunneled catheter removal (19%), followed by poor catheter blood flow (14%) and presence of a mature permanent vascular access (14%). Infection rates were compared by Poisson regression analysis. In this study catheter associated bacteremia was defined as one or more positive blood cultures in a patient with a tunneled catheter. In retrospect it was impossible to exclude other sources of infection and contamination and for this reason all positive blood culture results that were obtained in the presence of a tunneled catheter were included without discrimination. Blood cultures that were obtained after a tunneled catheter was removed were excluded per definition. Our institution is a tertiary care medical center that offered hemodialysis in two outpatient units, serving a population of about 400,000 people. Because of location in a rural area, limited availability of hemodialysis and other geographical factors limiting access to other institutions the long term follow up of patients was excellent. A proprietary medical record system integrated electronic inpatient and outpatient records with procedure notes and laboratory, radiological and microbiological test result and was ideally suited for a large retrospective study. As a result the fate of only 8 catheters (<0.5%) was unaccounted for.

The number of episodes and rates of catheter associated bacteria is shown in Table 1 which includes repeated episodes and polymicrobial infections with more than one bacterial isolate. As expected, Gram positive bacteria accounted for the majority of bacteremic episodes. When all bacteremic episodes were considered together, there was no difference between patients treated with aspirin or not. In fact, the only pathogen with a lower rate of catheter-associated bacteremia in patients treated with aspirin was *S.aureus* which caused only half as many episodes in the aspirin group compared to patients not treated with aspirin (0.17 versus 0.34 events/patient-catheter-years, p=0.003). In addition to blood cultures 369 catheter tip cultures were performed in the same time interval, albeit in a less systematic fashion. Of these 53 catheter tip cultures grew *S.aureus*. In such a case treatment is usually recommended because *S.aureus* bacteremia is considered more likely than contamination (Peacock et al., 1998). If these tip cultures were added to bona fide blood cultures in the analysis, the difference was statistically more significant: 83 instances (0.36 events per patient-catheter-year) of *S.aureus* in the non aspirin treated group versus 45 (0.18 event per patient-catheter-year) in the aspirin treated group (p=0.001).

Moreover, if we excluded repeated events in the same patient from our data and considered only first episodes of *S.aureus* bacteremia, the difference looked between the two groups looked even more impressive: 28 first episodes of *S.aureus* bacteremia in patients treated with aspirin (0.23 events per patient-catheter year) versus more than double, 64 first episodes of *S.aureus* bacteremia (0.57 events per patient catheter year) in patient not treated with aspirin ($p<0.001$).

We explored the association between aspirin dose and rates of catheter associated *S.aureus* and *MRSA* bacteremia in table 2. There was a dose effect as only a 325mg dose of Aspirin, but not an 81mg dose (common formulations in the United States), was associated with a decreased rate of *Staphylococcus aureus* infection compared to patients not treated with aspirin. Importantly there was a significantly lower rates of *Methicillin resistant Staphylococcus aureus* bacteremia (*MRSA*) in patients treated with 325mg of aspirin a day.

	No Aspirin		**Aspirin**		***P***
	978 Catheters/227.4 Patient-Catheter-Years		**875 Catheters/ 249.3 Patient-Catheter-Years**		
	No.	**Rate (/patient-catheter-y)**	**No.**	**Rate (/patient-catheter-y)**	
All positive	232	1.02	207	0.83	0.30
Gram-positive					
Coagulase-negative *Staphylococcus*	96	0.42	93	0.37	0.85
S aureus	77	0.34	43	0.17	0.003*
MRSA	19	0.08	11	0.04	0.16
Enterococcus species	21	0.09	30	0.12	0.18
Corynebacterium species	7	0.03	6	0.02	0.82
Streptococcus species	4	0.02	7	0.03	0.34
Bacillus species	4	0.02	4	0.02	0.97
Gram-negative					
Enterobacter species	20	0.09	21	0.09	0.81
Pseudomonas species	11	0.05	13	0.05	0.64
Serratia species	12	0.05	9	0.04	0.55
Klebsiella species	9	0.04	10	0.04	0.77
Escherichia coli	7	0.03	4	0.02	0.39
Acinetobacter species	4	0.02	4	0.02	0.97
Bacteroides species	3	0.01	3	0.01	0.78

Note: Multiple bacterial isolates and repeated episodes were included in this table. Fungal isolates and bacterial species found fewer than 5 times during the 10-year study period were omitted.
*Significant difference by Poisson regression.

Table 1. Number of Episodes and Rates of Catheter-Associated Bacteremia in a 10-Year Period from 1995 to 2005

Reprinted from Sedlacek et al.: "Aspirin Treatment Is Associated With a Significantly Decreased Risk of Staphylococcus aureus bacteremia in Hemodialysis Patients With Tunneled Catheters", Am J Kidney Dis Vol49, pp401-408 with permission from Elsevier

	No Aspirin		81 mg Aspirin		325 mg Aspirin	
	978 Catheters/227.4 Patient-Catheter-Years		367 Catheters/116.2 Patient-Catheter-Years		508 Catheters/133.1 Patient-Catheter-Years	
	No.	Rate (/patient-catheter-y)	No.	Rate (/patient-catheter-y)	No.	Rate (/patient-catheter-y)
S aureus	77	0.34	26	0.22	17	0.13
		No Aspirin vs 81 mg: $P = 0.26$				
		No Aspirin vs 325 mg: $P < 0.001$*				
MRSA	19	0.08	10	0.09	1	0.01
		No Aspirin vs 81 mg: $P = 0.62$				
		No Aspirin vs 325 mg: $P = 0.001$*				

Table 2. Association between Aspirin Dose and Rates of Catether-Associated *S aureus* and MRSA Bacteremia
Reprinted from Sedlacek et al.: "Aspirin Treatment Is Associated With a Significantly Decreased Risk of Staphylococcus aureus bacteremia in Hemodialysis Patients With Tunneled Catheters", Am J Kidney Dis Vol49, pp401-408 with permission from Elsevier

We used Cox proportional hazard analysis to study risk factors for developing a first episode of *S.aureus* bacteremia. Table 3 shows the patient characteristics and distribution of covariates that were used for this analysis. Patient treated with aspirin were on average 10 years older and had a higher prevalence of coronary artery disease, peripheral vascular disease, history of stroke, hypertension and diabetes mellitus than patients not treated with aspirin.
Table 4 shows the result of the Cox proportional hazard analysis. Aspirin decreased the odds of developing a first episode of *S.aureus* bacteremia by 54% (with a confidence interval of 72% to 24%, p=0.002). No other cardiovascular medication and neither clopidogrel nor Warfarin had a similar effect. Also, no beneficial effect of statins on the odds of *S.aureus* bacteremia was observed in this study. On the opposite side, the presence of diabetes mellitus increased the risk of developing a first episode of catheter associated *S.aureus* bacteremia, as was previous recognized (Breen et al. 1995). COPD decreased the odds of a first episode *S.aureus* bacteremia in this study. A potential explanation for this observation could be more frequent antibiotic use in this condition which might reduce nasal carriage. A greater incidence of *S.aureus* bacteremia was reported in patients with cardiovascular disease (K/DOQI, 2005) but the opposite, lower numbers of *S.aureus* bacteremia was observed in this sicker patient population which may be taken as a sign of the potential clinical importance of the anti staphylococcal effects of aspirin. Similar results were obtained when multiple logistic regression analysis was used instead of Cox analysis.
Data on metastatic infection (endocarditis, osteomyelitis, septic arthritis) was analyzed as well. There were significantly less events in patients treated with aspirin compared with events in patients not treated with aspirin (3 versus 11 events, p=0.04).
A Kaplan-Meier plot of cumulative catheter failure associated with *S.aureus* bacteremia is shown in Figure 1. Grouping by aspirin treatment resulted in two divergent graphs with catheter failure caused by *S.aureus* infection significantly more frequent in the non aspirin group (p<0.001). The two graphs diverge very early which is consistent with the clinical observation that almost a quarter of *S.aureus* infection occur very early within a week after catheter insertion (Little M.A. et al., 2001). Figure 1 also illustrates another measure of the beneficial anti staphylococcal effect of aspirin: delayed onset of infection.

	No Aspirin (454 patients)	Aspirin (418 patients)	*P*
Age (y)	59 ± 19*	68 ± 13*	<0.0001
Time on dialysis (d)	362 ± 810	346 ± 542	0.73
Catheter no.	1.8 ± 1.8	1.9 ± 1.7	0.70
Female sex	194 (42)	186 (44)	0.54
Tobacco use	205 (45)*	225 (54)*	0.01
Diabetes mellitus	170 (38)*	236 (56)*	<0.0001
Hypertension	333 (74)*	364 (87)*	<0.0001
COPD	92 (20)*	117 (28)*	0.009
Coronary artery disease	159 (35)*	309 (79)*	<0.0001
Peripheral vascular disease	113 (25)*	200 (48)*	<0.0001
Stroke	66 (15)*	99 (24)*	0.007
Arthritis	141 (31)*	164 (39)*	0.01
Cancer	102 (23)	80 (19)	0.24
Previous transplant	50 (11)*	14 (3)*	<0.0001
Clopidogrel	12 (3)*	40 (10)*	<0.0001
Warfarin	61 (14)	60 (14)	0.77
Statin	69 (15)*	172 (41)*	<0.0001
B-Blocker	248 (55)*	315 (75)*	<0.0001
ACE inhibitor/ARB	136 (30)*	187 (45)*	<0.0001
Calcium channel blocker	216 (48)	216 (52)	0.28
Aspirin	0	418	<0.0001

Note: Values expressed as mean ± SD or number (percent).
Abbreviations: ACE, angiotensin-converting enzyme; ARB, angiotensin receptor blocker.
*Statistically significant difference between aspirin-treated and non–aspirin-treated groups by means of Fisher exact test or unpaired Student *t*-test, as appropriate.

Table 3. Patient Characteristic and Distribution of Covariates for the Cox Proportional Hazard Analysis
Reprinted from Sedlacek et al.: "Aspirin Treatment Is Associated With a Significantly Decreased Risk of Staphylococcus aureus bacteremia in Hemodialysis Patients With Tunneled Catheters", Am J Kidney Dis Vol49, pp401-408 with permission from Elsevier

A second study that addressed the anti staphylococcal effects of aspirin in hemodialysis patients was published in abstract form (Sedlacek et al., 2008). We performed a historical cohort study of the United States Renal Data System (USRDS) Dialysis Morbidity and Mortality Study (DMMS) Wave II data, linking medication data to mortality data from the core files. The updated USRDS Wave II data comprise 4024 patients, 16% of which were treated with Aspirin at study start date and 2776 of whom died. 54 of 2262 deaths (2.39%) in patients not treated with aspirin were attributed to septicemia due to vascular access either as primary or secondary cause, while there were only 4 of 510 deaths (0.78%) in patients treated with aspirin that were attributed to this cause (p<0.02, 2-tailed Fisher's Exact Test). Although anti platelet agents and other cardiovascular medications are underused in dialysis patients, we still find a strong negative association between aspirin treatment and death from septicemia due to vascular access in USRDS data. These results provide a confirmation of a clinical anti-staphylococcal effect of aspirin in hemodialysis patient that is independent from the data pool used in our first study.

	Relative Risk (95% CI)	*P*
Age (y)	1.0 (1.0-1.0)	0.99
Time on dialysis (d)	1.0 (1.0-1.001)	0.88
Catheter no.	0.95 (0.83-1.09)	0.45
Female sex	1.19 (0.76-1.86)	0.45
Tobacco use	0.78 (0.49-1.24)	0.30
Diabetes mellitus	1.65 (1.02-2.67)	0.04*
Hypertension	1.36 (0.74-2.51)	0.33
COPD	0.49 (0.24-0.97)	0.04*
Coronary artery disease	0.80 (0.48-1.34)	0.40
Peripheral vascular disease	1.01 (0.62-1.65)	0.97
Stroke	1.11 (0.63-1.96)	0.72
Arthritis	1.22 (0.78-1.92)	0.39
Cancer	1.04 (0.59-1.83)	0.89
Previous transplant	1.19 (0.55-2.55)	0.66
Clopidogrel	1.06 (0.40-2.83)	0.91
Warfarin	1.79 (1.03-3.10)	0.04*
Statin	1.08 (0.63-1.85)	0.79
B-Blocker	1.13 (0.70-1.83)	0.62
ACE inhibitor/ARB	0.79 (0.50-1.25)	0.31
Calcium channel blocker	0.73 (0.46-1.15)	0.17
Aspirin	0.46 (0.28-0.76)	0.002*

Abbreviations: ACE, angiotensin-converting enzyme; ARB, angiotensin receptor blocker.
*Statistical significance in Cox proportional hazard model.

Table 4. Risk of First *S aureus* Bacteremia Episode in 872 Dialysis Patients with a Tunneled Catheter by using Cox Proportional Hazard Analysis
Reprinted from Sedlacek et al.: "Aspirin Treatment Is Associated With a Significantly Decreased Risk of Staphylococcus aureus bacteremia in Hemodialysis Patients With Tunneled Catheters", Am J Kidney Dis Vol49, pp401-408 with permission from Elsevier

3.5 Concerns about aspirin use in hemodialysis patients

The abuse of non steroidal inflammatory drugs is a well described risk factor for upper gastrointestinal bleeding. The concern has been raised that the use of aspirin in dialysis patients could be harmful by causing bleeding (Chan et al., 2003 and 2008). As noted in a recent metanalysis the available data is conflicting for a variety of reasons such as selection bias, insufficient length of follow up and concomitant treatment with proton pump inhibitors (Hiremath et al., 2009). In the study of Chan et al a trend towards a higher incidence of bleeding was observed which did not reach statistical significance as both the initial study as well as the subsequent post hoc analysis was underpowered to either

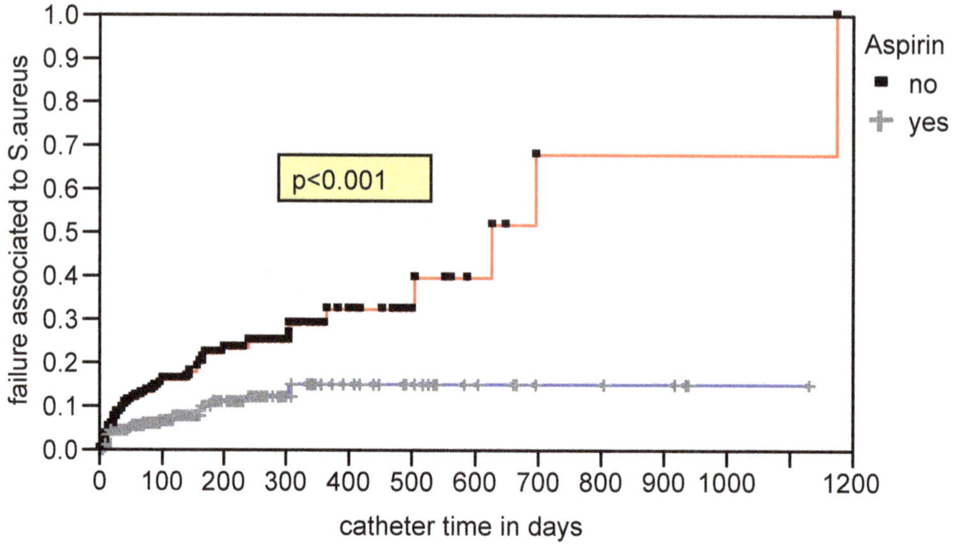

patients at risk:

ASA	417	142	66	35	25	16	9	6	5
no ASA	452	118	61	37	22	11	6	3	2

Fig. 1. Cumulative plot of tunneled catheter failure associated with *S aureus* bacteremia. The failure plot was obtained using the Kaplan-Meier method. Tics represent censoring of catheter removal unrelated to *S aureus* bacteremia. Log-rank test was used to calculate *P*. Reprinted from Sedlacek et al.: "Aspirin Treatment Is Associated With a Significantly Decreased Risk of Staphylococcus aureus bacteremia in Hemodialysis Patients With Tunneled Catheters", Am J Kidney Dis Vol49, pp401-408 with permission from Elsevier

support or refute this hypothesis. In our own study no increased risk of bleeding was observed (unpublished data, Sedlacek et al., 2008). A study on aspirin use in 28320 patients from the Dialysis Outcomes and Practice Patterns Study I and II found neither a decreased cardiovascular risk nor an increase in the gastrointestinal bleeding with the use of aspirin (Ethier J et al., 2007). (Of note, no data on infectious complications was included in this manuscript which why it was not discussed in the above sections.)

While there is no unequivocal proof that aspirin increases the risk of upper gastrointestinal bleeding in dialysis patients, it must not be forgotten that upper gastrointestinal bleeding is a well documented part of the uremic syndrome and that anticoagulation is routinely used during the hemodialysis procedure. It would thus seem reasonable to adopt a similar approach to high risk dialysis patients as has been recommended in high risk cardiac patients who would benefit from aspirin. Patients can be screened and treated for *H.pylorii* and proton pump inhibitors may be considered. Lastly it has to be noted that upper gastrointestinal bleeding is more amenable to treatment and represents a lesser risk to a high risk dialysis patient than for example cardiac stent occlusion.

4. Statins

Statins are cholesterol reducing medications that similarly to aspirin have become a cornerstone in the prevention and treatment of cardiovascular disease. The antimicrobial

effects of statins have been known for a long time. In fact, statins were discovered by searching for compounds that would inhibit HMG-CoA reductase in microbes that require sterols or other isoprenoids, which are part of bacterial cytoskeleton, for growth. The first statins were described as antibiotics secreted by Penicillium species. The first statin compound, mevastatin, is derived from a culture of *Pythium ultimum* and *Penicillium citrinum* and under the name compactin the same compound was isolated from a culture of *Penicillium brevicompactum* (Endo et al., 1976). A mevastatin analog currently in use, lovastatin, was isolated from a culture of *Aspergillus terreus.* (Endo A., 1992). The antimicrobial effects of statins were rediscovered at a later time and it was noted that the minimum inhibitory concentration of simvastatin for *S.aureus* was much higher than the serum levels that can be achieved during routine treatment at recommended doses (Jerwood S. & Cohen J., 2008). Direct antimicrobial effects with potential clinical relevance have been postulated for HIV, CMV, HCV, Salmonella and yeast (Gupta et al., 2007) but are perhaps less relevant for dialysis catheter associated infection. Newer laboratory evidence shows that the interferon response to viral infection of the innate immune immune system is coupled to the mevalonate-isoprenoid arm of the sterol pathway. These findings may explain the observation that the CMV and HCV viruses are sensitive to statin administration and that treatment with interferon decreases plasma cholesterol levels similar to treatment with statins (Blanc M et al., 2011).
Several observational studies in patients with severe bacterial infections have reported improved survival in patients treated with statins (Bjoerkheim-Bergman et al., 2010). These beneficial effects appear to be greater than what might be expected with lipid lowering alone and are attributed to pleiotropic effects of statins. Such effects involve improving endothelial function, decreasing oxidative stress and inflammation and inhibiting the thrombogenic response (Liao J.K. & Laufs U., 2005).
The hypothesis that treatment with statins could have an influence on the rate of septic events in dialysis patients was investigated by Gupta et al in 2007. The authors used data from a prospective study to investigate choices and outcomes of dialysis care, which enrolled 1041 patients from 1995 to 1998, the majority of which dialyzed in units associated with Dialysis Clinic Inc in Nashville TN. These patient data were linked to United States Renal Data System administrative data which included hospitalizations and data from other treatment settings, including outpatient and skilled nursing facilities. Primary outcome were sepsis events but "only episodes in which the primary event was sepsis were included (...) to avoid including cases in which infection was acquired as a secondary phenomenon" (Correction by the same authors in JAMA Vol 299 P 765). The correction to their method section published later by the authors raises the possibility that their data analysis could come to a different conclusion if all episodes of sepsis were considered, not only the events that were considered"primary". The authors found that 143 patients (14%) received statin treatment compared with 898 patients (86%) who were not. Among all 1041 patients there were a total of 303 events of primary sepsis during a mean follow up of 3.4 years. The crude incidence rate of sepsis events was 63% lower in patients treated with statins compared with the control group (41 events per 1000 patient-years compared with 110 events per 1000 patient years) The authors found that the odds ratio for a primary septic event in statin users was 0.38 (95% CI 0.21-0.67) with adjustments for demographics, dialysis modality, comorbidities and laboratory values. In a propensity-matched subcohort analysis statin use was even more protective with an odds ratio of 0.24 (CI 0.11-0.49) (Gupta et al., 2007). In

contrast to the results of this study no difference in the rate of death from fatal infection with the use of atorvastatin was found in the 4D study (Wanner et al., 2005).
An interesting question that is raised by the study by Gupta et al. is whether the observed benefit could be due to concomitant treatment with aspirin (Gupta et al., 2007). Both statins and aspirin are used for the treatment of coronary artery disease and a head to head comparison would be instructive. Our aspirin study did not find a beneficial effect of statins on the risk of septic events (Sedlacek et al., 2007) and the study by Gupta et al. did not control for aspirin use.
It has to be noted that the relation between lipid parameters and mortality in dialysis patients is complex, confounded by the fact that elevated serum cholesterol levels are paradoxically protective in this population, probably because they are a marker for the absence of malnutrition and inflammation. In practical terms it is advised to use low doses of statins to reduce side effects and to avoid the concomittant administration of other drugs metabolized by the cytochrome P-450 system such as cyclosporine, azole antifungals and fibrates (Olyaei et al., 2011).

5. Effects of other drugs used on dialysis

Several other drugs that are frequently used on dialysis have known interactions with microbes. Heparin is used frequently to block dialysis catheters when not in use to preserve their patency. Unfortunately, heparin has been found to promote growth of bacterial biofilm in dialysis catheters (Shanks et al., 2005). Citrate has been used as an alternative to heparin to block catheters and was found to have inhibitory effects on biofilms at elevated concentration. Reminiscent of the "Goldilocks effect" observed with aspirin, citrate stimulates biofilm formation at sub inhibitory concentrations, an effect which might have clinical relevance at catheter tips (Shanks et al., 2006). EDTA also has an inhibitory effect on biofilm. The mechanism for both EDTA and citrate is thought to be through chelation of divalent ions essential to the extracellular matrix structure of biofilm (Percival et al., 2005).
Diltiazem, Amlodipine and the angiotension converting enzyme inhibitor Zofenopril have modest in vitro antimicrobial activity against S.aureus. Most of these effects are bacteriostatic and occur at higher drug concentrations in vitro than the therapeutic concentrations that are usually achieved during therapy in vivo. It has to be noted however, that drug concentration can vary considerably throughout different organs and body compartments. In the case of Amiloride it has been determined that urine concentrations achieved in patients are not sufficient to replicate the antibacterial effects that are observed in vivo (Cederlund et al., 1993). The relevance of these observations probably concerns more microbial purity testing of drugs during the fabrication process rather than clinical effects.
Emla cream, a mixture of lidocaine, prilocaine and preservatives, which is used for topical anesthesia at the site of dialysis fistula puncture, has no effect on microbial growth (Kruszewska et al., 2010). Other drugs relevant to ESRD that have been tested and were found to be devoid of antimicrobial effects are the loop diuretics furosemide and bumetanide.
The antihistaminic drug diphenhydramine has been reported to be synergistic with the penicillins (Kristiansen, 1992) and amiloride reportedly enhances uptake of tobramycin in pseudomonas aeruginosa (Cederlund et al., 1993).

6. Last but not least: Honey

Honey has been used for the treatment of wounds since ancient times and its medicinal use is sanctioned by the Bible, Torah and Koran (Namias N., 2003). Johnson et al. conducted a prospective trial of topical honey versus topical Mupirocin ointment for the prevention of dialysis catheter associated infection. In a two year study period the authors enrolled 101 patients with tunneled dialysis catheters in their hospital based dialysis unit. Honey was applied three times a week to the dialysis catheter exit site in 51 patients while mupirocin ointment was used in 50 patients. No exit site infections were observed in either group and no difference in the rate of catheter associated bacteremia could be demonstrated. The cost of the Australian grown medicinal honey that the authors used was equivalent to mupirocin. As the authors noted, it is interesting that at the time of the study about 2% of staphylococcal isolates in their hospital were resistant to mupirocin while no bacterial resistance to honey has yet been reported despite millennia of being around (Johnson D.W. et al., 2005).

7. Conclusion

In summary, a couple of observational studies have shown that both aspirin and statins might have significant salutatory effects on infectious complications in hemodialysis patients. Of note, aspirin does not have growth inhibitory or bactericidal activity at pharmacologically relevant concentrations and thus may be less likely to promote bacterial resistance as traditional antimicrobials do (Eisen et al., 2009). The same might apply for statins as well (Jerwood & Cohen, 2008). However, retrospective and observational studies are prone to multiple sources of bias that are unquantifiable and of indeterminate direction. Thus, randomized prospective trials are needed to further investigate this exciting new approach to the prevention of infectious complications in dialysis patients.

8. References

Alvarez, L.P.; Barbagelata, M.S.; Gordiola M.; Cheung A.L.; Sordelli D.O.& Buzzola F.R. (2010). Salicylic acid diminishes staphylococcus aureus capsular polysaccharide Type 5 expression. *Infection Immunology,* Vol.78, (2010), pp. 1339-1344

Anavekar, N.S.; Tleyjeh, M.; Anavekar, N.S.; Mirzoyev, Z.; Steckeleberg, J.M.; Haddad, L.; Khandaker, M.H.; Wilson, W.R.; Chandrasekaran, K.& Baddour, L.M. (2007). Impact of prior antiplatelet therapy on risk of embolism in infectious endocarditis. *Clinical Infectious Disease,* Vol. 44, (2007), pp.1180-1186

Bjoerkhem-Bergman, L.; Bergman, P.; Andersson, J. & Lindh, J. (2010). Statin treatment and mortality in bacterial infections - a systematic review and meta-analysis. *PlosONE,* Vol5, No5, (2010), e10702

Blanc, M.; Hsieh, W.Y.; Robertson, K.A.; Watterson, S.; Shui, G.; Lacaze, P.; Khondoker, M.; Dickinson, P.; Sing, G.; Rodrigues-Martin, S.; Phelan, P.; Forster, T.; Strobl, B.; Mueller, M.; Riemersma, R.; Osborne, T.; Wenk, M.R.; Angulo, A. & Ghazal, P. (2011). Host Defense against viral infection involves interferon mediated down-regulation of sterol biosynthesis. Plos *Biology,* Vol 9,(2011) e1000598

Boelaert, J.R.; Van Landuyt, H.W.; De Baere, Y.A; Deruyter, M.M.; Daneels, R.F.; Schurgers, M.L.; Matthys, E.G.& Gordts,B.Z. (1950). Staphylococcus aureus infections in haemodialysis patients: pathophysiology and use of nasal mupirocin for prevention. *Journal of Chemotherapay,* Vol.7, Suppl. 3, (1950), pp.43-53

Breen, J.D. & Karchmer, A.W. (1995). Staphylococcus aureus infections in diabetic patients. *Infectious Disease Clinic of North America,* Vol.9, (1995), pp. 11-24

Cederlund H., Mardh P.A. (1993). Review: Antibacterial activities of non-antibiotic drugs. *Journal of Antimicrobial Chemotherapy* Vol. 32, (1993) pp.355-365

Chan, KL., Dumesnil, J.G., Cujec, B., Sanfilippo, A., Jue, J., Turek, M., Robinson, T., & Moher, D.(2003). A randomized trial of aspirin on the risk of embolic events in patients with infective endocarditis. *Journal of the American College of Cardiology,* Vol. 42, No 5, (2003), pp.775-780

Chan, K.L.; Tam, J.; Dumesnil, J.G.; Cujec, B.; Sanfilippo, A.J.; Jue, J,; Turek, M.; Robinson, T.& Williams, K. (2008). Effect of long-term aspirin use on embolic events in infective endocarditis. *Clinical Infectious Disease,* Vol46, (2008), pp. 37-41

Endo, A.; Kuroda, M. & Tsujita, Y. (1976). ML-236A, ML-236B and ML-236C, new inhibitors of cholesterogenesis produced by Penicillium citrinium. *Journal of Antibiotics,* Vol29. (1976) pp. 1346-1348

Endo, A. (2004) The origin of the statins. *Artherosclerosis Supplemen,t* Vol.5, (2004), pp. 67-80

Eisen, D.; Corey,G.,;McBryde,E.; Flowler, V.; Miro, J.; Cabell, C.; Street, A.; Goulart Paiva, M.; Ionac, A.; Tan, R.; Tribouilloy, C.; Pachirat, O.; Braun Jones, S.; Chipina, N.; Naber, C.; Pan, A.; Ravasio, V.; Gattringer, R.; Chu, V. &Bayer, A. (2009). Reduced valve replacement surgery and complication rate in Staphylococcus aureus endocarditis patients receiving acetyl-salicylic acid. *Journal of Infection,* Vol.58, No.5,(2009), pp.332-338

Eisen, D.P. & Bayer, A.S. (2008). Aspirin use in infective endocarditis. *Clinical Infectious Disease,* Vol. 46, (2008), pp. 1481-1482

Ethier, J.; Bragg-Gesham, J.L.; Piera, L.; Akizawa, T.; Asano, Y.; Mason, N.; Gillespie, B.W.& Young, E.W. (2007). Aspirin prescription and outcomes in hemodialysis patients: the dialysis outcomes and practice patterns study (DOPPS). *American Journal of Kidney Diease,* Vol.50, (2007), pp.602-611

Foley, R.N.; Guo, H.; Snyder, J.J.; Gilbertson, D.T. & Collins, A.J. (2004). Septicemia in the United States dialysis population, 1991 to 1999. *Journal of the American Society of Nephrology,* Vol. 15, (2004), pp. 1038-1045

Gupta, R.; Plantinga, L.; Fink, N.; Melamed, M., Coresh, J., Fox, C., Levin, N. & Powe,N. (2007). Statin use and hospitalization for sepsis in patients with chronic kidney disease. *Journal of the American Medical Association,* Vol. 297, No.13, (2007), pp. 1455-1464

Gupta, R.; Plantinga, L.; Fink, N.; Melamed, M.; Coresh, J.; Fox, C.; Levin, N. & Powe,N. (2008). Corrections. *Journal of the American Medical Association,* Vol. 299, No.7, (2008), p.765

Hiremath, S.; Holdren, R.M.; Fergusson, D. & Zimmerman, D.L. (2009). Antiplatelet medications in hemodialysis patients: a systematic review of bleeding rates. *Clinical Journal of the American Society of Nephrology,* Vol.4, (2009), pp1347-1355

Jerwood, S. & Cohen, J. (2008). Unexpected antimicrobial effects of statins. *Journal of Antimicrobial Chemotherapy,* Vol.61, No.2, (2008), pp.362-364

Johnson, D.W.; van Eps, C.; Mudge, D.W.; Wiggins, D.W.; Armstrong, K.; Hawley, C.M.; Campbell, S.B.; Isbel, N.M.; Nimmo, G.R. & Gibbs, H. (2005). Randomized controlled trial of topical exit-site application of honey (Medihoney) for the prevention of catheter-associated infections in hemodialysis patients. *Journal of the American Society of Nephrology*, Vol. 16, (2005), pp. 1456-1462

Karabay, O.; Arinc, H.; Gundu, Z.; Tamer, A.; Ozhan, H. & Uyan, C. (2006). A new effect of acetylsalicylic acid? Significantly lower prevalence of nasal carriage of staphylococcal aureus among patients receiving orally administered acetylsalicylic acid. *Infection Control Hospital Epidemiology*, Vol 27, (2006),pp. 317-319

National Kidney foundation: K/DOQI Clinical Practice guidelines for cardiovascular diease in dialysis patients. (2005) *American Journal of Kidney Diseases*, Vol. 45, Suppl.3, (2005), pp. S1-S153

Kristinasen, J.E. (1992). The antimicrobial activity of non-antibiotics. Report from a congress on the antimicrobial effect of drugs other than antibiotics on bacteria, viruses, protozoa and other organisms. *APMIS* Suppl.30, Vol.100, (1992), pp.7-14

Kristiansen, J.E.; Hendricks, O.; Delvin, T.; Butterworth, T.S.; Aagaard, L.; Christensen, J.B.; Flores, V.C. & Keyzer, H. (2007). Reversal of resistance in microorganisms by help of non-antibiotics. *Journal of Antimicrobial Chemotherapy*, Vol.59, (2007), pp 1271-1279

Kruszewska, H.; Zareba, T. & Tyski, S. (2010). Examination of antimicrobial activity of selected non-antibiotic products. *Acta Poloniae Pharmaceutica Drug Research*, Vol.67 No.6, (2010), pp.733-736

Kupferwasser, L.I.; Yeaman, M.R. & Shapiro, S.R. (1999). Acetylsalicylic acid reduces vegetation, bacterial density, hematogenous bacterial dissemination and frequency of embolic events in experimental staphylococcus aureus endocarditis through antiplatelet and antibacterial effects. *Circulation*, Vol.99, (1999),pp. 2791-2797

Kupferwasser, L., Yeaman,M.R., Nast, C., Kupferwasser,D.; Xiong,Y., Palma, M., Cheung,A., & Bayer, A. (2003). Salicylic acid attenuates virulence in endovascular infections by targeting global regulatory pathways in staphylococcus aureus. Journal of *Clinical Investigation*, Vol.122, No.2, (2003),pp. 222-233

Laupland, K.B.;Gregson ,D.B.; Zygun, D.A.; Doig, C.J,.; Mortis, G. & Church, D.L. (2004). Severe blood stream infections: a population based assessment. *Critical Care Medicine*, Vol. 32, (2004), pp. 992-997

Liao, J.K. & Laufs, U. (2005) Pleiotropic effects of statins. *Annual Review of Pharmacology and Toxicology*, Vol.45, (2005), pp. 89-118

Little, M.A.; O'Riordan, A.; Lucey, B. et al. (2001). A prospective study of complications associated with cuffed tunneled haemodialysis catheters. *Nephrology Dialysis Transplantation*, Vol 16,(2001), pp. 2194-2200

Liu, G.Y. & Nizrt, V. (2009). Colour me bad: microbial pigments as virulence factors. *Trends in Microbiology*, Vol. 17, (2009), pp. 406-413

Namias, N. (2003) Honey in the management of infections. *Surgical Infection*, Vol.4, (2003), pp. 219-226

Nicolau, D.P.; Freeman, C.D.; Nightingale, C.H.; Quintiliani, R.; Coe, C.J.; Maderazo, E.G. & Cooper, B.W. (1993). Reduction of bacterial titers by low-dose aspirin in experimental aortic valve endocarditis. *Infection and Immunity*, Vol.61, (1993), pp. 1593-1595

Nicolau, D.P.; Marangos, M.N.; Nightingale, C.H. & Quintiliani, R. (1995). Influence of Aspirin on development and treatment of experimental Staphylococcus aureus endocarditis. *Antimicrobial Agents and Chemotherapy*, Vol.39, (1995), pp. 1748-1751

Olyaei, A.; Greer, E.; Delos Santos, R. & Rueda, J. (2011) The efficacy and safety of 3-hydroxy-3-methylglutaryl-CoA esterase inhibitors in chronic kidney disease, dialysis and transplant patients. *Clinical Journal of the American Society of Nephrology*, Vol6, (2011), pp. 664-678

Paterson, J.R. & Lawrence, J.R. (2001), Salicylic acid: a link between aspirin, diet and the prevention of colorectal cancer. *Quarterly Journal of Medicine*, Vol. 94, (2001), pp. 445-448

Peacock, S.J.; Eddleston, M.; Emptage, A.; King, A. & Crook, D.W. (1998) Positive intravenous line tip cultures as predictors of bacteremia. *Journal of Hospital Infection*, Vol. 40, (1998), pp. 35-38

Percival, S.L.; Kite, P.; Eastwood, K.; Murga, R.; Carr, J.; Arduino, M.J. & Donlan, R.M. (2005). Tertrasodium EDTA as a novel central venous catheter lock solution against biofilm. *Infection Control Hospital Epidemiology* Vol. 26 (2005), pp.511-514

Pujadas, R.E.; Escriva, F.; Jane, J.; Argimon, J.; Fava, P. & Calera, M.C. (1988). Effect of various doses of aspirin on the development of aseptic thrombotic aortic endocarditis experimentally induced in the rabbit. *Revista Espanola de Cardiologia,* Vol. 41,(1988), pp 31-34

Rayner, H.C.; Besarab, A.; Brown, W.; Disney, A.; Saito, A. & Pisoni, R.L. (2004). Vascular access results from the Dialysis Outcomes and Practice Patterns Study (DOPPS): performance against kidney disease outcomes quality initiative (K/DOQI) clinical practice guidelines. *American Journal of Kidney Disease*, Vol. 44, Suppl.2, (2004), pp. S22-S26

Ruder, E.H.; Layemo, A.O.; Graubard, B.I.; Hollenbeck, A.R.; Schatzkin, A & Cross, A.J. (2011). Non steroidal anti-inflammatory drugs and colorectal cancer risk in a large prospective cohort. *American Journal of Gastroenterology*, (2011), (e-published before print)

Sedlacek, M.; Gemery, J.; Cheung, A.; Bayer, A. & Remillard, B. (2007). Aspirin Treatment is associated with a significantly decreased risk of Staphylococcus aureus bacteremia in Hemodialysis patients with tunneled catheters. *American Journal of Kidney Diseases*, Vol. 49, No.3, (2007), pp. 401-408

Sedlacek, M.; Kaneko, T.; Schoolwerth, A. & Remillard, B.(2008) Septicemia due to vascular access is a rare cause of death in dialysis patients treated with aspirin. *Journal of the American Society of Nephrology*, Vol.19, (2007), abstract F-PO1586

Schunemann, S.; Werner, G.S.; Schulz, R.; Bitsch, A.; Prange, H.W. & Kreutzer, H. (1997). Embolische Komplikationen bei bacterieller Endokarditis. *Zeitschrift fuer Kardiologie*, Vol.86,(1997), pp1017-1025

Shanks, R.M.Q.; Donegan, N.P.; Graber, M.L.; Buckingham, S.E.; Zegans, M.; Cheung, A.L. & O'Toole, G.A. (2005). Heparin stimulates staphylococcus aureus biofilm formation. *Infection and Immunity*, Vol. 73, No 8, (2005), pp. 4596-4606

Shanks, R.M.Q.; Sargent, J.L.; Martinez, R.M.; Graber, M.L. & O'Toole, G.A. (2006). Catheter lock solutions influence staphylococcal biofilm formation on abiotic surfaces. *Nephrology Dialysis Transplantation*, Vol. 21, (2006), pp. 2247-2255

Taha, T.H.; Durrant, S.S.; Mazeika, P.K.; Nihoyannopoulos,P. & Oakley, C.M. (1992). Aspirin to prevent growth of vegetations and cerebral emboli in infective endocarditis. *Journal of Internal Medicine,* Vol. 231, (1992), pp. 543-546

Vandecasteele, S.J.; Boelaert , J.R. & De Vriese, A.S. (2009). Staphylococcus aureus infections in hemodialysis: what a nephrologist should know. *Clinical Journal of the American Society of Nephrology,* Vol.4, (2009), Pp. 1388-1400

VanderBergh, M.F.; Yzerman, E.P.; van Belkum, A.; Boelens, H.A;, Sijmons, M. & Verbrugh, H.A (1999). Follow up of Staphylococcus aureus nasal carriage after eight years: redefining the persistent carrier state. *Journal of Clinical Microbiology,* Vol 37, (1999), pp .3133-3140

Von Eiff, C.; Becker, K.; Machka, K.; Stammer, H. & Peters, G. (2001). Nasal carriage as a source of staphylococcus aureus bacteremia. *New England Journal of Medicine,* Vol. 344, (2001), pp11-16

Williams J.D. (1995). The Garrod lecture: Selective toxicity and concordant pharmacodynamics of antibiotics and other drugs. *Journal of Antimicrobial Chemotherapy,* Vol35, (1995), pp.721-737

Wanner, C.; Kanne, V. & Marz, W. (2005). Atorvastatin in patients with type 2 diabetes mellitus undergoing hemodialysis. *New England Journal of Medicine,* Vol. 353, (2005), pp 238-248

12

Identification of Hemodialysis Patients' Physical and Psychosocial Problems Using the International Classification of Functioning, Disability and Health (ICF)

Hideyo Tsutsui, Teruhiko Koike and Yoshiharu Oshida
Research Center of Health, Physical Fitness and Sports, Nagoya University
Japan

1. Introduction

We aimed to identify hemodialysis (HD) patients' physical and psychosocial problems using the International Classification of Functioning, Disability and Health (ICF)-based checklist we developed. The ICF belongs to the WHO's family of international classifications, and it is the instrument for comprehensive understanding of patients. HD patients have diverse physical and psychosocial problems, and ICF-based approach may be useful to improve management and quality of life (QOL) of patients on HD. In this article, we introduced the new data associated with physical and psychosocial problems of 222 patients in HD, which extends our previous report (Tsutsui et al. 2009).

In Japan, the number of patients on HD was 36,397 in 1980 and increased to 290,675 in 2009 (Patient Registration Committee, Japanese Society for Dialysis Therapy, 2010). In addition to the physical limitations in functioning caused by renal failure and its comorbidities, HD patients have various restrictions resulting from HD therapy requiring radical lifestyle changes. Therefore, HD patients tend to have both physical and psychosocial problems. Thus, evaluation of QOL is especially important, and the Kidney Disease Quality of Life (KDQOL™) (Hays et al, 1994) and the Kidney Disease Quality of Life-Short Form (KDQOL-SF™) (Hays et al, 1994) have been widely used. The KDQOL-SF™ includes multi-item scales targeted at the particular health-related concerns of individuals who have kidney disease and are on dialysis. In the present study, we aimed to investigate the use of the International Classification of Functioning, Disability and Health (ICF) (WHO 2001), which is the instrument for comprehensive understanding of patients. In addition to evaluate physical and psychosocial problems of patients, ICF can be used as a tool for team medical treatment to make plans for treatment and care of patients. We have reported the checklist for HD patients based on ICF (Tsutsui et al. 2009). The data in this article include those of patients on HD with diabetic nephropathy, which was excluded in the previous report.

2. International classification of functioning, disability and health

The ICF was published by the World Health Organization (WHO) in 2001 to standardize descriptions of health and disability. The ICF and International Classification of Disease-10th

Revision (ICD-10) constitute the core classification in the WHO's family of international classifications, which provides a valuable tool to describe and compare the health of populations in an international context. The information on mortality (provided by ICD-10) and on health outcomes (provided by ICF) may be combined in summary measures of population health.

The overall aim of the ICF classification is to provide a unified and standard language and framework for the description of health and health-related states. It defines components of health and some health-related components of well-being (such as education and labor). An ICF-based approach can also be useful to collect information on a broad set of impairments, activity limitations and environmental factors that contribute to improve or worsen patients' functioning and disability status. Such information could provide a common framework for research, clinical work and social policy and help in improving the identification of needs related to health and social services, and related interventions.

The ICF provides a description of situations about human functioning and its restrictions and serves as a framework to organize this information. The ICF is based on the biopsychosocial model, an integration of medical and social models. The patient's functioning is conceived as a dynamic interaction between the underlying health condition and specific personal and environmental factors. The following diagram is one representation of model of disability that is the basis for ICF (Figure 1).

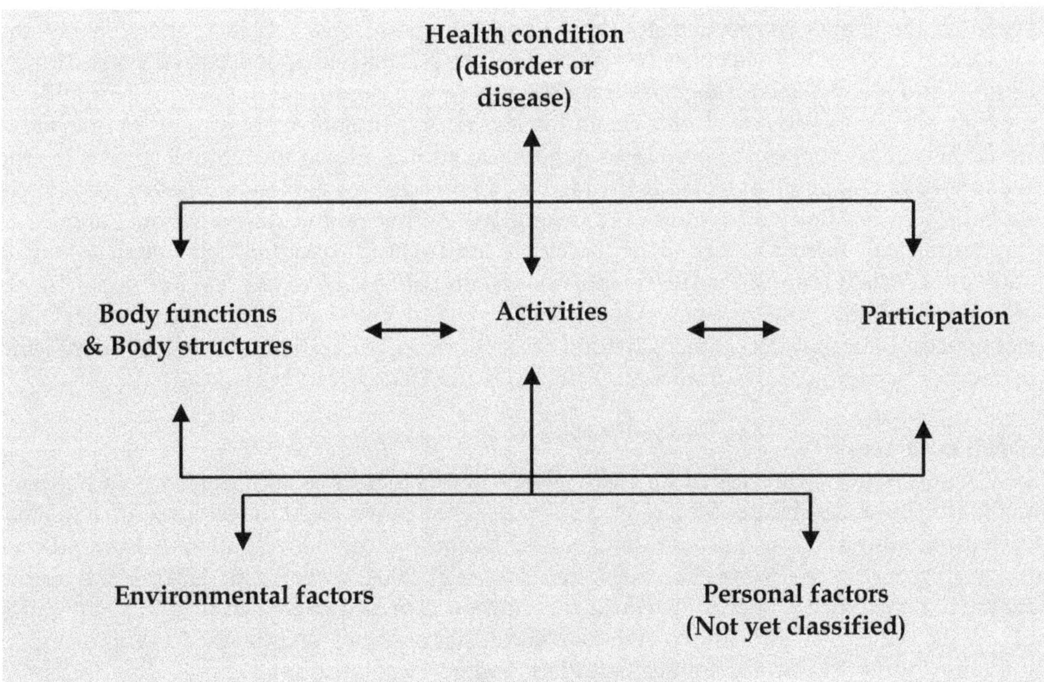

Fig. 1. Interactions between the components of ICF (WHO, 2001)

The ICF organizes information in the two main subdivisions: Part 1 covers functioning and disability and Part 2 covers contextual factors. Each of these two parts is divided into components. Components of functioning and disability consist of "Body functions and structures" and "Activities and participation". Components of contextual factors consists of

"Environmental factors" and "Personal factors". "Body functions" relate to the physiological and psychological functions of the body. "Body structures" are anatomic parts of the body such as organs, limbs and their components classified according to body systems. "Activities" is the execution of a task or action by an individual. It represents the individual perspective of functioning. "Participation" is a person's involvement in a life situation. It represents the societal perspective of functioning. "Environmental factors" refer to all aspects of the external or extrinsic world that from the context of an individual's life such as social attitudes and values, social systems and services, policies, rules and laws. "Personal factors" are those related to the individual such as age, gender, social status, and life experiences, which are not currently classified in ICF, although users may incorporate in their applications of the classification (WHO 2001).

Every component of the ICF has a hierarchical structure. The categories of ICF are classified by the code in which the letters (b, s, d, and e) is combined with the number. The letters b, s, d and e refer to the components "Body functions" (b), "Body structures" (s), "Activities and participation" (d), and "Environmental factors" (e). The letters are followed by a numeric code that defines the chapter number (first digit) and the category levels up to the fourth level (suffix of two, three, or four digits).

2.1 ICF checklist

The ICF in its current version consists of 1424 codes. Therefore, it is necessary to select a subset of the codes as needed for any given purpose. One of such activities is the development of the ICF checklist (WHO, 2003). The ICF checklist consists of a selection of 128 first- and second-level categories from the whole ICF classification system. It provides a relatively simple-to-use questionnaire, and is a generic template for a structured interview. The ICF checklist makes it possible to generate a profile of the individual patient on the functioning and disability in clinical practice. Of the 128 categories, 32 belong to "Body functions", 16 to "Body structures", 48 belong to "Activities and participation", and 32 to "Environmental factors". The ICF checklist utilizes a "qualifier" to evaluate each component, which is considered to be positive when patients have any level of impairments (i.e. mild, moderate, severe, or complete) in "Body functions" and "Body structures"; any level of activity limitations or participation restrictions in "Activities and participation"; and any level of barrier in "Environmental factors" (WHO 2003, Ewert et al. 2004).

2.2 ICF core sets

The ICF core sets are developed for medical conditions that have high impact on a patient's functioning and disability (Stucki et al. 2002). They have been developed in a formal decision making and consensus-based process integrating evidence gathered from studies for chronic conditions (Weigl et al. 2004, Brockow et al. 2004, Ewert et al. 2004). The ICF core sets for patients with a determined health condition represent a selection of ICF categories out of the whole classification that can serve as minimal standards for reporting of functioning and health for clinical studied and clinical encounter or as standards for multiprofessional. The ICF core sets contain categories not only on anatomic and pathophysiologic changes but also on functioning in every-day activities and relevant environmental factors.

These ICF core sets are to be developed in two levels: A brief and comprehensive ICF core sets. The brief ICF core sets includes only the most important ICF-categories and is intended to be rated in all patients of a clinical study. However, the comprehensive ICF core sets

include all categories that are typically limited in the selected health condition, and are created to guide multidisciplinary assessment (Stucki et al. 2002).
The ICF core sets have been developed for many health conditions including diabetes mellitus (Ruof et al. 2004), obesity (Stucki et al. 2004), and stroke (Geyh et al. 2004).

3. Identification of HD patients' physical and psychosocial problems

The process of developing the checklist for the HD treatment is briefly described.
Initially, we interviewed 32 HD patients using ICF checklist. They were interviewed for each category of the ICF checklist whether they had problems since starting HD treatment. For example, in the category of *b134 Sleep*, patients were interviewed "Have you ever experienced insomnia, nocturnal awakening, or hypersomnia since starting HD treatment?" The interviewer questioned about the details of their problems when patients answered "yes". The interview was done by the first author who was the medical social worker. All categories that at least 1 patient reported a problem were selected as problem categories. As a result, 57 categories of the ICF checklist were selected for the checklist for the HD treatment. Thirty-five categories in the ICF that were not included in the ICF checklist were chosen based on the consensus of the conference that included physician, nurses, and medical social worker. These 92 categories consisted of 39 categories from the "Body functions" component, 13 from the "Body structures" component, 20 categories from the "Activities and participation" component, and 20 categories from the "Environmental factors" component. Finally, we added 8 categories that are not included in the ICF categories considering the specificities of HD. These categories are following; *Functions of vascular access* in "Body functions" component, *Vascular access* in "Body structures" component, *Going to hospital, Managing weight, Angiostasis by oneself after drawing out needle,* and *Preparing a dialysis diet* in "Activities and participation" component, *Dialysis professionals* in "Environmental factors" component. Taken together, the checklist for the HD comprises 100 categories.

	Body Functions	Body Structures	Activities and Participation	Environmental Factors	Total
ICF checklist Version2.1α	19	8	15	15	57
Additional ICF categories for HD	20	5	5	5	35
Categories specific for HD	1	1	5	1	8
Final Checklist for HD	40	14	25	21	100

Table 1. Component of checklist.

3.1 Physical and psychosocial problems of maintenance HD patients

We interviewed 222 maintenance HD patients using the checklist for HD patients. The characteristics of them are shown in Table 2.

3.1.1 Body functions

The percentage of patients on maintenance HD who reported problems in each category of "Body functions" component is described in Table 3.

	Total n=222
Sex (men/women)	152/70
Age (years)	61±11
Age of HD introduction (years)	52±13
Duration of HD (years)	9.1±8.0
Underlying disease	
Diabetic nephropathy	86
Chronic glomerulonephritis	46
Nephrosclerosis	44
Polycystic kidney	9
Gouty kidney	6
Interstitinal nephritis	2
Obstructive urinary disorder	2
Reflux nephropathy	1
Cystinuria	1
Pregnancy-induced kidney disease	1
Pyelonephritis	1
Systemic lupus erythematosus	1
Unidentified	22

Table 2. Maintenance HD patients' characteristics.

Body Functions	%
b110 Consciousness functions	25.7
b1300 Energy level	39.2
b1302 Appetite	26.6
b134 Sleep functions	46.4
b140 Attention functions	32.9
b152 Emotional functions	26.6
b210 Seeing functions	50.9
b240 Sensations associated with hearing and vestibular function	37.8
b250 Taste function	20.7
b260 Proprioceptive function	36.9
b265 Touch function	16.7
b270 Sensory functions related to temperature and other stimuli	12.2
b280 Sensation of pain	45.9
b410 Heart functions	45.9
b415 Blood vessel functions	22.5
§ Functions of vascular access	27.2
b420 Blood pressure functions	75.7
b430 Haematological system functions	14.0
b440 Respiration functions	26.6
b4550 General physical endurance	50.5

Body Functions	%
b4551 Aerobic capacity	45.9
b4552 Fatigability	57.2
b515 Digestive functions	24.8
b525 Defecation functions	51.4
b530 Weight maintenance functions	22.5
b535 Sensations associated with the digestive system	33.8
b545 Water, mineral and electrolyte balance functions	26.6
b555 Endocrine gland functions	14.0
b610 Urinary excretory functions	61.3
b620 Urination functions	47.7
b64 Sexual functions	18.0
b670 Sensations associated with genital and reproductive functions	12.6
b710 Mobility of joint functions	43.2
b730 Muscle power functions	12.6
b735 Muscle tone functions	40.5
b780 Sensations related to muscles and movement functions	64.4
b810 Protective functions of the skin	59.9
b820 Repair function of the skin	36.9
b840 Sensation related to the skin	74.8
b850 Functions of hair	29.7

§; Categories specific for HD (Not ICF categories)

Table 3. Percentage of maintenance HD patients who reported impairment in each category of "Body functions" component.

In the "Body functions" component, problems of patients on maintenance HD are associated with sleep, fatigue, defecation, blood pressure, urination, muscle, skin, and those related to the symptoms or complication of kidney disease. Itching of the skin (Danquah et al. 2010, Caplin et al. 2011), sleep (Čengić et al. 2010, Danquah et al. 2010), blood pressure (Van Buren et al. 2011, Caplin et al. 2011), muscle cramps (Danquah et al. 2010, Weisbord et al. 2008), and constipation (Wu et al. 2004, Yasuda et al. 2002) have been reported as significant problems in patients with maintenance HD. According to the interview, these patients tend to have problems such as itching, muscle cramp, or low blood pressure not only in everyday life but also during HD treatment, which seem worry them substantially.

3.1.2 Body structures

The percentage of maintenance HD patients who reported problems in each category of component of "Body structures" component is described in Table 4.

In the "Body structures" component, a high percentage of patients on maintenance HD reported problems related to nail, disorder of urinary system, and eye disease. Disorder of nail structure such as half-and-half nail and tinea unguium (Saray et al. 2004, Dyachenko et al. 2007), disorder of urinary system such as pyuria and loss of urination (Vij et al. 2009, Fasolo et al. 2006), and eye disease such as diabetic retinopathy and glaucoma (Chiu et al. 2008, Varbec et al. 2005) have been reported.

Body structures	%
s220 Structure of eyeball	41.0
s410 Structure of cardiovascular system	30.2
s4100 Heart	9.5
§ Vascular access	33.8
s550 Structure of pancreas	0.9
s5801 Thyroid gland	12.1
s5802 Parathyroid gland	14.7
s610 Structure of urinary system	61.3
s6100 Kidneys	100.0
s630 Structure of reproductive system	6.8
s730 Structure of upper extremity	28.4
s750 Structure of lower extremity	13.5
s770 Additional musculoskeletal structures related to movement	5.0
s830 Structure of nails	56.3

§; Categories specific for HD (Not ICF categories)

Table 4. Percentage of maintenance HD patients who reported impairment in each category of "Body structures" component.

3.1.3 Activities and participation

The percentage of maintenance HD patients who reported restrictions in each category of "Activities and participation" component is described in Table 5.

In the "Activities and participation" component, a high percentage of patients reported restrictions related to actions that use upper limbs, job, and hobby. Consistently, actions that use upper limbs (Tander et al. 2007, Namazi et al. 2007), job (Panagopoulou et al. 2009, Kutner et al. 2010), and hobby (Al Eissa et al. 2010) have been reported to be highly restricted. The time restriction due to the regular dialysis and the need to protect vascular access seem to be major factors to affect patients' restriction in activities and participation.

3.1.4 Environmental factors

The percentage of maintenance HD patients who reported barriers in each category of "Activities and participation" component is described in Table 6.

In the "Environmental factors" component, a high percentage of paients reported as barriers in categories related to transportation service, social security, and labor. Transportation (Diamant et al. 2010, Gorden et al. 2003), social security such as medical fee (Holley et al. 2006, Gracia-Gracia et al. 2005) and labor (Neri et al. 2009, Muehrer et al. 2011) have been reported as barriers. Maintaining employment is one of the most serious problems. We reported that 41% of the patients in the previous study (Tsutsui et al, 2009) were terminated, transferred to a different position, demoted, or changed their employment agreement (from

Activities and Participation	%
d220 Undertaking multiple tasks	14.0
b240 Handling stress and other psychological demands	17.1
d430 Lifting and carrying objects	35.1
d440 Fine hand use	23.0
d450 Walking	13.1
d465 Moving around using equipment	9.9
d470 Using transportation	15.8
d475 Driving	19.4
§ Going to hospital	5.4
d510 Washing oneself	9.9
d520 Caring for body parts	9.5
d550 Eating	7.2
d570 Looking after one's health	15.8
§ Managing weight	14.0
§ Confirmation of vascular access	0.5
§ Angiostasis by oneself after drawing out needle	9.9
d630 Preparing meals	7.2
§ Preparing a dialysis diet	17.1
d640 Doing housework	9.5
d660 Assisting others	2.7
d845 Acquiring, keeping and terminating a job	24.8
d850 Remunerative employment	21.6
d9201 Sports	18.5
d9204 Hobbies	32.0
d9205 Socializing	24.8

§; Categories specific for HD (Not ICF categories)

Table 5. Percentage of maintenance HD patients who reported restrictions in each category of "Activities and participation" component.

full-time to part-time employment). According to Japanese statistics, 37.7% of men HD patients and 43% of women HD patients were terminated or retired in the past 5 years (Japan Association of Kidney Disease Patients, Japanese Association of Dialysis Physician. 2007). The problem related to the payment of medical fees is another serious concern for patients. Patients on HD had received a total exemption of medical fees until the coming into force of the "Law for Independence of Persons With Disabilities" in 2006. According to a report (Japan Association of Kidney Disease Patients, Japanese Association of Dialysis Physician. 2007), 75.2% of Japanese HD patients greatly hope for "continuation of medical security of HD treatment".

Environmental Factors	%
e110 Products or substances for personal consumption	27.5
e310 Immediate family	8.1
e320 Friends	7.7
e325 Acquaintances, peers, colleagues, neighbors and community members	5.0
e330 People in positions of authority	5.9
e350 Domesticated animals	14.4
e355 Health professionals	16.7
§ Dialysis professionals	5.4
e410 Individual attitudes of immediate family members	4.1
e420 Individual attitudes of friends	4.1
e425 Individual attitudes of acquaintances, peers, colleagues, neighbors and community members	6.3
e430 Individual attitudes of people in positions of authority	3.6
e440 Individual attitudes of personal care providers and personal assistants	2.3
e450 Individual attitudes of health professionals	18.5
e465 Social norms, practices and ideologies	17.1
e540 Transportation services, systems and policies	10.4
e555 Associations and organizational services, systems and policies	14.9
e560 Media services, systems and policies	23.4
e570 Social security services, systems and policies	23.8
e580 Health services, systems and policies	32.4
e590 Labour and employment services, systems and policies	35.1

§; Categories specific for HD (Not ICF categories)

Table 6. Percentage of the maintenance HD patients who reported barriers in each category of "Environmental factors" component.

4. Conclusion

We developed the ICF-based checklist for the HD treatment, and identified the physical and psychosocial problems that the HD patients had. We showed the features of HD patients with problems associated with disease or impairments as well as daily life activities. The checklist based on ICF, which is an integrated model of the medical and the social models, enables us to understand HD patients comprehensively. We will continue efforts to identify more relevant ICF categories to complete the final version of the checklist.

5. Acknowledgments

The authors would like to thank: Dr. F Kato, nephrologist, Dr. A Ito, hospital director, and H Sato, director of nursing department, at the Masuko Memorial Hospital; Dr. C Yamazaki, hospital director, and M Imai, chief nurse at the Masko Clinic Subaru; and Dr. H Tawada, hospital director, and S Sekine, medical social worker, at the Tawada Hospital; and Dr. H

Tawada, hospital director, K Moriya, medical social worker, and A Nakanishi, manager; and Dr. Y Hatanaka, hospital director, and H Kozakai, medical social worker, at the Sakashita Clinic, for their support with respect to the interviews.

6. References

Al Eissa M, Al Sulaiman M, Jondeby M et al. (2010) Factors affecting hemodialysis patients' satisfaction with their dialysis therapy. *Int J Nephrol.* Vol. 2010, pp.342901-342901, ISSN 2090-2158.

Brockow T, Cieza A, Kuhlow H et al. (2004) Identifying the concepts contained in outcome measures of clinical trials on musculoskeletal disorders and chronic widespread pain using the International Classification of Functioning, Disability and Health as a reference. *J Rehabil Med.* Vol. 44, No. Suppl., pp. 30-36, ISSN 1650-1969.

Caplin B, Kumar S, Davenport A. (2011) Patients' perspective of haemodialysis-associated symptoms. *Nephrol Dial Transplant.* Epub ahead of print, ISSN 1460-2385.

Čengić B, Resić H, Spasovski G et al. (2010) Quality of sleep in patients undergoing hemodialysis. *Int Urol Nephrol.* Epub ahead of print, ISSN 1573-2584.

Chiu E, Markowitz SN, Cook WL et al. (2008) Visual impairment in elderly patients receiving long-term hemodialysis. *Am J Kidney Dis.* Vol. 52, No. 6, pp. 1131-1138, ISSN 1523-6838.

Cieza A, Bickenbach J, Chatterji S. (2008) The ICF as a conceptual platform to specify and discuss health and health-related concepts. *Gesundheitswesen.* Vol. 70, No.10, pp. e47-56, ISSN 1439-4421.

Danquah FVN, Zimmerman L, Diamond PM et al. (2010) Frequency, severity, and distress of dialysis-related symptoms reported by patients on hemodialysis. *Nephrol Nurs J.* Vol. 37, No. 6, pp. 627-638, ISSN 1526-744X.

Diamant MJ, Harwood L, Movva S et al. (2010) A comparison of quality of life and travel-related factors between in-center and satellite-based hemodialysis patients. Clin J Am Soc Nephrol. Vol. 5, No. 2, pp. 268-274, ISSN 1555-905X.

Dyachenko P, Monselise A, Shustak A et al. (2007) Nail disorders in patients with chronic renal failure and undergoing haemodialysis treatment: a case-control study. *J Eur Acad Dermatol Venereol.* Vol. 21, No. 3, pp. 340-344, ISSN 1468-3083.

Ewert T, Fuessl M, Cieza A, et al. (2004) Identification of the most common patient problems in patients with chronic conditions using the ICF checklist. *J Rehabil Med.* Vol. 44, No. Suppl, pp. 22-29, ISNN 1650-1969.

Fasolo LR, Rocha LM, Campbell S et al. (2006) Diagnostic relevance of pyuria in dialysis patients. *Kidney Int.* Vol. 70, No. 11, pp. 2035-2038, ISSN 1523-1755.

Garcia-Garcia G, Monteon-Ramos JF, Gracia-Bejarano H et al. (2005) Renal replacement therapy among disadvantaged populations in Mexico: A report from the Jalisco dialysis and transplant registry (REDTAL). *Kidney Int.* Vol. 68, No. 97, pp. s58-s61, ISSN 0098-6577.

Geyh S, Cieza A, Schouten J et al. (2004) ICF core sets for stroke. *J Rehabil Med.* Vol. 44, No. suppl., pp. 135-141, ISSN 1650-1969.

Gorden EJ, Leon JB, Sehgal AR et al. (2003) Why are hemodialysis treatments shortened and skipped? Development of a taxonomy and relationship to patient subgroups. *Nephrol Nurs J.* Vol. 30, No. 2, pp.209-217, ISSN 1526-744X.

Hays RD, Kallich JD, Mapes DL et al. (1994) Development of the Kidney Disease Quality of Life (KDQOL™) instrument. *Qual Life Res.* Vol. 5, No. 3, pp. 329-338, ISSN 1573-2649.

Hays RD, Kallich JD, Mapes DL, et al. (1997) Kidney Disease Quality of Life Short Form (KDQOL-SF™) version 1.3: A for use and scoring. 7994, Santa Monica, CA, Rand

Holley JL, De Vote CC. (2006) Why all prescribed medications are not taken: Results from a survey of chronic dialysis patients. *Adv Perit Dial.* Vol. 22, pp. 162-166, ISSN 1197-8554.

Japan Association of Kidney Disease Patients, Japanese Association of Dialysis Physician (2007) Report of research on patients with dialysis treatment in 2006., Tokyo (Japanese)

Koskinen S, Hokkinen EM, Sarajuuri J et al. (2007) Applicability of the ICF checklist to traumatically brain-injured patients in post-acute rehabilitation settings. *J Rehab Med.* Vol. 39, No. 6, pp. 467-472, ISSN 1651-2081.

Kutner NG, Zhang R, Huang Y et al. (2010) Depressed mood, usual activity level, and continued employment after starting dialysis. *Clin J Am Soc Nephrol.* Vol. 5, No. 11, pp. 2040-2045, ISSN 1555-905X.

Muehrer RJ, Schatell D, Witten B et al. (2011) Factors affecting employment at initiation of dialysis. *Clin J Am Soc Nephrol.* Epub ahead of print, ISSN 1555-905X.

Namazi H, Majd Z. (2007) Carpal tunnel syndrome in patients who are receiving long-term renal hemodialysis. *Arch Orthop Trauma Surg.* Vol. 127, No. 8, pp. 725-728, ISSN 1434-3916.

Neri L, Rocca Rey LA, Gallieni M et al. (2009) Occupational stress is associated with impaired work ability and reduced quality of life in patients with chronic kidney failure. *Int J Artif Organs.* Vol. 32, No. 5, pp. 291-298, ISSN 1724-6040.

Panagopoulou A, Hardalias A, Berati S et al. (2009) Psychosocial issues and quality of life in patients on renal replacement therapy. *Saudi J Kidney Dis Transpl.* Vol. 20, No. 2, pp. 213-218, ISSN 1319-2442.

Patient Registration Committee, Japanese Society for Dialysis Therapy (2010). An overview of regular dialysis treatment in Japan, As of 31 December 2009. Available from http://docs.jsdt.or.jp/overview/index.html

Ruof J, Cieza A, Wolff B et al. (2004) ICF core sets for diabetes mellitus. *J Rehabil Med.* Vol. 44, No.Suppl, pp. 100-106, ISSN 1650-1969.

Saray Y, Seçkin D, Güleç AT et al. (2004) Nail disorders in hemodialysis patients and renal transplant recipients: a case-control study. *J Am Acad Dermatol.* Vol. 50, No. 2, pp. 197-202, ISSN 1097-6787.

Stucki A, Daansen P, Fuessl M et al. (2004) ICF core sets for obesity. *J Rehabil Med.* Vol. 44, No.Suppl, pp. 107-113, ISSN 1650-1969.

Stucki G, Ewert T, Cieza A (2002) Value and application of the ICF in rehabilitation medicine. *Disabl Rehabil.* Vol. 24, No. 17, pp. 932-938, ISSN 1464-5165.

Tander B, Akpolat T, Durmus D et al. (2007) Evaluation of hand functions in hemodialysis patients. *Ren Fail.* Vol. 29, No. 4, pp.477-480, ISSN 1525-6049.

Tenorio-Martinez R, Del Carmen Lara-Munoz M, Mrdina-Mora ME. (2009) Measurement of problems in activities and participation in patients with anxiety, depression and schizophrenia using the ICF checklist. *Soc Psychiatry Psychaoatr Epidemiol.* Vol. 44, No. 5, pp.377-384, ISSN 1433-9285.

Tsutsui H, Koike T, Yamazaki C et al. (2009) Identification of hemodialysis patients' common problems using the International Classification of Functioning, Disability and Health. *Ther Apher Dial.* Vol. 13, No. 3, pp.186-192, ISSN 1744-9987.

Van Buren PN, Inrig JK. (2011) Hypertension and hemodialysis: pathophysiology and outcomes in adult and pediatric populations. *Pediatr Nephrol.* Vol. 6, No. 3, pp. 489-496, ISSN 1432-198X.

Vij R, Nataraj S, Peixoto AJ. (2009) Diagnostic utility of urinalysis in detecting urinary tract infection in hemodialysis patients. *Nephron Clin Pract.* Vol. 113, No. 4, pp. c281-c285, ISSN 1660-2110.

Vrabec R, Vatavyk Z, Pavlović D et al. (2005) Ocular findings in patients with chronic renal failure undergoing haemodialysis. *Coll Antropol.* Vol. 29, No. Suppl. 1, pp.95-98, ISSN 0350-6134.

Weigl M, Cieza A, Andersen C et al. (2004) Identification of relevant ICF categories in patients with chronic health conditions: A Delphi exercise. *J Rehabil Med.* Vol. 44, No. Suppl, pp.12-21, ISSN 1650-1969.

Weisbord SD, Bossola M, Fried LF et al. (2008) Cultural comparison of symptoms in patients on maintenance. *Hemodial Int.* Vol. 12, No. 4, pp.434-440, ISSN 1542-4758.

World Health Organization (2001) International Classification of Functioning, Disability and Health: ICF. ISBN 92-4-154741-3, Geneva: WHO

World Health Organization (2003) ICF checklist version 2.1α, Clinician form for International Classification of Functioning, Disability and Health. Available from http://www.who.int/classifications/icf/training/icfchecklist.pdf

Wu MJ, Change CS, Cheng CH et al. (2004) Colonic transit in long-term dialysis patients. *Am J Kidney Dis.* Vol. 44, No. 2, pp. 322-327, ISSN 1523-6838.

Yasuda G, Shibata K, Takizawa T et al. (2002) Prevalence of constipation in continuous ambulatory peritoneal dialysis patients and comparison with hemodialysis patients. *Am J Kidney Dis.* Vol. 39, No. 6, pp. 1292-1299, ISSN 1523-6838.

13

Choice of Renal Replacement Therapy and Role of Hemodialysis in the Intensive Care Unit

Marlies Ostermann
King's College London, Guy's & St Thomas' Hospital
United Kingdom

1. Introduction

Renal replacement therapy (RRT) has become an established component of modern critical care. Approximately 60 - 70% of critically ill patients with severe acute kidney injury (AKI) are treated with RRT which represents ~5% of all intensive care unit (ICU) admissions (Ostermann & Chang, 2008; Uchino et al., 2005). Thirty years ago, intermittent haemodialysis for the critically ill patient with AKI was typically delivered three times weekly using dialysis machines without accurate volumetric control, acetate-based dialysate and unmodified cellulosic membrane dialysers. Peritoneal dialysis was performed with hard catheters and low dwell volumes. Since then, the types of RRT used in ICU and the available kits have advanced significantly.

Despite its worldwide use, the practice of RRT is variable. The main reasons are differences in expertise of nursing and medical staff, local availability of machines and lack of robust clinical data to support one technique over another (Pannu et al., 2008). Several important aspects related to the management of RRT, including mode, optimal indications and timing are the focus of ongoing discussion and opposing views.

2. Aims of RRT

AKI in critically ill patients manifests itself with varying degrees of uraemia, fluid accumulation, acid base disturbance and non-renal dysfunction. The clinical course can be very variable. RRT for AKI is predominantly supportive with the aim to maintain metabolic and volume haemostasis and to prevent uraemic complications and dysfunction of other organs during the critical illness until renal function recovers. It is important that these benefits of RRT are balanced by potential harm, including risks related to central venous access, infections and anticoagulation (Oudemans-van Straaten, 2007).

3. Practice of RRT

3.1 Indications for RRT

In the setting of chronic kidney disease, the European Best Practice Guidelines recommend starting chronic dialysis when a patient with an estimated glomerular filtration rate (GFR) of $<15 ml/min/1.73m^2$ has symptoms or signs of uraemia, fluid overload or malnutrition in spite of medical therapy or before estimated GFR has fallen to

<6ml/min/1.73m^2 in an asymptomatic patient (European Best Practice Guidelines, 2005). The overall aim is to replace renal function. The situation is very different in the acute setting where RRT for AKI is predominantly viewed as organ support until kidney function recovers. Although acute RRT should be started before the onset of any potentially life threatening complications of uraemia, the optimal time and indications remain controversial. Potential benefits of early initiation are more rapid metabolic/uraemic control and more effective prevention and management of fluid overload (Gibney et al., 2008). Some data also suggest that RRT before the onset of severe AKI may attenuate kidney-specific and non-kidney organ injury from acidemia, uremia, fluid overload, and systemic inflammation, and potentially translate into improved survival and earlier recovery of kidney function (Clark et al., 2006; Matson et al., 2004). The obvious counterargument is that early RRT might subject patients who would recover renal function with conservative treatment alone, to the potential risks associated with RRT (Vinsonneau & Monchi, 2011). Delay of RRT until AKI is severe avoids treatment in patients with potentially recoverable AKI but increases the risk of uraemic complications and fluid overload.

3.1.1 Indicators for initiation of RRT

Studies exploring the optimal indication for starting RRT have used different parameters, including arbitrary cut-offs for serum creatinine, serum urea or urine output, fluid balance, time from ICU admission or time after onset of AKI. Several retrospective studies have shown an association between lower serum urea levels at time of RRT and better outcomes (Gettings et al., 1999; Liu et al., 2006; Shiao et al., 2009). Liu et al reported a lower mortality in 122 patients in a mixed ICU who had serum urea levels ≤27 mmol/L (≤76 mg/dL) on the day when RRT was started compared to 121 patients with higher urea values (Liu et al., 2006). When adjusted for age, hepatic failure, sepsis, thrombocytopenia and serum creatinine, the relative risk of death with a higher urea level at time of RRT was 1.85 (95% CI 1.16 - 2.96). Improved mortality was also reported in other retrospective studies when RRT was instituted with serum urea <21 mmol/L (Gettings et al., 1999) or <23 mmol/L (Shiao et al., 2009) compared to higher levels. The authors made the conclusion that "early RRT may be better than late RRT". However, 2 larger studies did not find any correlation between serum urea at time of RRT and outcome (Bagshaw et al., 2009; Ostermann & Chang, 2009). Instead, they showed that patients who had a serum creatinine < 309 µmol/L at time of RRT had a greater risk of dying compared to those with higher serum creatinine levels. Other studies found a better outcome in patients with a shorter time from ICU admission (Payen et al., 2008; Piccinni et al., 2006), a higher urine output at time of RRT (Sughara & Suzuki, 2004), and a shorter time between onset of AKI and RRT (Ostermann & Chang, 2009).

Despite the perception that early RRT may be better, the data are conflicting (Bagshaw et al., 2009; Bouman et al., 2002; Demirkilic et al., 2004; Elahi et al., 2004; Gettings et al., 1999; Liu et al, 2006; Ostermann & Chang, 2009; Payen et al., 2008; Piccinni et al., 2006; Shiao et al., 2009; Sughara et al., 2004). There are only 2 randomized controlled trials (RCTs) exploring the impact of timing of RRT (Bouman et al., 2002; Sughara & Suzuki, 2004). The majority of data stem from retrospective analyses with different biochemical cut-offs to distinguish between early and late treatment. Therefore, it cannot be excluded that patients in the "early" RRT group simply had less severe AKI and that patients in the "late" group received RRT too late, ie. after the onset of uraemic complications. Finally, the interpretation of non-randomized studies is limited by the exclusion of patients who met criteria for early RRT but never received it.

In the largest prospective RCT investigating the role of timing, 106 predominantly cardiac surgical patients with AKI were randomized to three groups: early high-volume continuous venovenous haemofiltration (CVVHF) (n=35), early low-volume CVVHF (n=35) and late low-volume CVVHF (n=36) (Bouman et al., 2002). There were no significant differences in 28 day mortality or duration of AKI between the groups. All hospital survivors recovered renal function except for one patient in the early low volume CVVH group. Of interest, 4 patients in the late arm recovered renal function spontaneously and 2 patients died before the criteria for CVVH were met. The authors came to the conclusion that there was no significant benefit with either early CVVH or high filtration rates for patients with oliguric AKI. A large retrospective analysis of 1,847 ICU patients treated with RRT for AKI demonstrated that the most important independent risk factors for ICU mortality were mechanical ventilation, associated organ failure, pre-existing chronic health problems, acidosis, oliguria and age (Ostermann & Chang, 2009). There was no association between serum urea and creatinine at time of RRT and outcome. The paper concluded that the decision to start RRT should depend less on classic renal parameters but more on the clinical status of the patient, degree of acidosis, risk of fluid overload and associated organ failure.

The negative impact of fluid overload is increasingly being recognised (Bouchard et al., 2009; Payen et al., 2008). In a retrospective analysis of 398 ICU patients, Bouchard et al found a significantly higher ICU mortality in patients who had gained 1-20% or more in body weight between ICU admission and day of RRT compared to patients without any weight gain (Bouchard et al., 2009). Oliguria and fluid overload in the context of AKI should be viewed as triggers for RRT independent of actual serum urea and creatinine results.

In summary, based on the existing data in the literature, the decision when to start RRT should take into account the patient's severity of illness and its trends, degree of fluid overload and number and types of associated organ failure. Individual serum creatinine or urea parameters are not adequate in identifying the optimal time for RRT. Obviously, in patients with a futile prognosis RRT may not be appropriate. In this case, withholding RRT constitutes good end-of life care (Gabbay & Meyer, 2009).

3.2 Choice of RRT modality

Current RRT options for ICU patients with AKI are continuous modes [continuous haemofiltration (CVVHF), continuous haemodialysis (CVVHD) and continuous haemodiafiltration (CVVHDF)], intermittent haemodialysis (HD), hybrid techniques like slow extended haemodialysis (SLED) or prolonged intermittent renal replacement therapy (PIRRT) and acute peritoneal dialysis. Some characteristics of the different modalities are listed in Table 1.

Continuous RRT is often perceived to offer greater cardiovascular stability compared to traditional intermittent HD. However, intermittent techniques have evolved over the last 20 years. HD machines now have accurate fluid balance control modules with real-time indirect assessment of relative changes in blood volume which allow rapid fluid removal with less haemodynamic instability. A switch towards bicarbonate-based dialysate and less bioincompatible membranes, together with a recognition of the importance of higher dialysate sodium concentrations and cooled dialysate have also led to a reduced the risk of intradialytic hypotension. Advantages of intermittent HD are the reduced need for anticoagulation, lower financial costs and greater flexibility which ultimately allows more time for investigations and therapies, including active rehabilitation. Small solutes such as potassium are removed more efficiently with HD which may be particularly beneficial in the setting of acute life threatening hyperkalaemia.

	CVVH	CVVHD	CVVHDF	Intermittent HD	SLED / PIRRT	PD
Solute transport	Convection	Diffusion	Convection + diffusion	Diffusion	Diffusion	Diffusion
Therapy time/day	24 hours	24 hours	variable	4 - 6 hours	6 – 12 hours	24 hours
Blood flow (ml/min)	100 - 250	100 - 250	100 - 250	200 - 350	100 - 300	none
Urea clearance (ml/min)	20- 40	25 – 45	25 – 45	150 – 180	90 – 140	15 - 35
Need for Anticoagulation	Yes	Yes	Yes	Not absolutely	Not absolutely	No

Table 1. Comparison between different modes of RRT (adapted from Mehta et al., 1993)

In addition to potentially better haemodynamic stability, continuous RRT offers the advantage of more sustained fluid removal and less fluctuations in fluid status and metabolic control. Obvious disadvantages are the need for continuous anticoagulation and less flexibility, including less time for the patient to participate in active rehabilitation. The rate of solute removal is lower than with intermittent HD. Over the last few years, there has been much debate whether haemofiltration offers additional benefits for patients with AKI and severe sepsis / septic shock beyond solute clearance (Peng Z et al., 2010). Proponents argue that RRT in the context of severe sepsis contributes to removal of soluble inflammatory mediators of sepsis and restores immune function through improved antigen-presenting capability and leukocyte responsiveness (Honoré et al., 2007). Although this concept of "blood purification" is conceptually appealing, the evidence is limited to data from animal models and small human studies (Bouman et al., 2007).

Although there are differences in capillary fibre structure and design, most ICUs use the same dialysers for CRRT, PIRRT and IHD. The resurgence of batch dialysis systems (for instance, Genius® , NxStage®) and the use of individual water purification systems (microfilters, water softeners, multiple pass reverse osmosis) coupled with endotoxin filters has made it possible to provide haemodialysis even without access to ultrapure water supply as in chronic haemodialysis units.

3.2.1 Continuous versus intermittent RRT

It is widely perceived that continuous modes may be better for critically ill patients with AKI. However, prospective randomised clinical trials have failed to confirm this. Based on 4 different systematic reviews, there is no convincing evidence that continuous RRT is superior to intermittent HD in terms of mortality or renal recovery (Bagshaw et al., 2008; Kellum et al., 2002; Rabindranath et al., 2007; Tonelli et al., 2002). Although these analyses included different studies of varying methodological quality and size, the authors came to similar conclusions. The Hemodiafe Study, a multicenter RCT comparing intermittent HD versus CVVHDF in patients with AKI and multiple-organ dysfunction syndrome (MODS), showed that it is possible to treat almost all critically ill patients with AKI with intermittent HD, provided strict guidelines to improve tolerance and metabolic control are adhered to (Vinsonneau et al., 2006). In the intermittent HD group, haemodynamic stability was maintained by using a high dialysate sodium concentration and dialysate cooled to 35^{0}C. There was no difference in outcome between both groups.

Despite the lack of data that continuous RRT is superior to intermittent HD with regards to mortality or renal recovery, there is some evidence that fluid overload may be easier to control with continuous RRT compared to intermittent modalities. Retrospective analysis of data collected as part of the Program to improve Care in Acute Renal Disease (PICARD) study showed that patients treated with intermittent RRT continued to gain fluid in the subsequent days in contrast to patients on continuous RRT in whom the fluid balance was significantly better controlled (Bouchard et al., 2009). This observation makes intermittent HD less suitable for patients with major fluid overload and supports the recommendation to use continuous RRT for this patient group (Vanholder et al., 2011).

Comparative studies of continuous and hybrid techniques are limited (Abe et al., 2010; Kielstein et al., 2004; Kumar et al., 2000; Kumar et al., 2004; Marshall et al., 2004). In a small trial, 39 patients were randomised to either CVVHF or 12-hour SLED (Kielstein et al., 2004). Cardiovascular tolerability and urea clearances were equivalent. However, less heparin was needed and acidosis was corrected faster in patients treated with SLED. In another randomised trial in 60 patients, CVVHDF was compared to 6 - 8 hours of SLED (Abe et al., 2010). There was no difference in ICU or 30 day mortality but survivors in the SLED group had higher renal recovery rates and a shorter length of stay in ICU.

3.2.2 Peritoneal dialysis versus continuous RRT

Acute peritoneal dialysis in the ICU is possible but requires the insertion of a peritoneal dialysis catheter and relies on an intact peritoneum and adequate bowel movement. It is contraindicated in patients with abdominal pathology. Solute clearance and fluid removal are generally less predictable and controllable and may be reduced in patients with impaired mesenteric blood flow. Removal of large volumes of fluid may not be possible with small dwell volumes, especially in the first 2 weeks after insertion of the peritoneal catheter.

There are only limited data comparing peritoneal dialysis to continuous RRT in adults (Gangji et al., 2005; Swartz et al., 2005). In a Vietnamese study in patients with infection associated AKI, CVVHF was superior but the applied peritoneal dialysis strategies were different from current practice (Phu et al., 2002). Another study showed not difference but the clearance delivered by peritoneal dialysis was low (Gabriel et al., 2008).

In summary, analysis of the currently published studies shows no clear advantage of one modality over the other in terms of mortality or renal recovery. The decision regarding type of RRT should take into account the individual patient's clinical condition, medical and nursing expertise, and the availability of RRT machines. Regular education and training of those who provide RRT is essential with emphasis on the characteristics and values of each RRT technique. During the dynamic course of critical illness the type of RRT modality may have to change in response to the varying needs of the patient. Most clinicians choose continuous RRT for patients with cardiovascular compromise, significant fluid overload and multi-organ failure, and an intermittent mode for cardiovascularly stable patients

(Kanagasundaram, 2007; VA NIH Acute Renal Failure Trial Network et al., 2008) Although the risk of hypotension is increased during intermittent HD, the Hemodiafe study showed that the introduction of a relatively simple treatment algorithm including use of a high dialysate sodium concentration of 145 mmol/L in combination with cooled dialysate and stopping vasodilator infusions, markedly reduced the risk of intradialytic hypotension (Vinsonneau et al., 2006). Hybrid techniques like SLED / PIRRT offer the advantages of both CRRT and intermittent HD, including haemodynamic stability, increased patient mobility and reduced financial costs.

3.3 General care

Severe AKI results in hypercatabolism and altered drug metabolism. Provision of adequate nutrition and attention to drug dosing are essential when looking after patients on RRT. While no particular mode or filter is recommended, it is important to understand the characteristics of these different RRT techniques and potential differences in drug removal. Both, under-treatment and drug toxicity have been reported in patients on RRT.

4. Conclusions

RRT is a form of organ support for critically ill patients with AKI. The most commonly used modalities are continuous haemo(dia)filtration and intermittent modes. There is no evidence that one mode is superior to another in terms of mortality or renal recovery. Except for a few specific indications, each modality can be considered a valid RRT option for critically ill patients with AKI. The choice should depend on the patient's clinical condition, medical and nursing expertise and local availability of machines. Intermittent HD is an acceptable option for critically ill patients with AKI, including patients with MODS provided clear guidelines are adhered to in order to prevent haemodynamic instability. For patients with significant fluid overload, continuous RRT appears more appropriate.

It is widely acknowledged that the way RRT is delivered has an impact on quality and outcome of patients with severe AKI. The value of regular education and training of those who deliver RRT, and attention to concurrent interventions (drug dosing, nutrition, fluid management) cannot be emphasized enough. There is a clear role for each different modality in the management of AKI in ICU. RRT should be individualised depending on the patient's varying needs during the critical illness.

5. References

Abe, M., Okada, K., Suzuki, M., Nagura, C., Ishihara, Y., Fujii, Y., Ikeda, K., Kaizu, K. & Matsumoto, K. (2010). Comparison of sustained hemodiafiltration with continuous venovenous hemodiafiltration for the treatment of critically ill patients with acute kidney injury. *Artificial Organs,* Vol, 34, pp. 331-338

Bagshaw, S.M., Berthiaume, L.R., Delaney, A. & Bellomo, R. (2008). Continuous versus intermittent renal replacement therapy for critically ill patients with acute kidney injury: a meta-analysis. *Critical Care Medicine, Vol.* 36, pp. 610-617

Bagshaw, S.M., Uchino, S., Bellomo, R., Morimatsu, H., Morgera, S., Schetz, M., Tan, I., Bouman, C., Macedo, E., Gibney, N., Tolwani, A., Oudemans-van Straaten, H.M., Ronco, C., Kellum, J.A. & Beginning and Ending Supportive Therapy for the Kidney (BEST Kidney) Investigators (2009). Timing of renal replacement therapy and clinical outcomes in critically ill patients with severe acute kidney injury. *Journal of Critical Care*, Vol. 24, pp. 129-140

Bouchard, J., Soroko, S.B., Chertow, G.M., Himmelfarb, J., Ikizler, T.A., Paganini, E.P., Mehta, R.L. & Program to Improve Care in Acute Renal Disease (PICARD) Study Group. (2009). Fluid accumulation, survival and recovery of kidney function in critically ill patients with acute kidney injury. *Kidney International*, Vol. 76, pp. 422-427

Bouman, C.S., Oudemans-Van Straaten, H.M., Tijssen, J.G., Zandstra, D.F. & Kesecioglu, J. (2002). Effects of early high-volume continuous veno-venous hemofiltration on survival and recovery of renal function in intensive care patients with acute renal failure: a prospective, randomized trial. *Critical Care Medicine*, Vol. 30, pp. 2205-2211

Bouman, C.S., Oudemans-van Straaten, H.M., Schultz, M.J. & Vroom, M.B. (2007). Hemofiltration in sepsis and systemic inflammatory response syndrome: the role of dosing and timing. *Journal of Critical Care*, Vol. 22, pp. 1-12

Clark, W.R., Letteri, J.J., Uchino, S., Bellomo, R. & Ronco, C. (2006). Recent clinical advances in the management of critically ill patients with acute renal failure. *Blood Purification*, Vol. 24, pp. 487-498

Demirkiliç, U., Kuralay, E., Yenicesu, M., Cağlar, K., Oz, B.S., Cingöz, F., Günay, C., Yildirim, V., Ceylan, S., Arslan, M., Vural, A. & Tatar, H. (2004). Timing of replacement therapy for acute renal failure after cardiac surgery. *Journal of Cardiac Surgery*, Vol. 19, pp. 17-20

Elahi, M.M.,Lim, M.Y., Joseph, R.N., Dhannapuneni, R.R. & Spyt, T.J. (2004). Early hemofiltration improves survival in post-cardiotomy patients with acute renal failure. *European Journal of Cardiothoracic Surgery*, Vol. 26, pp. 1027-1031

European Best Practice Guidelines 2 (2005). The initiation of dialysis. *Nephrol Dial Transplant, Vol.* 20, pp. ix3-ix7

Gabbay, E. & Meyer, K.B. (2009). Identifying critically ill patients with acute kidney injury for whom renal replacement therapy is inappropriate: an exercise in futility? *Nephrology Dialysis Transplantation Plus*, Vol. 2, pp. 97-103

Gabriel, D.P., Caramori, J.T., Martim, L.C., Barretti, P. & Balbi, A.L. (2008). High volume peritoneal dialysis vs daily hemodialysis: a randomized, controlled trial in patients with acute kidney injury. Kidney International Supplement, Vol. 73 (Suppl), pp. S87-S93

Gangji, A.S., Rabbat, C.G. & Margetts, P.J. (2005). Benefit of continuous renal replacement therapy in subgroups of acutely ill patients: A retrospective analysis. *Clinical Nephrology*, Vol. 63, pp. 267-275

Gettings, L.G., Reynolds, H.N. & Scalea, T. (1999). Outcome in posttraumatic acute renal failure when continuous renal replacement therapy is applied early versus late. *Intensive Care Medicine*, Vol. 25, pp. 805–813

Gibney, N., Hoste, E., Burdmann, E.A., Bunchman, T., Kher, V., Viswanathan, R., Mehta, R.L. & Ronco, C. (2008). Timing of initiation and discontinuation of renal replacement therapy in AKI: unanswered key questions. *Clinical Journal of American Society of Nephrology*, Vol. 3, pp. 876-880

Honoré, P., Joannes-Bovau, O. & Gressens, B. (2007). Blood and plasma treatments: high-volume hemofiltration - a global view. *Contributions to Nephrology*, Vol. 156, pp. 371-386

Kanagasundaram, N.S. (2007). Renal replacement therapy in acute kidney injury: An overview. *British Journal of Hospital Medicine*, Vol, 68, pp. 292-297

Kellum, J.A.,Angus, D.C., Johnson, J.P., Leblanc, M., Griffin, M., Ramakrishnan, N. & Linde-Zwirble, W.T. (2002). Continuous versus intermittent renal replacement therapy: a meta-analysis. *Intensive Care Medicine*, Vol. 28, pp. 29-37

Kielstein, J.T., Kretschmer, U., Ernst, T., Hafer, C., Bahr, M.J., Haller, H. & Fliser, D. (2004). Efficacy and cardiovascular tolerability of extended dialysis in critically ill patients: A randomized controlled study. *American Journal of Kidney Diseases*, Vol.43, pp. 342-349

Kumar, V.A., Craig, M., Depner, T.A. & Yeun, J.Y. (2000). Extended daily dialysis: a new approach to renal replacement for acute renal failure in the intensive care unit. *American Journal of Kidney Diseases*, Vol. 36, pp. 294-300

Kumar, V.A., Yeun, J.Y., Depner, T.A. & Don, B.R. (2004). Extended daily dialysis vs continuous hemodialysis for ICU patients with acute renal failure: a two year single center report. *International Journal of Artificial Organs*, Vol. 27, pp. 371-379

Liu, K.D., Himmelfarb, J., Paganini, E., Ikizler, T.A., Soroko, S.H., Mehta, R.L. & Chertow, G.M. (2006). Timing of initiation of dialysis in critically ill patients with acute kidney injury. *Clinical Journal of the American Society of Nephrology*, Vol. 1, pp. 915-919

Marshall, M.R., Ma, T., Galler, D., Rankin, A.P. & Williams, A.B. (2004). Sustained low-efficiendy daily diafiltration (SLEDD-f) for critically ill patients requiring renal replacement therapy: towards an adequate therapy. *Nephrology Dialysis Transplantation*, Vol. 19, pp. 877-884

Matson, J., Zydney, A. & Honore, P.M. (2004). Blood filtration: new opportunities and the implications of systems biology. *Critical Care Resuscitation*, Vol, 6, pp. 209-217

Mehta, R.L. (1993). Renal replacement for acute renal failure: matching the method to the patient. *Semin Dial*, Vol. 6, pp. 253-259

Ostermann, M., Chang, R. & Riyadh ICU Program Users Group (2008). Correlation between the AKI classification and outcome. *Critical Care*, Vol. 12, pp. R144

Ostermann, M. & Chang, R.W.S. (2009). Correlation between parameters at initiation of renal replacement therapy and outcome in patients with acute kidney injury. *Critical Care*, Vol. 13, pp. R175

Oudemans-van Straaten, H.M. (2007). Primum non nocere, safety of continuous renal replacement therapy. *Current Opinion in Critical Care*, Vol. 13, pp. 635-637

Pannu, N., Klarenbach, S., Wiebe, N., Manns, B., Tonelli, M. & Alberta Kidney Disease Network (2008). Renal replacement therapy in patients with acute renal failure: a systematic review. *Journal of American Medical Association*, Vol. 299, pp. 793-805

Payen, D., de Pont, A.C., Sakr, Y., Spies, C., Reinhart, K., Vincent, J.L. & Sepsis Occurrence in Acutely Ill Patients (SOAP) Investigators (2008). A positive fluid balance is associated with a worse outcome in patients with acute renal failure. *Critical Care*, Vol., 12, pp. R74

Peng, Z., Singbartl, K., Simon, P., Rimmelé, T., Bishop, J., Clermont, G. & Kellum, J.A. (2010). Blood purification in sepsis: a new paradigm. *Contributions to Nephrology*, Vol. 165, pp. 322-328

Phu, N.H., Hien, T.T., Mai, N.T., Chau, T.T., Chuong, L.V., Loc, P.P., Winearls, C., Farrar, J., White, N. & Day, N. (2002). Hemofiltration and peritoneal dialysis in infection associated acute renal failure in Vietnam. *New England Journal of Medicine*, Vol. 347, pp. 895-902

Piccinni, P., Dan, M., Barbacini, S., Carraro, R., Lieta, E., Marafon, S., Zamperetti, N., Brendolan, A., D'Intini, V., Tetta, C., Bellomo, R. & Ronco, C. (2006). Early isovolaemic haemofiltration in oliguric patients with septic shock. I*ntensive Care Medicine*, Vol. 32, pp. 80-86

Rabindranath, K., Adams, J., Macleod, A.M. & Muirhead, N. (2007). Intermittent versus continuous renal replacement therapy for acute renal failure in adults. *Cochrane Database Systematic Reviews*, Vol. 3, pp. CD003773

Shiao, C.C., Wu, V.C., Li, W.Y., Lin, Y.F., Hu, F.C., Young, G.H., Kuo, C.C., Kao, T.W., Huang, D.M., Chen, Y.M., Tsai, P.R., Lin, S.L., Chou, N.K., Lin, T.H., Yeh, Y.C., Wang, C.H., Chou, A., Ko, W.J., Wu, K.D. & National Taiwan University Surgical Intensive Care Unit-Associated Renal Failure Study Group (2009). Late initiation of renal replacement therapy is associated with worse outcomes in acute kidney injury after major abdominal surgery. *Critical Care*, Vol. 13, pp. R71

Sughara, S. & Suzuki, H. (2004). Early start on continuous hemodialysis therapy improves survival rate in patients with acute renal failure following coronary bypass surgery. *Hemodialysis International*, Vol. 8, pp. 320-325

Swartz, R.D., Bustami, R.T., Daley, J.M., Gillespie, B.W. & Port, F.K. (2005). Estimating the impact of renal replacement therapy choice on outcome in severe acute renal failure. *Clinical Nephrol*ogy, Vol. 63, pp. 335-345

Tonelli, M., Manns, B. & Feller-Kopman, D. (2002). Acute renal failure in the intensive care unit: a systematic review of the impact of dialytic modality on mortality and renal recovery. *American Journal of Kidney Diseases*, Vol. 40, pp. 875-885

Uchino, S., Kellum, J.A., Bellomo, R., Doig, G.S., Morimatsu, H., Morgera, S., Schetz, M., Tan, I., Bouman, C., Macedo, E., Gibney, N., Tolwani, A., Ronco, C. & Beginning and Ending Supportive Therapy for the Kidney (BEST Kidney) Investigators (2005). Acute renal failure in critically ill patients: a multinational, multicenter study. *Journal of American Medical Association*, Vol. 294, pp. 813-818

VA/NIH Acute Renal Failure Trial Network, Palevsky, P.M., Zhang, J.H., O'Connor, T.Z., Chertow, G.M., Crowley, S.T., Choudhury, D., Finkel, K., Kellum, J.A., Paganini, E., Schein, R.M., Smith, M.W., Swanson, K.M., Thompson, B.T., Vijayan, A., Watnick, S., Star, R.A. & Peduzzi P. (2008). Intensity of renal support in critically ill patients with acute kidney injury. *New England Journal of Medicine*, Vol. 359, pp. 7-20

Vanholder, R.,Van Biesen, W., Hoste, R. & Lameire, N. (2011). Pro/con debate: Continuous versus intermittent dialysis for acute kidney injury: a never-ending story yet approaching the finish? *Critical Care*, Vol. 15, pp. 204-210

Vinsonneau, C., Camus, C., Combes, A., Costa de Beauregard, M.A., Klouche, K., Boulain, T., Pallot, J.L., Chiche, J.D., Taupin, P., Landais, P., Dhainaut, J.F. & Hemodiafe Study Group. (2006). Continuous venovenous haemodiafiltration versus intermittent haemodialysis for acute renal failure in patients with multiple-organ dysfunction syndrome: a multicentre randomised trial. *Lancet*, Vol. 368, pp. 379-385

Vinsonneau, C. & Monchi, M. (2011). Too early initiation of renal replacement therapy may be harmful. *Critical Care*, Vol. 15, pp. 11

Permissions

All chapters in this book were first published by InTech Open; hereby published with permission under the Creative Commons Attribution License or equivalent. Every chapter published in this book has been scrutinized by our experts. Their significance has been extensively debated. The topics covered herein carry significant findings which will fuel the growth of the discipline. They may even be implemented as practical applications or may be referred to as a beginning point for another development.

The contributors of this book come from diverse backgrounds, making this book a truly international effort. This book will bring forth new frontiers with its revolutionizing research information and detailed analysis of the nascent developments around the world.

We would like to thank all the contributing authors for lending their expertise to make the book truly unique. They have played a crucial role in the development of this book. Without their invaluable contributions this book wouldn't have been possible. They have made vital efforts to compile up to date information on the varied aspects of this subject to make this book a valuable addition to the collection of many professionals and students.

This book was conceptualized with the vision of imparting up-to-date information and advanced data in this field. To ensure the same, a matchless editorial board was set up. Every individual on the board went through rigorous rounds of assessment to prove their worth. After which they invested a large part of their time researching and compiling the most relevant data for our readers.

The editorial board has been involved in producing this book since its inception. They have spent rigorous hours researching and exploring the diverse topics which have resulted in the successful publishing of this book. They have passed on their knowledge of decades through this book. To expedite this challenging task, the publisher supported the team at every step. A small team of assistant editors was also appointed to further simplify the editing procedure and attain best results for the readers.

Apart from the editorial board, the designing team has also invested a significant amount of their time in understanding the subject and creating the most relevant covers. They scrutinized every image to scout for the most suitable representation of the subject and create an appropriate cover for the book.

The publishing team has been an ardent support to the editorial, designing and production team. Their endless efforts to recruit the best for this project, has resulted in the accomplishment of this book. They are a veteran in the field of academics and their pool of knowledge is as vast as their experience in printing. Their expertise and guidance has proved useful at every step. Their uncompromising quality standards have made this book an exceptional effort. Their encouragement from time to time has been an inspiration for everyone.

The publisher and the editorial board hope that this book will prove to be a valuable piece of knowledge for researchers, students, practitioners and scholars across the globe.

List of Contributors

Olimpia Ortega
Hospital Severo Ochoa, Leganés, Madrid, Spain

Parin Makadia, Payam Benson, Filberto Kelly and Joshua Kaplan
New Jersey Medical School, United States of America

Emanuel Zitt
Department of Nephrology and Dialysis, Academic Teaching Hospital Feldkirch, Austria
Vorarlberg Institute for Vascular Investigation and Treatment (VIVIT), Feldkirch, Austria

Ulrich Neyer
Vorarlberg Institute for Vascular Investigation and Treatment (VIVIT), Feldkirch, Austria

Mukadder Mollaoğlu
Cumhuriyet University, Turkey

Aysegul Zumrutdal
Baskent University, Adana Teaching and Research Hospital, Turkey

Eiji Takeda, Hironori Yamamoto, Hisami Yamanaka-Okumura and Yutaka Taketani
University of Tokushima Graduate School, Japan

Susanne Heiwe
Dept of Physiotherapy, Karolinska Institutet, Dept of Medicine & Dept of Clinical Sciences, Sweden

Andrej Ekholm
Karolinska Institute, Sweden

Ingela Fehrman-Ekholm
Dept of Renal Medicine, Karolinska University Hospital, Sweden
Stockholm and Transplantation Centre, Sahlgrenska Academy, Göteborg, Sweden

Oliver Rácz
Šafárik University, Medical School, Košice, Slovak Republic

Rudolf Gaško
Railway Hospital, Košice, Slovak Republic

Eleonóra Klímová
University of Prešov, Faculty of Health Care, Prešov, Slovak Republic

Rodney G. Bowden, Neil A. Schwarz and Brian D. Shelmadine
Baylor University, Waco, TX, USA

Timmy Lee
Assistant Professor of Medicine Department of Internal Medicine and Division of Nephrology and Hypertension, University of Cincinnati and Veterans Affairs Medical Center, Cincinnati, OH; United States of America

Hideyo Tsutsui, Teruhiko Koike and Yoshiharu Oshida
Research Center of Health, Physical Fitness and Sports, Nagoya University, Japan

Martin Sedlacek
Dartmouth Hitchcock Medical Center, One Medical Center Drive, Lebanon

Marlies Ostermann
King's College London, Guy's & St Thomas' Hospital United Kingdom

Index

www.ingramcontent.com/pod-product-compliance
Lightning Source LLC
Chambersburg PA
CBHW081212180926
51613CB00003B/215
* 9 7 8 1 6 4 6 4 7 5 7 5 9 *